C000230488

Cancer Epidemiology:
Principles and Methods

International Agency for Research on Cancer

The International Agency for Research on Cancer (IARC) was established in 1965 by the World Health Assembly, as an independently financed organization within the framework of the World Health Organization. The headquarters of the Agency are at Lyon, France.

The Agency conducts a programme of research concentrating particularly on the epidemiology of cancer and the study of potential carcinogens in the human environment. Its field studies are supplemented by biological and chemical research carried out in the Agency's laboratories in Lyon, and, through collaborative research agreements, in national research institutions in many countries. The Agency also conducts a programme for the education and training of personnel for cancer research.

The publications of the Agency are intended to contribute to the dissemination of authoritative information on different aspects of cancer research. Information about IARC publications and how to order them is also available via the Internet at: **http://www.iarc.fr/**

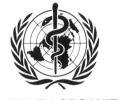

WORLD HEALTH ORGANIZATION
INTERNATIONAL AGENCY FOR RESEARCH ON CANCER

Cancer Epidemiology: Principles and Methods

By
Isabel dos Santos Silva

International Agency for Research on Cancer
Lyon, France
1999

Published by the International Agency for Research on Cancer,
150 cours Albert Thomas, 69372 Lyon cédex 08, France

© International Agency for Research on Cancer, 1999

Distributed by IARCPress (fax: +33 04 72 73 83 02; E-mail: press@iarc.fr)
and by the World Health Organization Distribution and Sales, CH-1211
Geneva 27 (fax: +41 22 791 4857)

Publications of the World Health Organization enjoy copyright protection in
accordance with the provisions of Protocol 2 of the Universal Copyright Convention.
All rights reserved.

The designations employed and the presentation of the material in this publication do not imply
the expression of any opinion whatsoever on the part of the Secretariat of the World Health
Organization concerning the legal status of any country, territory, city, or area or of its authorities,
or concerning the delimitation of its frontiers or boundaries.

The mention of specific companies or of certain manufacturers' products does not imply
that they are endorsed or recommended by the World Health Organization in preference to others
of a similar nature that are not mentioned. Errors and omissions excepted,
the names of proprietary products are distinguished by initial capital letters.

The authors alone are responsible for the views expressed in this publication.

The International Agency for Research on Cancer welcomes requests for permission to
reproduce or translate its publications, in part or in full. Applications and enquiries should be
addressed to the Editorial & Publications Service, International Agency for Research on Cancer,
which will be glad to provide the latest information on any changes made to the text, plans for new
editions, and reprints and translations already available.

IARC Library Cataloguing in Publication Data

dos Santos Silva, I.
    Cancer epidemiology: principles and methods / Isabel dos Santos Silva

    1. Neoplasms – epidemiology   I. Title

    ISBN 92 832 0405 0   (NLM Classification W1)

Printed in Spain

Printing by: THAU S.L.
Aristides Maillol, 5. C 1 08028 Barcelona

Contents

Foreword

Within the IARC programme of training courses, high priority is given to courses on cancer epidemiology, particularly in countries of the developing world. Population-based epidemiological studies are the only reliable source on the occurrence and outcome of cancer and inform the basis of any national or regional cancer control programme. Over the years, the International Agency for Research on Cancer has been faced with the problem of selecting an appropriate textbook for its courses. To resolve this difficulty, we decided to publish a textbook suitable for the course faculty and the non-initiated reader. Isabel dos Santos Silva, from the London School of Hygiene and Tropical Medicine, a prominent epidemiologist with extensive teaching experience, has accomplished this task admirably, in close consultation with external experts and an IARC Advisory Board (see below).

We hope that this textbook will guide students and health professionals wishing to understand the basic principles and methods used in cancer epidemiology.

P. Kleihues
Director, IARC

IARC Advisory Board

Nubia Muñoz
D. Maxwell Parkin
Jacques Estève
Paolo Boffetta

About this book

This book is addressed primarily to medical and public health students, clinicians, health professionals and all those seeking to understand the principles and methods used in cancer epidemiology. Its aim is not to convert the readers into epidemiological experts but to make them competent in the use of basic epidemiological tools and capable of exercising critical judgement when assessing results reported by others.

The book is designed to provide an easy understanding of the basic concepts and methods through the use of illustrative examples, often using real research data. It was my intention to ensure that the material would be accessible to everyone new to the field. Knowledge of statistics is indispensable to the proper conduct, analysis and interpretation of epidemiological studies. Thus, statistical concepts (and formulae) are also presented but the emphasis is on the interpretation of the data rather than on the actual calculations.

The book is divided into 18 chapters. The first six introduce the basic principles of epidemiology and statistics. Chapters 7–13 deal in more depth with each of the study designs and interpretation of their findings. Chapters 14 and 15 cover more complex statistical concepts and can be omitted at a first reading. Chapter 16 deals with methodological issues in cancer prevention, including primary prevention, early detection (screening activities) and tertiary prevention. Chapter 17 reviews the role of cancer registries in cancer epidemiology and prevention. Finally, Chapter 18 discusses logistic issues and practical considerations that should be taken into account in the design, planning and conduct of any type of epidemiological research.

Few, if any, of the ideas and concepts in this book are original. Many of them derive from my own teaching experience at the London School of Hygiene and Tropical Medicine and, in particular, to my role as the organizer of the School's intensive course in epidemiology and medical statistics. I am deeply indebted to many colleagues and students with whom I have worked over the past years for all I have learnt from them. It would be impossible for me to name all who, in one way or another, helped me to write this book—I can only hope that they are aware of my appreciation. I am, however, particularly grateful for the help of my colleagues (and good friends) Bianca De Stavola and Esä Läärä for the long hours they spent reading earlier drafts and for their helpful comments, suggestions and stimulating discussions—I certainly learnt a lot from them! I would also like to thank IARC for giving me the opportunity to write this book and, in particular, the members of the editorial committee (Drs Jacques Estève, Nubia Muñoz, Max Parkin and Paolo Boffetta), Dr. Rengaswami Sankaranarayanan and Dr. Martyn Plummer, for their suggestions and comments in the earlier stages of the project. I am also grateful for all the support and encouragement given by my colleagues at the London School of Hygiene and Tropical Medicine and, in particular, to the thoughtful comments on earlier versions of various chapters provided by Professor Peter Smith, Dr Noreen Maconochie and Dr Punam Mangtani. I also wish to thank Ms Maria Quigley and Mr. Craig Higgins for giving permission to include some of their teaching examples in Chapter 14. Part of the material presented in Chapters 6 and 12 was initially developed as teaching material for our intensive course in collaboration with Dr Maconochie and Mr Jerry Wheeler—the stimulating discussions we had at that time and the feedback received from our students were very helpful in shaping those chapters. Lastly, I would like to thank Dr John Cheney and Ms Helis Miido for all their editorial assistance.

Isabel dos Santos Silva

Chapter 1
Introduction to cancer epidemiology

Interest in cancer has grown during the past century as infectious diseases have increasingly been controlled as the result of improved sanitation, vaccination and antibiotics. Although this interest is relatively recent, cancer is not a new disease. Autopsies of ancient Egyptian mummies have shown the presence of bone tumours and possibly other neoplasias (Brothwell, 1967). Symptoms of what can be assumed to be malignant diseases were also described in Chinese and Arabic medical writings. By the time of Hippocrates in the 4th century BC, many types of tumour were clinically recognized and described. Hippocrates introduced the term carcinoma from the Greek word *karkinos*, for crab: he saw cancer as crablike in its spread through the body and in its persistence (Long, 1928). Some 600 years later, Galen distinguished three types of tumour: 'tumours according to nature', which included all normal physiological swellings, such as enlargement of the breast with normal female maturation; 'tumours exceeding nature', which included the productive process following injury, such as the proliferation of bone that occurs during the reuniting of a fracture; and 'tumours contrary to nature', which included what we now define as neoplastic growths, as well as many inflammatory lesions (Long, 1928).

However, it was not until the end of the 18th century that cancer began to be studied systematically and intensively. Bichat (1771–1802) described the pathology of many neoplasms in humans and suggested that cancer was an 'accidental formation' of tissue built up in the same manner as any other part of the organism. Some decades later, Müller (1801–58) and Virchow (1821–1902) extended Bichat's findings, using the microscope to show that cancerous tissue was made up of cells (Long, 1928).

Ever since, pathologists and clinicians have considered cancers in the various organs of the body as being in many respects completely different diseases with distinct morphologies, clinical manifestations and prognoses. But only during the past few decades has it emerged that their causes also differ enormously. As a discipline, epidemiology has been crucially important in defining the causes of different cancers and in evaluating preventive measures.

1.1   What is cancer epidemiology?

A recent definition of epidemiology is given in the dictionary compiled by Last (1995):

"Epidemiology is the study of the distribution and determinants of health-related states or events in specified populations, and the application of this study to control of health problems."

Cancer epidemiology is the branch of epidemiology concerned with the disease cancer. Therefore, this definition is as valid to cancer epidemiology as it is to epidemiology in general.

The first thing to note in the above definition is that epidemiology is concerned with events that occur in populations: the primary units of concern are groups of people, not separate individuals. This is what differentiates epidemiology from clinical medicine. Epidemiological studies are concerned not only with people who get a disease, but also with those who do not, and in particular how these two groups may differ. Thus, unlike a doctor in clinical practice, who is usually concerned only with patients, the epidemiologist is concerned equally with the population from which the patients came. Whereas clinicians direct their questions towards a particular patient—'What is wrong with this patient? What treatment is appropriate?'—the epidemiologist asks similar questions about whole communities—'What are the leading causes of death or disability in this population? What can be done to reduce them?' Thinking in epidemiological terms often seems foreign to clinicians and other health-care professionals, who are used to thinking of the problems of each individual patient.

While it seems obvious that cancer epidemiology should focus on the disease known as cancer, this is not necessarily the case. In fact, cancer epidemiological studies may focus on precursors of cancer; for example, on cervical intraepithelial neoplasia (CIN) as a precursor of invasive cervical cancer, or on chronic atrophic gastritis as a precursor of stomach cancer. Alternatively, the object of the study may be a characteristic that is related to cancer, such as growth or fertility. Thus, epidemiologists are concerned not only with illness, disability and death, but also with health and with preventing disease.

The epidemiologist is interested in the distribution of disease in a population. Which types of people are at a higher risk? How does the disease frequency change over time? How much does it vary from place to place? These are summarized as 'Who?', 'When?' and 'Where?'. The most basic task of cancer epidemiology is to describe the occurrence of human cancer, noting differences, for example, between males and females, between people of different ages, between socioeconomic classes, between occupations, between time periods, between areas of a country, and between countries. These observations are the starting points in epidemiological research. Like a detective, the epidemiologist then pursues the most promising clues.

Epidemiology aims to answer not only 'Who has what, when, and where?', but also to find out why. Why are some at higher risk than others? Are associations between certain factors and increased risk of disease causal or spurious? Epidemiologists seek to address such basic issues, viewing their work as the search for a relationship between two factors. The first, called exposure (or risk factor), refers to any factor that can affect a person's health: such factors include environmental agents, such as sunlight, air pollution and occupational exposures; lifestyle variables like diet, smoking and physical exercise; and constitutional factors, such as blood type and other genetic traits. The second is the disease itself (or other health-related event of interest). The epidemiologist must examine whether there is an association between an exposure and a disease, and decide whether the observed relationship is likely to be causal. Questions to be addressed might be 'Is lung cancer associated with cigarette smoking?' or 'Does cigarette smoking cause the disease?'.

Epidemiology is the only source of direct scientific evidence about exposure effects and the preventability of disease within human populations. Laboratory scientists have identified carcinogenic compounds in tobacco smoke and have been able to produce respiratory cancers in experimental animals by forcing them to inhale cigarette smoke (IARC, 1986). However, the argument that cigarette smoking causes lung cancer in humans would remain unconvincing if epidemiologists had not also demonstrated that lung cancer occurs much more often in smokers than in non-smokers. But, in contrast to the laboratory-based sciences, the strategy in epidemiology is usually to observe and compare, rather than to experiment, as major ethical and practical considerations limit the possibilities for experimental studies upon humans.

In addition to establishing whether particular exposure–disease associations exist, epidemiology attempts to measure their strength. Thus, after finding an association, the next stage is always to determine the magnitude of the possible effects. To do so, epidemiologists ask questions such as 'By how much does cigarette smoking increase the risk of lung cancer?' or 'By how much does hepatitis B vaccination reduce the risk of liver cancer?'.

One of the most important roles of epidemiology is to learn about the causes of disease, or its natural history, knowledge that can lead to the introduction of preventive measures. Even when the biology of a disease is not fully understood, epidemiology can identify a cause and a means of prevention. Complete knowledge of causal mechanisms is not essential for effective preventive strategies, although in the spirit of scientific enquiry accepted in western culture, knowledge of the mechanisms involved is desirable in itself. We can greatly reduce our risk of developing lung cancer if we do not smoke cigarettes, without knowing what specific component of cigarettes is carcinogenic, nor precisely how these substances affect the control of cell growth.

The epidemiologist is to society what the doctor is to the patient, and epidemiology is thus part of the foundations of public health. Epidemiology describes and measures the occurrence of disease in the community, so that questions can be addressed such as 'Is the disease (or condition) a priority for health intervention?' and 'Why do cases occur and why does the condition persist in the community?'. Epidemiology also helps in choosing the health programmes that are most likely to control a particular health problem and in evaluating their impact in the community.

1.2   A brief history of cancer epidemiology

Epidemiology has its origins in the idea present in many ancient civilizations that environmental factors can influence the occurrence of disease. This idea was clearly expressed about 2400 years ago by Hippocrates:

"Whoever wishes to pursue properly the science of medicine must proceed thus. First he ought to consider what effects each season of the year can produce; for the seasons are not all alike, but differ widely both in themselves and at their changes. The next point is the hot winds and the cold, especially those that are universal, but also those that are peculiar to each particular region. He must also consider the properties of the waters (...) and how the natives are off for water, whether they use marshy, soft waters, or such as are hard and come from rocky heights, or brackish and harsh. The soil too, whether bare and dry or wooded and watered, hollow and hot or high and cold. The mode of life also of the inhabitants that is pleasing to them, whether they are heavy drinkers, taking lunch, and inactive, or athletic, industrious, eating much and drinking little.(...) Using this evidence he must examine the several problems that arise. For if a physician know these things well, by preference all of them, but at any rate most, he will not, on arrival at a town with which he is unfamiliar, be ignorant of the local diseases, or of the nature of those that commonly prevail; so that he will not be at a loss in the treatment of diseases, or make blunders, as is likely to be the case if he have not this knowledge before he consider his several problems." (Translated into English by Jones, 1923)

Despite his emphasis on the role of environmental factors in causing human disease, Hippocrates believed that cancer was a disease caused by an excess of 'black bile', which was manufactured by both the spleen and stomach, but not the liver. His ideas dominated medical practice during the Middle Ages, and it was only with the advent of the Renaissance that they began to be disputed by a number of physicians. Ramazzini was among these. In his book entitled *De Morbis Artificum* (1713) (translated into English by Wright, 1964), he suggested that the high occurrence of breast cancer among nuns was due to their celibate life, an observation that has withstood the test of time. This observation was confirmed by Rigoni-Stern in a paper published in 1842 (translated into English by De Stavola, 1987).

In 1775, Percival Pott described the relationship between scrotal cancer in chimney sweeps and soot in his *Chirurgical Observations*. His work is now considered a milestone in epidemiology. Pott was the first to attribute an occupational cause to this disease, raising the possibility of prevention.

"The fate of these people seems singularly hard; in their early infancy they are most frequently treated with great brutality, and almost starved with cold and hunger; they are thrust up narrow, and sometimes hot chimneys, where they are buried, burned and almost suffocated; and when they get to puberty, become liable to a most noisome, painful and fatal disease." (Pott, 1775)

Pott's work was continued by Henry Butlin (1845–1912), a surgeon at St Bartholomew's Hospital in London. An interesting account of this is given by Waldron (1983):

"A feature of the disease which exercised those interested in it, and which was connected with its aetiology, was that chimney sweeps' cancer seemed to be almost exclusively an English disease. Cases were virtually unknown on the Continent, in America, or even in Scotland. This problem was fully investigated by Henry Butlin. Butlin took himself to the Continent during the course of his researches and, as the result of meeting and talking to Continental sweeps, he considered that he had established the reasons for the virtual absence of scrotal cancer among them. In part it was due to the protective clothing they wore. As early as 1785, the German sweep is depicted in a close fitting suit complete with head covering [Figure 1.1]. There are no openings for the soot to penetrate nor any loose clothing in which it can lodge. The London sweep, as late as 1851 stands in sharp contrast, a waif-like boy, dirty and in loose smock and trousers. [Figure 1.2]"

Butlin made use of a 'natural experiment' to observe that protective clothing seems to be associated with a reduction in the risk of scrotal cancer.

The development and growth of the field of vital statistics in the 19th century made it possible to study the patterns of cancer occurrence in specific populations. William Farr (1807–83) in England, in collaboration with Marc d'Espine in Geneva, developed a nomenclature system for grouping diseases (Farr, 1975), which formed the basis for the *International Classification of Diseases* (see Appendix 2.2). The adoption of this classification by many countries to code causes of death recorded on death certificates greatly improved the comparability of international mortality statistics. One of the earliest and most extensive reports on international cancer mortality statistics was published by Hoffman in 1915 in a book entitled *The Mortality from Cancer Throughout the World*. A graph from this book is reproduced in Figure 1.3. The first population-based cancer registries, which collect information on all new cases of cancer that occur in a well defined population, were also set up in the first decades of this century (Wagner, 1991) (see Chapter 17).

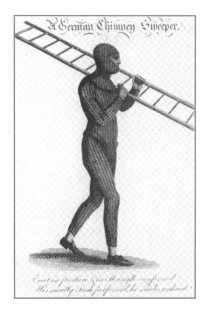

Figure 1.1.
Protective clothing worn by a German sweep in 1785 (reproduced, by permission of BMJ Publishing Group, from Waldron, 1983).

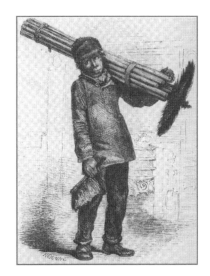

Figure 1.2.
An English chimney sweep in 1851 (reproduced, by permission of BMJ Publishing Group, from Waldron, 1983).

Figure 1.3.
Mortality from all malignant neoplasms for certain countries and cities, 1908–1912 (reproduced from Hoffman, 1915).

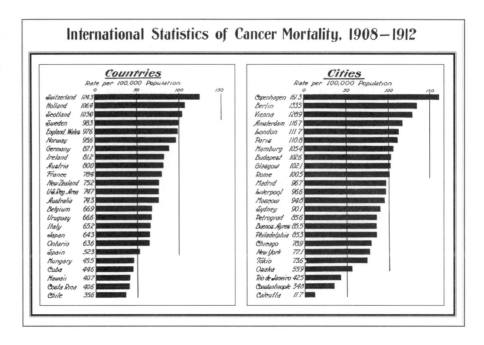

Although several studies that would now be considered examples of cancer epidemiology were conducted before the 20th century, the growth of this discipline (and of epidemiology in general) did not begin until the end of the Second World War. In 1954, results from two important cohort studies, now considered as classical, were published. One was the British Doctors' Study (Doll & Hill, 1954), designed to investigate the relationship between tobacco smoking and lung cancer. The other had been set up to determine the risk of bladder cancer in the British chemical industry (Case *et al.*, 1954; Case & Pearson, 1954).

Cohort studies of human populations, particularly of industrial workers, patients treated with radiation and cytotoxic chemotherapy, and victims of nuclear and other disasters, have provided the most convincing evidence of links between exposure to specific agents and cancer.

In cohort studies, the epidemiologist assembles a group of people and collects information to identify those who are exposed to a particular agent (e.g., smokers) and those who are not (e.g., non-smokers). The group is then followed over time, and the disease occurrence (e.g., lung cancer) in exposed individuals is compared with the disease occurrence in the non-exposed group (see Chapter 8). However, the follow-up and observation of disease occurrence in a population is not a simple task. Many diseases, including cancer, occur rarely, so that large numbers of people must be followed up for long periods to observe enough cases with the disease. This requires a great deal of effort from the researchers, cooperation from the study subjects and, above all, a sizeable budget. The high costs and the logistic difficulties involved mean that cohort studies have been favoured in settings where exposure and medical records and vital statistics are carefully collected and available for use, or where society can support the expense of gathering the necessary information. Despite this, a considerable number of cohort studies have been carried out in developing countries (e.g., Geser *et al.*, 1982; Gupta *et al.*, 1984; Ross *et al.*, 1992). One of the most impressive was the seven-year follow-up of a cohort of 42 000 Ugandan children in an investigation of the etiological role of Epstein–Barr virus in Burkitt's lymphoma (Geser *et al.*, 1982). This study design has also been widely used in developing countries to examine the health effects (including cancer) of exposure to a large number of occupational (Pearce *et al.*, 1994) and other environmental hazards.

The logistic problems and costs encountered with cohort studies have led to the development and increase in popularity of another type of study: the case–control study. In these studies, the epidemiologist compares a group of individuals who have the disease under investigation (termed 'cases'—e.g., persons with lung cancer) with a group without that disease (termed 'controls'), to see whether the groups differ in their past history of exposures (e.g., smoking habits) (see Chapter 9). This type of study is uniquely well suited to studying cancer and other diseases with a long induction period, allowing the epidemiologist to look through time, retrospectively tracing the path back from effect to cause. This is the reverse of the time-sequence adopted in cohort studies. This technique of looking retrospectively is used daily by clinicians when they take case histories. However, case–control studies differ from case series in that they use a control group for drawing comparisons with the group of cases.

One of the earliest studies to make use of the case–control approach was that reported by Broders (1920) on squamous cell epithelioma of the lip in relation to pipe smoking. Unfortunately, Broders failed to describe the method by which he selected the controls. In 1926, Lane-Claypon reported a case–control study of the role of reproductive experience in the etiology of breast cancer. This report is particularly important because it emphasized the need to use a control group for comparison with the cases, and discussed methods for selecting hospital controls to address specific hypotheses. Thereafter until the late 1940s, no further case–control studies of comparable quality were published. There were, however, studies in which the characteristics of cancer patients were compared with those of a group of non-cancer patients; an example, on betel chewing and oral cancers in India, was published by Orr (1933). In 1947, Schrek & Lenowitz reported a case–control study of the relationship between carcinoma of the penis and poor sexual hygiene. In the early 1950s, results from four case–control studies linking cigarette smoking to lung cancer were reported (Schrek *et al.*, 1950; Levin *et al.*, 1950; Wynder & Graham, 1950; Doll & Hill, 1950, 1952), and the following years saw numerous similar studies of many cancers. The 1950s also brought the first methodological developments of the case–control approach (e.g., Cornfield, 1951; Mantel & Haenszel, 1959).

The case–control study has revealed or clarified our understanding of such associations as late first birth and breast cancer (MacMahon *et al.*,

1970); diethylstilbestrol and vaginal clear-cell adenocarcinoma in young women (Herbst *et al.*, 1971); exogenous estrogens and cancer of the endometrium (Ziel & Finkle, 1975; Smith *et al.*, 1975); alcohol and tobacco consumption and cancer of the oesophagus (Tuyns *et al.*, 1977); chronic infection with hepatitis B virus and liver cancer (Prince *et al.*, 1975; Trichopoulos *et al.*, 1978); and human papillomavirus infection and cervical cancer (Muñoz *et al.*, 1992a). The case–control study is particularly appropriate for investigating causal relationships where resources are relatively scarce, such as in developing countries.

A more recent development has been the application of epidemiological principles and methods to the design, conduct and analysis of intervention trials. These are studies in which the exposures being studied are allocated to participants by the investigators themselves (see Chapter 7). This type of controlled experiment has become an integral part of the evaluation of new preventive and therapeutic agents and procedures. For instance, the intervention trial has been used to evaluate the impact of anti-smoking advice on health (Rose & Colwell, 1992), to assess the role of health education programmes in preventing oral cancer in India (Gupta *et al.*, 1986), to evaluate screening programmes for breast cancer (e.g., Shapiro *et al.*, 1971), and to assess the efficacy of hepatitis B vaccination in preventing liver cancer (e.g., Gambia Hepatitis Study Group, 1987).

It is obvious from the low survival from many cancers that if these diseases are to be controlled, we cannot rely solely on increasing the availability of medical care. It is vital to increase our understanding of the genetic, environmental and social factors that foster these diseases, with the aim of applying this knowledge to effective preventive measures. The ultimate goal of cancer epidemiology is to identify risk factors so as to allow the early introduction of effective preventive measures. To achieve this goal, however, cancer epidemiology requires a multidisciplinary approach, bringing together clinicians, laboratory and social scientists, and public health and other health-related professionals.

The contribution of epidemiology to strategies for preventing certain types of cancer was until recently well in advance of our biological knowledge of the disease. However, advances in biology are now providing new tools and directions for epidemiological investigations into the occurrence and distribution of cancer in populations. Incorporation of biological markers into epidemiological research and development of genetic epidemiology are just some examples of this multidisciplinary approach.

Box 1.1. Key issues

- Cancer epidemiology is concerned with the study of the distribution of the disease cancer in populations. Its ultimate goal is to identify risk factors that may lead to early introduction of effective preventive measures.

- Cancer epidemiology, and epidemiology in general, is based on the comparison of groups of people. For ethical reasons, however, epidemiological methods are predominantly observational (i.e., non-experimental). The major challenge for epidemiologists is to identify and make use of 'natural experiments' that will help to answer the question under investigation.

- Cancer epidemiology is a relatively new science, which has matured only in the last half of the 20th century. Despite its youth, it has already contributed greatly to our understanding of the causes of different types of cancers and the evaluation of preventive measures.

Further reading

* Buck *et al.* (1988) compiled and discussed a collection of classic epidemiological papers, including many of those quoted in Section 1.2.

Chapter 2
Measurement of exposures and outcomes

2.1   Introduction

Most epidemiological research involves the study of the relationship of one type of event or characteristic to another. Consider the following questions as examples:

> *   *Does alcohol intake increase the risk of lung cancer?*
>
>   Alcohol ⎯⎯⎯⎯⎯⎯⟶ lung cancer
>   (exposure)   (outcome)

> *   *Does hepatitis B vaccination protect against liver cancer?*
>
>   Hepatitis B vaccine ⎯⟶ liver cancer
>   (exposure)   (outcome)

In these relationships, we assume that one event—exposure—affects the other—outcome.

The *exposure* of interest may be associated with either an increased or a decreased occurrence of disease or other specified health outcome, and may relate to the environment (e.g., air pollution, indoor radon), lifestyle (e.g., smoking habits, diet), or inborn or inherited characteristics (e.g., blood group A, fair skin). The term risk factor is often used to describe an exposure variable.

The *outcome* of a study is a broad term for any defined disease, state of health, health-related event or death. In some studies, there may be multiple outcomes.

The exposures and outcomes of interest are specific to study hypotheses and should always be clearly defined before the study starts. The exposure of interest in one study may be the outcome in another. For example, smoking is clearly the exposure of interest in a study that examines whether smokers are more likely to develop lung cancer than non-smokers, but would be the outcome in a study examining the effectiveness of an anti-smoking intervention programme in reducing the frequency of smoking in a certain population.

In most instances, it is not sufficient to collect information only on the exposure and outcome of interest. This is because their relationship may be mixed up with the effect of another exposure on the same outcome, the two exposures being correlated. This phenomenon is known as confounding. Consider again the relationship between alcohol intake and lung cancer.

* *Does alcohol intake increase the risk of lung cancer?*

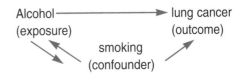

Suppose that a researcher observes that lung cancer occurs more often in people who drink alcohol than in those who do not. It would not be possible to conclude from this observation that exposure to alcohol increases the probability of developing lung cancer, unless the researcher can show that the observed relationship cannot be due to the fact that those who drink alcohol smoke more heavily than non-drinkers. In this example, smoking is acting as a *confounder*. Confounding can be dealt with when designing studies or when analysing the results provided that the relevant data have been collected. These issues are discussed in detail in Chapters 13 and 14.

Thus, most epidemiological studies must collect information on three types of variable:

(1) the primary exposure(s) of interest,
(2) other exposure(s) that may influence the outcome (potential confounders), and
(3) the outcome(s).

It is impossible to select appropriate measurements for a particular investigation unless a specific and detailed statement of research objectives has been made. Without such a statement, information on key variables may be inadequate or missing.

This chapter discusses different ways of collecting data on exposures and outcomes.

2.2   Types of exposure

A wide range of exposures may be of interest in cancer epidemiology. These include genetic traits (e.g., blood group), demographic variables (e.g., sex, age, ethnicity, socioeconomic status), reproductive and sex-related variables, diet and body build, physical activity, smoking and alcohol habits, past medications (e.g., oral contraceptive use), environmental and occupational exposures, and infectious agents.

The characteristic of interest, the true exposure, may not be directly measurable, or it may be difficult or impossible to define. Socioeconomic status is an example of such an abstract concept. Epidemiologists commonly measure socioeconomic status using proxy variables such as occupation, income, education, and place of residence. Moreover, socioeconomic status is not *per se* a cause of disease, but rather an indicator of the level or probability of exposure to some underlying cause, which is often unknown.

2.3. Measurement of exposure

Data on the exposures of interest may be obtained through personal interviews (either face-to-face or by telephone), self-administered questionnaires, diaries of behaviour, reference to records, biological measurements and measurements in the environment. If a subject is too young, too ill, or dead, it is also common to obtain data from a proxy respondent, usually a member of their family.

The method chosen to collect data depends on many factors: the type of study; the type and detail of data required; availability of existing records collected for other purposes; lack of knowledge or poor recall of the exposure by subjects; sensitivity of the subjects to questioning about the exposure; frequency and level of the exposure, and their variability over time; availability of physical or chemical methods for measuring the exposure in the human body or in the environment; and the costs of the various possible methods. Often, more than one approach is used. Different components of the data often require different collection methods, and using several methods of data collection can help to validate data and to reduce error in measurement (see Section 2.6).

The information obtained should include details of the exact nature of the exposure, its amount or dose, and its distribution over time.

2.3.1 Nature of the exposure

The information collected should be as detailed as possible. For instance, it is better to enquire about different forms of tobacco smoking separately (cigarettes, pipes, cigars), rather than to enquire simply about 'smoking'. Questions on types of cigarette may also be asked to obtain information on their tar content. Enquiries should also be made about the route of exposure to the agent (for example, in a study of contraceptives and breast cancer, it is important to distinguish oral contraceptives from other types of contraceptive), as well as about any behaviour that may protect against exposure (for example, in an occupational study, it is important to ask about any behaviour that may have protected the workers from being exposed to hazards, such as use of protective clothing).

2.3.2 Dose

Exposure is seldom simply present or absent. Most exposures of interest are quantitative variables. Smokers can be classified according to the number of cigarettes smoked daily; industrial exposures by the extent of exposure (often achieved by classifying workers according to the duration of employment and type of job); infections by dose of agent or age at exposure; breast-feeding by duration; and psychological exposures by some arbitrary scale of severity. Thus the simple situation of two groups, one exposed and one unexposed, is rare, and the conclusions of a study are greatly strengthened where there is a trend of increasing disease incidence with increasing exposure—an exposure–response relationship.

Dose may be measured either as the total accumulated dose (cumulative exposure), for example, the total number of packets of cigarettes ever smoked, or as the dose or exposure rate, for example, the number of cigarettes smoked daily. Exposure rate is a measurement of dose per unit time.

It is important to realize that although measurements of dose are usually made in the subject's external environment (e.g., levels of environmental pollution), this is not the dose that matters in biological terms. The biologically effective dose is the amount of the external agent or its active metabolite that affects cellular mechanisms in the target organs. The biologically effective dose cannot usually be measured directly, but it may be possible to obtain an estimate, an example being the measurement in humans of DNA adducts with nitrosamines or aflatoxins. Nevertheless, such measurements have their limitations: for instance, they may be useful markers of current or recent, but not of past, exposure (see Section 2.4.4).

2.3.3 Time

As far as possible, each exposure should be characterized as to when it began, when it ended (if at all), and how it was distributed during the intervening period (was it periodic or continuous? did the dose vary over time?). Similar details should also be obtained for any behaviour that may protect against the exposure.

There is thought to be a restricted period, the critical time window, during which the exposure could have caused cancer. Unfortunately, the beginning and end of this critical time window are not known, and its length is likely to vary between individuals. Collecting data on the timing of exposure allows the possible extent of this window to be estimated. Analyses may include examination of the effects of time since first exposure and time since last exposure.

Pattern of exposure may also be important. Exposure that occurs periodically in intense bursts may have a different effect from a similar total amount of exposure that occurs continuously at low intensity (e.g., constant versus intermittent exposure to sunlight; chronic exposure to low levels of ionizing radiation versus acute exposure to high levels).

2.4 Sources of exposure data

2.4.1 Questionnaires

Questionnaires are used to collect exposure data in epidemiological studies by putting the same set of questions to each study participant in a standardized form. Questionnaires can be self-administered or may be administered by an interviewer.

The aim of a research questionnaire is to obtain, with minimal error, measurements of the exposure variables of interest for the study. Thus, the questions to be included in a questionnaire should relate directly to the objectives of the study. Some basic principles that should be taken into account when designing a questionnaire are discussed in Appendix 2.1. To ensure that the questions are properly understood and will elicit appropriate answers, questionnaires should be pre-tested on a sample of subjects from the population to be studied.

Self-administered questionnaires

Self-administered questionnaires are distributed to study subjects who are asked to complete them. They can be delivered and returned either personally or by mail if this is feasible and more convenient. Such questionnaires are particularly appropriate when small amounts of reasonably simple data are required, or for documenting sensitive or socially undesirable behaviour. They are one of the cheapest ways of collecting information, but have the limitation that they can be used only in literate populations. The investigator also has relatively little control on the quality of the data collected.

Personal interviews (interviewer-administered questionnaires)

Using an interviewer to administer a questionnaire may reduce error by increasing the subjects' participation and motivating them to respond adequately. Moreover, an interviewer may probe to obtain more complete data. However, interviewers may also increase error if they influence the subject's responses, either directly or indirectly.

As an interview is a conversation between interviewer and respondent, it is essential that a rapport is established right from the start. Interviewers should be selected taking into account the cultural norms of the study population, so that they will be trusted by the study subjects. As a simple example, in some societies, male interviewers will not be allowed to interview women. Cultural characteristics of interviewers may also influence the degree of participation of respondents, and/or the accuracy of the information they give. The respondent must feel that the interviewer understands him or her and that there are no barriers to communication.

For collecting large amounts of complex data, face-to-face interviews are clearly best. However, when subjects are widely dispersed and the questionnaire is relatively brief, interviewing by telephone may be a better approach. Of course, this is feasible only where the telephone is widely used, which is not always the case. Even in societies where there is widespread use of telephones, certain groups of people will be excluded from the study either because they do not have a telephone or because they do not like to provide personal information over the telephone.

Proxy or *surrogate respondents* are people who provide information on exposure in place of the study subjects themselves (index subjects). They are used in epidemiology when the index subjects are for any reason unable to provide the data required. Studies involving children normally also rely on proxy respondents. Proxy respondents usually provide less valid information than the index subjects; for instance, they often tend to under-enumerate occupational exposures and to report the index subject as having a job of higher status than is actually the case. Closeness to the study subject is an important determinant of the quality of information obtained; in general, the most accurate information tends to come from spouses and, in the case of children, mothers.

2.4.2 Diaries

Diaries are detailed records of exposure kept by the subject. They are generally open-ended and take the form of a booklet in which the subject records each occurrence of a particular behaviour such as physical exercise, alcohol consumption, dietary intake, sexual activity, use of medication, etc. Diaries are assumed to be highly accurate in measuring current behaviour, because they do not rely on memory. They also allow more detailed information about the exposure to be collected than with a questionnaire. For example, foods can be weighed by the subject before being eaten.

The main limitation of diaries is that only current exposures can be measured. In addition, diaries generally demand more of subjects in terms of time and skill than other methods, so compliance may be a problem. Training of subjects in the skills needed to keep an accurate diary can be time-consuming for both subjects and investigators. Thus, diaries are rarely used in countries in which many people are illiterate.

2.4.3 Records

Data on the exposure of interest may be available from census, employment, medical (in- and out-patient), cancer registry, birth certification and death certification records. Typically, as the data have already been collected for purposes other than epidemiological research, the researcher has no control over what items were recorded, how questions were phrased, and so on. Records are also often produced by a large number of people with little uniform training. Moreover, the availability and quality of records in many countries tends to be poor.

Despite these limitations, the use of records has several advantages over other methods of data collection. Study costs are usually low, and the duration of the study is shorter because some or all of the data have already been collected. Records can also provide near-complete data on a well defined population, and information can be obtained without contacting the subjects or their relatives. Certain data items (for example, intake of medications or occupational exposures) may be recorded more accurately than information obtained in a personal interview; for instance, errors caused by poor recall or lack of knowledge of the exposure are eliminated.

Characteristics and limitations of some such routine data-collection systems are discussed in more detail in Section 2.9 and Chapter 11.

2.4.4 Biological measurements

In principle, the ideal approach to determining exposure involves measurements made directly on the human body or its products. Biological measurements will be more objective, in that they are independent both of the subjects' perceptions and, where instrumental or laboratory methods are used, of the researcher. Biological measurements may also reflect more closely the biologically effective dose, i.e., the level of exposure that affects cells in the target organ(s).

Interest in the epidemiological application of measurements of exposure in the human body has recently been growing, with the development of increasingly refined laboratory techniques for measuring active metabolites of carcinogens and the products of their interaction with DNA or proteins (adducts). The term 'molecular epidemiology' has been coined to describe epidemiological approaches that incorporate a laboratory component.

An example of the successful application of molecular epidemiology is the measurement of aflatoxin in the human diet. Aflatoxin is produced by the mould *Aspergillus flavus*, which grows on stored foods such as groundnuts in tropical climates, in particular in eastern Asia and sub-Saharan Africa. Although experiments have shown that aflatoxin is a potent inducer of liver cancer in laboratory animals, most epidemiological research has been hampered by the difficulty of measuring the amount of aflatoxin consumed by humans. Recently, biological markers for estimating current or recent aflatoxin consumption have been established, involving measurement of metabolites of aflatoxin and DNA adducts in the urine. Such measurements were made in a study undertaken in Shanghai (Qian *et al.*, 1994), in which the incidence of liver cancer in approximately 18 000 Chinese men was related to urinary measurements of their exposure to aflatoxin. Results from this study have provided the most direct evidence that aflatoxin has an etiological role in human hepatocellular carcinogenesis. These biological markers are, however, not ideal, as they cannot measure past exposure, which may be crucial in studying the role of aflatoxin in liver cancer.

Laboratory assays have also been developed to ascertain exposure to infectious agents such as human papillomavirus (HPV) (Muñoz *et al.*, 1992b) and *Helicobacter pylori* (IARC, 1994a). These assays have helped to clarify the role of HPV infection in the etiology of cervical cancer, and that of *H. pylori* in stomach cancer.

The possibility of using laboratory measurements in an epidemiological study is determined mainly by the availability of a suitable test, its feasibility (e.g., availability of laboratory equipment) and the cost. Moreover, most laboratory measurements are limited in that they can assess only current exposures, while past exposure is generally more relevant in cancer epidemiology. Thus, laboratory measurements are particularly useful when they assess attributes that remain stable, for example, genetic traits. One way in which this limitation can be overcome is to use banks of biological specimens. Biological samples collected some time before the study subjects develop the outcome of interest can be analysed with the latest laboratory techniques. For instance, blood and urine samples may be collected from all individuals in a particular cohort at the time they enter the study and an aliquot stored frozen. These samples can be re-analysed later when more sophisticated techniques become available.

2.4.5 Measurements in the environment

Measurements in the environment include those of agents in the air (e.g., air pollutants, dust), water (e.g., fluoride), soil (e.g., elements), foods (e.g., nutrient composition), etc. The samples may come from homes, workplaces, recreational sites, or the ambient environment in general. Such measurements are particularly useful when the subjects are unaware of the exposure (e.g., indoor radiation levels) or cannot recall it accurately.

The value of environmental measurements depends on the procedures used both for sampling and for analysis. Ideally, environmental agents should be assessed for each study subject throughout the etiologically relevant period, so as to reflect as accurately as possible personal attributes. For example, individual measurements of exposure to ionizing radiation can be made by each study subject wearing a film-badge throughout the study period and individual nutrient intake can be measured by analysing identical portions of all foods and beverages consumed by a subject during the study period. However, this approach is generally not feasible because of time and cost constraints, technical concerns and lack of subject compliance. Usually it is only possible to make measurements in a sample of study subjects at certain defined time points. The choice of the sample and the timing of the measurements is obviously of crucial importance to the validity of the measurements.

One limitation of environmental measurements is that they usually reflect only current exposure levels. In certain situations, it may be reasonable to assume that measurements made in the present environment are highly correlated with the exposure levels at etiologically relevant periods in the past. Records of previous exposure measurements may be available, but should be used with caution: such measurements were usually made for other purposes using methods that may now be considered inadequate. When no such measurements are available, proxy measures of past exposures may be used. For example, in a study of occupational exposures, information on 'type of job', 'year of employment' and 'duration of employment' may be used to classify workers according to exposure status. This information may be extracted from employment records or obtained through questionnaires.

2.5 Measurement of outcome

As for measurements of exposure, data on the outcome(s) of interest may be obtained from various sources. Regular questionnaires or telephone calls may be used to ascertain subjects' health status. Periodic personal interviews with clinical check-ups may be arranged, which may include biological measurements and any other appropriate diagnostic procedures (e.g., radiography, endoscopy, ultrasound, etc.). Alternatively, information on the outcomes, and in particular on the occurrence of cancer, may be obtained from records, such as hospital records, cancer registrations, death certificates or some other specialized surveillance method (see Section 2.9). When records are used, the data available are limited to outcomes that are recorded routinely, their completeness, and the way in which they are coded.

Because malignancies develop slowly and are relatively rare, studies of the relationship between suspected carcinogenic exposures and cancer may require the observation of many participants over a long period. One way to avoid this is to use intermediate end-points as cancer surrogates: that is, to use as an outcome a biological event that is believed to lie on the causal pathway between exposure and cancer. Studies that use intermediate end-points are, in principle, quicker, smaller and less expensive than those using malignancy as the outcome. For instance, a study of the relationship between diet and estrogen metabolism could be carried out on several dozen patients, whereas a dietary intervention study with breast cancer as the end-point would require tens of thousands of women with many years of follow-up (Schatzkin *et al.*, 1990). The underlying assumption in these studies is that the observed relationship between exposure (e.g., diet) and the intermediate end-point (e.g., estrogen metabolism) reflects a similar relationship between exposure and the cancer of interest. Clearly, this assumption must be validated before the intermediate end-point can be used as a cancer surrogate (Toniolo *et al.*, 1997).

2.6 Validity and reliability of measurements of exposure and outcome

2.6.1 Validity

Validity is defined as the extent to which an instrument (for example, a questionnaire or a laboratory test) measures what it is intended to measure. Validity can be determined only if there is a reference procedure or 'gold standard': a definitive procedure to determine the characteristic being measured. For example, information on birth weight obtained from an interview can be validated against hospital records, and food-frequency questionnaires against food diaries and biological measurements. However, in some circumstances there is no obvious reference procedure and the best available method must be taken as the standard.

Consider the simple example of a test that can give only a positive or negative (i.e., binary) result. When the same subjects have been examined by both the study test and the gold standard, the findings can be expressed in a 2×2 table, as in Table 2.1.

The *sensitivity* of the study test is the proportion of individuals classified as positives by the gold standard who are correctly identified by the study test:

Sensitivity = $a/(a+c)$

		Gold standard	
		Positive	Negative
Study	Positive	*a*	*b*
test	Negative	*c*	*d*

a, true positives; *b*, false positives; *c*, false negatives; *d*, true negatives .

Table 2.1.
General layout of a 2 x 2 table to assess the validity of a test that can give only a binary result.

The *specificity* of the study test is the proportion of individuals classified as negatives by the gold standard who are correctly identified by the study test:

Specificity = $d/(b+d)$

The *predictive value of a positive study test result* represents the probability that someone with a positive study test result really has the characteristic of interest as determined by the gold standard:

Predictive value of a positive study test result = $a/(a+b)$

The *predictive value of a negative study test result* represents the probability that someone with a negative study test result does not have the characteristic of interest as determined by the gold standard:

Predictive value of a negative study test result = $d/(c+d)$

Example 2.1. *A variety of laboratory methods have been developed for detecting human papillomavirus (HPV) infection of the cervix uteri. In a study conducted some years ago, the performance of a new commercially available dot-filter hybridization test (ViraPap®) was assessed by comparing its results with those obtained using a gold standard test in a sample of 450 women who attended a clinic for sexually transmitted diseases in Washington state, USA during 1987–88 (Kiviat et al., 1990). The Southern hybridization test, which is expensive and time-consuming, was taken as the gold standard in this study. The results are shown in Table 2.2.*

Table 2.2.
Comparison of ViraPap® and Southern hybridization methods in the diagnosis of cervical HPV infection in a sample of women who attended a sexually transmitted disease clinic.[a]

		Southern hybridization (gold standard test)		
		Positive	Negative	Total
ViraPap® (new test)	Positive	62	22	84
	Negative	7	359	366
	Total	69	381	450

[a] Modified from Kiviat *et al.*, 1990

These data yield the following for the ViraPap® test:
Sensitivity = 62/69 = 90%
Specificity = 359/381 = 94%
Predictive value of a positive ViraPap® test = 62/84 = 74%
Predictive value of a negative ViraPap® test = 359/366 = 98%

An ideal test has high sensitivity (correctly identifies a high proportion of truly exposed or diseased individuals) and high specificity (gives few positive results in unexposed or non-diseased individuals). In Example 2.1, the ViraPap® test had both high sensitivity and high specificity, indicating that the test was highly valid in the detection of cervical HPV infection (as compared to the Southern hybridization test) and therefore that its results would be little affected by measurement error.

While the predictive value of a study test result strongly depends upon the frequency of the disease (or other characteristic of interest) in the population, sensitivity and specificity are essentially unaffected. When the disease frequency changes, the numbers of diseased people as determined by the gold standard (left-hand column) change in proportion to the numbers of non-diseased people (right-hand column). Unlike sensitivity and specificity, the predictive value of a study test result depends on the numbers in both columns, and will change if the frequency of the disease changes.

Example 2.2. Suppose that the same ViraPap® test was used in a sample of 450 apparently healthy women who visited their general practitioners for a regular check-up. The results are given in Table 2.3.

		Southern hybridization (gold standard test)		
		Positive	Negative	Total
ViraPap® (new test)	Positive	21	26	47
	Negative	2	401	403
	Total	23	427	450

Table 2.3.
Comparison of ViraPap® and Southern hybridization methods in the detection of cervical HPV infection among apparently healthy women: hypothetical data.

These data yield the following for the ViraPap® test:
Sensitivity = 21/23 = 91%
Specificity = 401/427 = 94%
Predictive value of a positive ViraPap® test = 21/47 = 45%
Predictive value of a negative ViraPap® test = 401/403 = 100%

In Example 2.2, the predictive value of a positive ViraPap® test is markedly decreased (from 74% to 45%). This is because the proportion of HPV-infected women (as determined by the gold standard) was much higher (69/450 = 15%) in the sample of women who attended the clinic for sexually transmitted disease (Table 2.2) than among the group of apparently healthy women (23/450 = 5%). Thus, diagnostic tests which are useful in clinical medicine may perform poorly in epidemiological surveys or in population screening programmes. In clinical medicine, diagnostic tests are applied to patients in populations already selected as having a high occurrence of the condition. In this situation, the test may have high predictive value. In an epidemiological survey of an unselected population, the same test may have poor predictive value because the frequency of the condition is much lower. For example, mammography has high predictive value as a test for breast cancer in women who consult doctors because of a lump in the breast, but low predictive value when used to screen apparently healthy women in the population. These issues are discussed further in Chapter 16.

The selection of a gold standard is a crucial aspect of evaluating the validity of any measurement. Unfortunately, in many cases there is no appropriate gold standard, and the investigator has to rely on the best available method. For instance, for many years, Southern hybridization was regarded as the gold standard method for detecting cervical HPV infection. However, with the development in recent years of polymerase chain reaction (PCR) to amplify HPV-specific DNA sequences, these newer methods have become the accepted gold standard.

Example 2.3. *The performance of the ViraPap® test was compared with that of the polymerase chain reaction (PCR) in newly diagnosed cervical cancer patients. Results are shown in Table 2.4.*

Table 2.4.
Comparison of ViraPap® and polymerase chain reaction (PCR) in the detection of cervical HPV infection.[a]

		PCR (gold standard test)		
		Positive	Negative	Total
ViraPap® test	Positive	163	11	174
	Negative	120	79	199
	Total	283	90	373

[a] From Muñoz *et al.* (unpublished)

These data yield the following for the ViraPap® test:
Sensitivity = 163/283 = 58%
Specificity = 79 / 90 = 88%

In Example 2.3 the validity of the ViraPap® test (as measured by its sensitivity and specificity) was much lower than when Southern hybridization was used as the gold standard method (Example 2.1). This is because the PCR method is more sensitive and more specific than the Southern hybridization technique.

Not all tests give a simple yes/no result. Some yield results that are numerical values along a continuous scale of measurement. In these situations, high sensitivity is obtained at the cost of low specificity and vice versa. For example, the higher the blood pressure, the more probable is hypertensive disease. If a diagnostic or screening test for hypertension is set at a diastolic pressure of 90 mmHg, most hypertensive patients would be detected (high sensitivity) but many non-diseased subjects (with diastolic blood pressure higher than 90 mmHg) will be wrongly classified as hypertensive (low specificity). If the screening level for hypertensive disease is set at 110 mmHg for diastolic blood pressure, most non-diseased individuals would be excluded (high specificity), but many hypertensive patients (with diastolic blood pressures lower than 110 mmHg) would be missed (low sensitivity).

Example 2.4. A new laboratory assay measuring the concentration of a particular enzyme in the blood is developed. To assess its value in the diagnosis of a specific cancer, the new test is applied to 360 hospital patients and the results are compared with those from anatomo-pathological examination. Blood concentrations of the enzyme ≥40 IU are taken as positive results. The results are shown in Table 2.5.

		Anatomo-pathological examination (gold standard test)		
		Positive	Negative	Total
Blood assay	Positive (≥40 IU)	190	80	270
	Negative (<40 IU)	0	90	90
	Total	190	170	360

Table 2.5.
Comparison of a new laboratory assay with anatomo-pathological examination in the diagnosis of a specific cancer: hypothetical data.

The following can be calculated for the new laboratory assay:
Sensitivity = 190/190 = 100%
Specificity = 90 / 170 = 53%

In Example 2.4, other blood concentration values could be taken as cut-off values to define the assay results as 'positive' or 'negative'. Table 2.6 gives the sensitivity and specificity of the blood assay for different cut-off values. The sensitivity of the laboratory assay decreases as the cut-off value increases, whereas the reverse is true for specificity. This is clearly illustrated in Figure 2.1.

One way to summarize the validity of a continuous measurement is to plot sensitivity against (1 – specificity) for different cut-off values. This curve is called the receiver operating characteristic (ROC) curve. The ROC curve corresponding to the data in Table 2.6 is shown in Figure 2.2.

The closer the ROC curve of a particular test is to the top left-hand corner of the box, where both the sensitivity and specificity are maximized, the better the test. A test with a curve that lies on the diagonal is for practical purposes useless, and no better than a complete guess.

Table 2.6.
Sensitivity and specificity of the blood assay for different cut-off values: hypothetical data.

Cut-off value (IU)	Result of blood assay	Result of anatomo-pathological examination	Number of patients
40[a]	+	+	190
	+	−	80
	−	+	0
	−	−	90
80[a]	+	+	188
	+	−	42
	−	+	2
	−	−	128
120[a]	+	+	173
	+	−	25
	−	+	17
	−	−	145
280[a]	+	+	95
	+	−	0
	−	+	95
	−	−	170

[a] Blood assay results equal to or greater than the cut-off value were taken as positive: +, positive result; −, negative result

40 IU: sensitivity = 190 / 190 = 100%   specificity = 90 / 170 = 53%
80 IU: sensitivity = 188 / 190 = 99%   specificity = 128 / 170 = 75%
120 IU: sensitivity = 173 / 190 = 91%   specificity = 145 / 170 = 85%
280 IU: sensitivity = 95 / 190 = 50%   specificity = 170 / 170 = 100%

Figure 2.1.
The upper curve describes the distribution of results of the blood assay among healthy individuals and the lower curve the distribution among cancer patients (as defined by the anatomo-pathological examination). Different cut-off values are used to classify the results of the blood assay as 'positive' or 'negative'.

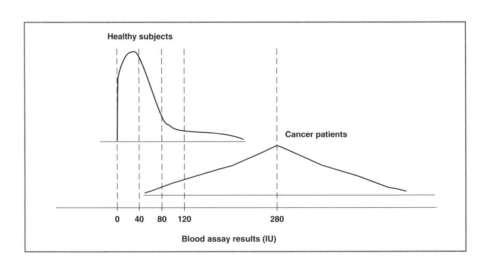

2.6.2 Reliability

Reliability, sometimes also called repeatability or reproducibility, is a measure of the consistency of the performance of a test when used under similar circumstances. To be valid, a measurement must be reliable. However, reliability is not in itself sufficient for validity: in other words, a test may yield the same result consistently, but the result may not be the true (valid) one. Poor reliability of a measurement may be due to variation when a subject is tested on different occasions (biological variation), or to errors in the measurement technique (observer and instrument variation). Checks of the repeatability of measurements of the main exposures and outcomes should usually be included in an epidemiological study. These checks can take various forms.

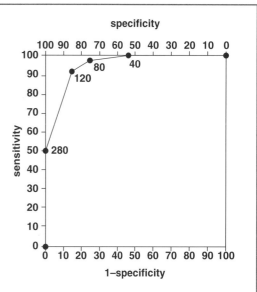

Figure 2.2.
Receiver operating characteristic (ROC) curve for the data in Table 2.6 and Figure 2.1.

(1) Intra-observer or intra-measurement reliability

Intra-observer or intra-measurement reliability can be determined by having the same observer perform the same measurements on the same subjects on two or more separate occasions. For example, data from medical records may be extracted by the same abstractor on two occasions; the same interviewer may re-interview subjects after a time interval; duplicate biological samples may be re-processed by the same laboratory technician. These separate measurements are then compared. The appropriate time interval between measurements varies according to the type of outcome or exposure measurement. If it is too short, subjects and/or observers may recall the previous result; if it is too long, the subject's exposure or outcome status may have changed (of course, this is not a problem when data are extracted from medical records).

(2) Inter-observer reliability

Inter-observer reliability can be assessed by having the same subjects measured by two or more independent observers. For example, the performance of two or more data abstractors may be compared using information extracted independently from the same medical records, or the performance of two or more interviewers may be compared using independent interviews of the same subjects on two different occasions. Again, the interval used between measurements needs careful consideration.

Consider the simple example of a test that can give only a positive or negative (i.e. binary) result. The agreement between pairs of measurements carried out by two independent observers on the same subjects can be presented as a 2×2 table (Table 2.7).

One measure of repeatability is the observed agreement (O) or mean pair agreement index, which can be calculated as:

(No. of agreements/Total no. of pairs) = $(a + d) / N$

Table 2.7.
General layout of a table to assess reliability between two observers for a binary test. *a*, *b*, *c* and *d* refer to the numbers of pairs of observations where the observers gave the indicated result.

		Observer B		
		Positive	Negative	Row total
Observer A	Positive	*a*	*b*	*a+b*
	Negative	*c*	*d*	*c+d*
Column total		*a+c*	*b+d*	
			Grand total	*N*

This index has the disadvantage that some agreement would be expected even if both observers simply guessed the result. The kappa statistic (κ) is an alternative measure that takes account of the agreement expected solely on the basis of chance.

To calculate the kappa statistic, the number of pairs of observations that would be expected on the basis of chance in cells (++) and (– –) must first be calculated. The expected value in any cell is given by:

[(Total of relevant row) × (Total of relevant column)]/Grand total

Thus for cell (++), the expected value will equal:

$[(a+b) \times (a+c)]/N$

and for cell (– –), the expected value will equal:

$[(c+d) \times (b+d)]/N$

The expected agreement on the basis of chance (*E*) can now be calculated as:

[Expected value for cell (++) + Expected value for cell (– –)] / *N*

The actual agreement beyond chance is therefore:

Observed agreement (*O*) – Expected agreement (*E*)

This value is, however, difficult to interpret, as similar results may be obtained for different values of *O* and *E*. For instance, the actual agreement beyond chance is equal to 0.20 for values of $O = 0.95$ and $E = 0.75$, and for $O = 0.75$ and $E = 0.55$. What we need to know is how much does it represent in relation to the maximum potential agreement beyond chance that could have been achieved. Complete agreement would imply that all the results would have fallen in cells (++) and (– –) and, therefore, $(a+d)/N$ would have equalled 1. Thus, the potential for agreement beyond chance is

$1 - E$

The kappa statistic indicates how much the actual agreement beyond chance (O–E) represents relative to this potential ($1 - E$).

Kappa (κ) = ($O - E$)/($1 - E$)

The kappa statistic can be used in a similar way to measure intra-observer variability. The values of this coefficient may vary from –1.0 to 1.0. A value of 1.0 indicates perfect agreement and a value of zero means agreement is no better than would be expected on the basis of chance alone; a negative value indicates that the level of disagreement is greater than that expected on the basis of chance. While there is no value of kappa that can be regarded universally as indicating good agreement, in practice, a κ value considerably less than 0.5 indicates poor agreement. Landis and Koch (1977) suggested the following guidelines: kappa values ≤0.40 represent poor-to-fair agreement; 0.41–0.60, moderate agreement; 0.61–0.80, substantial agreement; and 0.81–1.00, almost perfect agreement.

Use of the kappa statistic can be extended to situations where the results of the test are classified in more than two categories, as in Example 2.5. The kappa shows substantial agreement between observers A and B. Intra-observer agreement was calculated in a similar way: the kappa statistic equalled 0.83. In general, intra-observer agreement tends to be better than inter-observer agreement.

kappa values should not be presented alone, as they provide a summary measure of agreement without giving any indication where disagreements occurred. The results of a reliability study should therefore always be presented in a table similar to Table 2.8, so that the main areas of agreement and disagreement are apparent. If different importance is given to different types of agreement or disagreement, the kappa statistics may be weighted to take this into account (Landis & Koch, 1977).

Methods are also available for assessing the reliability of measurements that provide results on a continuous scale (e.g. blood pressure measurements, blood glucose levels): however, these are beyond the scope of this chapter. A discussion of these methods can be found in Bland & Altman (1986).

2.7 Consequences of measurement error

Errors in measurement can lead to individuals being misclassified and to spurious conclusions about the relationship between the exposure and the outcome. The impact of measurement errors on the results of an epidemiological study depends essentially on the nature of any misclassification.

Consider the following example. Suppose that to determine whether cigarette smoking is associated with lung cancer, we rely on a questionnaire that asks 'Have you ever smoked?' and 'Do you have lung cancer?'. The questionnaire is administered to 10 000 men. Assume that the 'true'

Example 2.5. In the study by Kiviat et al. *(1990) mentioned in Section 2.6.1, the authors state: 'To assess inter-observer variation all autoradiographs were initially reviewed independently by two observers without their knowledge of other laboratory and clinical data, and specimens were classified as positive, negative, or indeterminate according to the manufacturer's specifications. Intra-observer variation was assessed by having membranes re-read by observer A six months later without her knowledge of other (or previous) laboratory or clinical data'. The results for inter-observer variability are given in Table 2.8.*

Table 2.8.
Inter-observer variability in the reading of the ViraPap® test.[a]

	Observer B[b]			
	Positive	Negative	Indeterminate	Row total
Observer A[b]				
Positive	58 (a_1)	8 (a_2)	2 (a_3)	68 (a)
Negative	12 (b_1)	357 (b_2)	3 (b_3)	372 (b)
Indeterminate	0 (c_1)	0 (c_2)	7 (c_3)	7 (c)
Column total	70 (n_1)	365 (n_2)	12 (n_3)	447 (N)

[a] Data from Kiviat *et al.* (1990).
[b] Figures represent numbers of pairs of observations where the observers gave the indicated result; letters in parentheses indicate each specific cell in the table.

Observed agreement (O) = (a_1 + b_2 + c_3)/N = (58 + 357 + 7)/447 = 0.94
Expected value for cell a_1 = ($a \times n_1$)/N = (68 × 70)/447 = 10.65
Expected value for cell b_2 = ($b \times n_2$)/N = (372 × 365)/447 = 303.76
Expected value for cell c_3 = ($c \times n_3$)/N = (7 × 12)/447 = 0.19
Agreement expected on the basis of chance (E) = (10.65 + 303.76 + 0.19)/447 = 0.70
Actual agreement beyond chance (O − E) = 0.94 − 0.70 = 0.24.
Potential agreement beyond chance = 1 − 0.70 = 0.30.
Kappa (κ) = 0.24 / 0.30 = 0.80

Table 2.9.
Distribution of a population by smoking and disease status as determined by a perfect test for measuring smoking habits (sensitivity = 100%; specificity = 100%): hypothetical data.

		Cigarette smoking		
		Ever	Never	Total
Lung cancer	**Yes**	150	50	200
	No	1850	7950	9800
	Total	2000	8000	10 000

smoking status in this study population (as determined by a perfect test, having both a sensitivity and a specificity of 100%) is as indicated in Table 2.9. This table shows that lung cancer is more common among people who have smoked (ever smokers) (150 of 2000 = 7.5%) than among those who have never smoked (never smokers) (50 of 8000 = 0.63%). Thus, if a perfect method could be used to measure smoking habits in this example, ever smokers would be found to be 12 times (7.5% / 0.63% = 12) more likely to develop lung cancer than never smokers.

| | | Cigarette smoking | | |
		Ever	Never	Total
Lung cancer	Yes	$150 - 0.2 \times 150 = 120$	$50 + 0.2 \times 150 = 80$	200
	No	$1850 - 0.2 \times 1850 = 1480$	$7950 + 0.2 \times 1850 = 8320$	9800
	Total	1600	8400	10 000

Table 2.10.
Distribution of a population by smoking and disease status as determined by a test for measuring smoking habits that has a sensitivity of 80% and a specificity of 100%: hypothetical data.

Suppose now that when the questionnaire is applied, 20% of smokers, regardless of their disease status, answered that they had never smoked (sensitivity=80%), but that all men who have never smoked reported this accurately (specificity=100%). The results that would be obtained with this imperfect questionnaire are shown in Table 2.10.

Using this imperfect questionnaire, the proportion of lung cancers in 'smokers' is 120/1600=7.5%. This is about eight times the proportion in 'never smokers' (80/8400=0.95%). Despite the poor quality of the data on smoking elicited by the questionnaire, the relationship between cigarette smoking and lung cancer, while appearing weaker than it truly is, is still evident.

Non-differential misclassification occurs when an exposure or outcome classification is incorrect for equal proportions of subjects in the groups being compared. In other words, the sensitivity and specificity of the exposure (or outcome) measurement are equal for both the diseased and non-diseased (or exposed and unexposed). In these circumstances, the misclassification is random (i.e., all individuals have the same probability of being misclassified).

In non-differential misclassification, individuals are wrongly classified, reducing the confidence that can be placed in each particular test result. Although this random misclassification has important implications in clinical medicine, it is of less concern in epidemiology, where groups rather than individuals are the main interest. Herein lies a great strength of epidemiology. In the above example, the association between smoking and lung cancer was weakened because those classifying themselves as 'never smokers' were in fact a mixture of those who had never smoked and those who had. Although this type of misclassification makes it more difficult to reveal an association between the exposure and the outcome of interest, the problem can usually be overcome by increasing the sample size and/or replicating measurements (except, as discussed in Chapter 13, where there is non-differential misclassification of confounding variables). Thus, the epidemiologist can rely on simple, cheap and non-invasive tests which, despite being in general less valid than those used in clinical settings, are more appropriate for studies in the community.

This is an important aspect of epidemiological research that clinicians often find difficult to accept. Clinicians focus on individual patients, trying to obtain the most complete and valid information on which to base the most accurate diagnosis possible and the optimal treatment. Being accustomed to using specialized and high-technology procedures, they may find it hard to believe that one could undertake scientific studies based on relatively low-quality data such as those derived from questionnaires or death certificates.

Differential misclassification occurs when the sensitivity and/or specificity of the exposure measurement for the diseased group differs from that for the non-diseased group, or when the sensitivity and/or specificity of the outcome measurement for the exposed group differs from that for the unexposed group. In other words, differential misclassification may occur when errors in classification of outcome status are dependent upon exposure status, or vice versa. For example, clinicians may be more likely to diagnose leukaemia in children who live around nuclear power stations than in those living elsewhere, and women with breast cancer may be more likely to remember having taken oral contraceptives in the past than healthy women. In the example already considered, differential misclassification would have occurred if men with lung cancer were likely to report their smoking habits more or less accurately than men without lung cancer; in such circumstances, the resulting data could exaggerate, attenuate, or even reverse the relationship, and make the results misleading.

Differential misclassification is a consequence of defects in the design or execution of an epidemiological study. Unfortunately, it cannot be controlled for in the analysis, and its effect cannot be minimized by increasing the sample size.

A more detailed discussion of the consequences of errors in the measurement of exposure and outcome in the interpretation of epidemiological studies is given elsewhere in this book; in particular, in Chapter 13.

2.8 How can misclassification of exposure and outcome be reduced?

All procedures used in the measurements should be described in sufficient detail in the study protocol to allow reproduction of the measurements, within the limits of biological and physical variability, by other investigators. The protocol should include not only a description of the method of measurement, but also instructions for its application. All other procedures involved should also be specified.

For a personal interview, this will include:
- specifications for the training of interviewers and instructions given to them,
- instructions or explanations given by interviewers to subjects,
- the questionnaire used to elicit data from the subjects,
- quality-control procedures.

For a laboratory test, this will include:
- procedures for the preparation of subjects,
- procedures for the collection, manipulation, transport, and storage of the specimens,
- analytical procedures in the laboratory,
- quality-control procedures.

The epidemiologist should establish and maintain close contact with the specialists in the laboratory, so that standard criteria for collecting, storing and analysing specimens are established at the beginning of the study. Although most laboratories routinely apply intra- and inter-laboratory quality-control procedures, epidemiologists should send specimens without revealing the exposure (or disease) status of the subjects from whom they were collected. It is also advisable to send replicate samples without the laboratory staff being aware that they are replicates.

Measurement procedures should always be evaluated in a pilot study to identify any potential problems, gauge their validity and reliability, and determine in what way observers or responders may be biased. These issues are discussed further elsewhere in this book; in particular, in Chapters 13 and 18.

2.9 Sources of routine data

'Routine data' are derived from established data collection systems associated with the health and social services. In general, the data are not collected with the aim of answering any specific question. For whatever purpose they were collected, such data can often be used in epidemiological studies; these include data from censuses and population registers, birth and death certificates, cancer registrations, health information systems, medical and hospital records, etc. (see Chapter 11).

Routine data collection systems can provide information on the exposure(s) and outcome(s) of interest in an epidemiological study. Two such systems—death certification and cancer registration—are particularly important in cancer epidemiology.

2.9.1 Death certification

Mortality data are usually based upon a standard death certificate, which records the date of death, cause of death, age, sex, date of birth and place of residence of the deceased. In addition, occupation and other information may be recorded. In most countries, death certificates are usually completed by a doctor or other health worker but in some cases this is done by the police or other authorities. Once certificates are completed, the cause of death is coded according to the *International Classification of Diseases*, now in its tenth revision (WHO, 1992). This is a hierarchical classification of diseases, from broad categories down to a detailed four-character classification (see Appendix 2.2). Usually, only the underlying cause of death is coded and used in mortality statistics, although contributing causes may also be coded.

While more complete and reliable than many routine sources of morbidity data, mortality data are still subject to some misclassification (Cameron & McGoogan, 1981; Heasman & Lipworth, 1966). A large international study of 8737 cancer deaths in cities in England, USA and Latin America revealed that of deaths classified on the death certificate as caused by cancer, 20% were due to other causes (Puffer & Griffith, 1967). However, 24.6% of cancer deaths had been wrongly classified under other causes of death. On balance, therefore, total cancer mortality was only 4% underestimated in the official statistics derived from death certificates. The degree of misclassification varied with cancer site, being greater for those that are more difficult to diagnose, such as primary liver cancer and brain tumours.

International cancer mortality statistics are published regularly by the World Health Organization (*World Health Statistics Annual* series) and by Segi and his colleagues (Kurihara *et al.*, 1989).

2.9.2   Cancer registration

There are two types of cancer registry: hospital-based and population-based. Hospital-based cancer registries record all cancer patients seen in a particular hospital. Their main purpose is to contribute to patient care and administrative management, although they may be useful to a certain extent for epidemiological purposes. For instance, 'rolling' case–control studies may be set up to investigate the etiology of a particular cancer; this is achieved by comparing the characteristics of such cases with those of a control group, which may be made up of patients either with other types of cancer, or with other illnesses. Nevertheless, hospital-based registries cannot provide measures of the occurrence of cancer in the general population, because it is not possible to define the population from which cases arise.

Population-based cancer registries seek to record all new (incident) cancer cases that occur in a well defined population. As a result, they provide measures of the occurrence of cancer in their catchment population. Population-based cancer registration has been developed in many countries to provide reasonably comparable data on cancer incidence and as a resource for epidemiologal studies. Cancer incidence data from higher-quality registers are compiled by the International Agency for Research on Cancer in the series *Cancer Incidence in Five Continents* (Doll *et al.*, 1966; Waterhouse *et al.*, 1970, 1976, 1982; Muir *et al.*, 1987; Parkin *et al.*, 1992, 1997). Some indicators of data quality for the different registries included in this publication are tabulated in these volumes. However, these are mostly indirect indicators of data quality: proportion of registrations verified histologically; proportion of cases registered on the basis of information on the death certificate only; proportion of cases with missing information, etc. More systematic analyses of the validity of cancer registration data are available for certain registries, where a sample of cases was re-abstracted and re-coded (see Parkin *et al.*, 1994).

The majority of cancer registries collect information about cancer patients, such as their occupation, social class, country of birth, ethnicity, etc. Occurrence of cancer can therefore be examined in relation to these variables.

The role of cancer registries in cancer epidemiology is discussed in detail in Chapter 17.

2.9.3 Record linkage

Information on individuals from birth to death is available in the records of many institutions and agencies. These various records may be merged into a single comprehensive record using personal identifiers, in a process known as record linkage. The unified record can then be used in epidemiological and public health investigations. The potential for linkage between registers varies enormously between countries according to how the relevant information is collected and identified. Thus, in the Nordic countries, where everyone is assigned a personal number which is used for all social security, census and health records, mortality and cancer incidence data can readily be traced and linked to other data-sets of interest. In the United Kingdom, a national register linked to the health service is widely used for follow-up studies of cancer and mortality, and computerized linkage is now possible for people who were alive in January 1991, matching information such as name and date of birth.

Linkage of cancer registry records with records from other sources, such as census data and company records, has been undertaken in an attempt to investigate risk factors for occupational cancers and cancers of the reproductive system. Registries can also draw information on exposure from hospital records, as they often record hospital admission numbers. This linkage with hospital records has been used in studies of cancer risks associated with radiotherapy and other treatments (Day & Boice, 1983; Kaldor *et al.*, 1992).

The Oxford Record Linkage Study (ORLS) and the national Scottish medical record linkage system are two good examples of record linkage. The ORLS was established in Oxford, UK in 1962, to assess the feasibility, cost and methods of medical record linkage for an entire community. The system links morbidity and mortality data and provides information on a wide range of variables. Data in the system can be used to study etiological questions and to assess the natural history of various diseases (Acheson, 1967; Baldwin *et al.*, 1987). In Scotland, all births, deaths, hospitalizations, cancer incidence, school medical examinations and handicapped children's records can be linked (Heasman & Clarke, 1979). Similar record-linkage systems have been set up in the USA by the National Center for Health Statistics (Feinleib, 1984) and in many other developed countries.

Further reading

* Comprehensive coverage of principles and practical aspects of questionnaire design, the conduct of personal interviews, the abstraction of information from records, and the use of biological measurements and measurements in the environment, is given by Armstrong *et al.* (1992). Although this book focuses on exposure measurement, many of the principles presented are also relevant to the measurement of outcomes.

* An often-referenced paper on the validity and reliability of tests that yield results on a continuous scale (e.g., blood pressure measurements) is that by Bland & Altman (1986).

* For a further, more complex, discussion on the kappa statistic, see Feinstein & Cicchetti (1990), Cicchetti & Feinstein (1990) and Lantz & Nebenzahl (1996).

Box 2.1. Key issues

• In epidemiological studies, it is necessary to measure: (1) the primary exposure(s) of interest; (2) other exposure(s) that may influence the outcome (potential confounders); and (3) the outcome(s) of interest.

• Many approaches can be used to measure exposure and outcome. These include personal interviews, self-administered questionnaires, diaries, records, biological measurements and measurements in the environment. Each method has its own advantages and disadvantages.

• In any epidemiological study, it is important to assess the validity and reliability of the main measurements of exposure and outcome. This will provide an estimate of the magnitude of measurement errors and their probable impact on the study results. Measurement errors may be non-differential or differential.

• *Non-differential measurement error* occurs when the sensitivity and specificity of the exposure measurement for the diseased group equal those for the non-diseased group, or when the sensitivity and specificity of the outcome measurement is the same for both exposed and unexposed subjects. Non-differential measurement error generally leads to under-estimation of the association between the exposure and the outcome. Although non-differential measurement errors make it more difficult to reveal an association between the exposure and the outcome, this can usually be overcome by increasing the sample size and/or replicating measurements.

• *Differential measurement error* occurs when the sensitivity and/or specificity of the exposure measurement for the diseased subjects differs from that for the non-diseased subjects, or when the sensitivity and/or specificity of the outcome measurement is different for exposed and unexposed subjects. Differential measurement error can exaggerate, attenuate, or even reverse, the relationship between the exposure and the outcome, so that the results of the study can be misleading. Unfortunately, differential measurement errors cannot be controlled for in the analysis, and their effects cannot be lessened by increasing the sample size.

Appendix 2.1
Designing a questionnaire

Questionnaires are used in epidemiology to assess exposure levels to possible causal agents and, less often, to determine the presence or absence of disease, or another outcome of interest.

A2.1.1 Objectives of questionnaire design
(1) To provide valid measurements of the exposure(s) and outcome(s) being studied.
(2) To design a questionnaire that is easily completed by the interviewer and/or subject.
(3) To facilitate data-processing and analysis.

A2.1.2 General principles of questionnaire design
Content
The questionnaire should be as brief as possible, with every question being carefully justified in terms of the objectives of the study. It is important to ensure that the variables needed for the analysis can be easily obtained from the questionnaire.

Types of question
There are two main types of question: 'open-ended' and 'closed-ended'. *Open-ended questions* allow the respondents to answer on their own terms and should be recorded in the respondent's own words. Open-ended questions should be used for numerical data (for example, age, date of birth) and for questions having many possible answers (e.g. country of birth).

Example A2.1.1. *Example of an open-ended question.*

What is your mother tongue?.. ☐

Closed-ended questions allow only a limited range of answers. The questionnaire should specify in detail all the possible alternative answers. With multiple alternative answers, a final alternative 'Other: please specify...' should be provided unless it is certain that all possible answers have been provided. A 'Do not know' option should also be given for questions where it is possible that some subjects may not know (or may not remember) the answer. A 'Not applicable' option should be given if the question does not apply to all subjects.

> **Example A2.1.2.** *Example of a closed-ended question.*
>
> 7. If you have NEVER BEEN PREGNANT was it because:
>
> You never tried ☐ 1
>
> You tried but it never happened ☐ 2
>
> Other reasons: please specify .... ☐
>
> Not applicable ☐ 7

Epidemiological questionnaires usually contain a majority of closed-ended questions to reduce the possibility of interviewer, response, interpretation, and/or coding bias, and to facilitate data-processing.

Wording of questions

Questions must be written in simple, non-threatening language, avoiding the use of abbreviations and technical jargon. The wording should avoid any suggestion that a particular answer is preferred by the researcher(s). Each question should contain only one concept related to a clear time period.

Order of questions

Questions should follow a logical sequence resembling, as far as possible, the sequence that the respondents might expect to follow when thinking about the topic. Questions about a particular subject should be grouped together, and proceed from the general to the particular. When a response to a general question makes further responses on that topic irrelevant (e.g., a woman who has never been pregnant need not answer questions about number and characteristics of pregnancies), a branching of the question sequence may be introduced. This should be as simple as possible, with clear instructions given on the questionnaire (Example A2.1.3).

Questionnaire layout

Layout is important in both self- and interviewer-administered questionnaires. A pleasant appearance will arouse interest and encourage correct completion. A separate page with a brief introduction, explanatory notes and instructions should precede the first question. To help interviewers and subjects, long questionnaires may be subdivided into sections, each one corresponding to a specific topic. All questions should be assigned a number.

If some questions are optional, this should be indicated on the questionnaire with clear instructions and appropriate branch and jump expla-

Example A2.1.3. Example of instructions for omitting questions (jumping).

1. Have you ever been pregnant?

Yes ☐ 1

No ☐ 2

If No, please go to question 4.

If Yes,
2. How many pregnancies in total (including still births, miscarriages and abortions) have you had? ☐☐

nations. For questions that are repeated several times, such as questions about each pregnancy, a tabular layout may be used (Example A2.1.4).

Space should be provided at the end of the questionnaire for any information or comments that the subject may wish to add.

Example A2.1.4. Example of a question with a tabular layout.

3. Please indicate the characteristics of your pregnancies

	1st	2nd	3rd	4th	5th
Age at start of pregnancy (years)	☐☐	☐☐	☐☐	☐☐	☐☐
Outcome	Birth ☐1 Still birth ☐2 Miscarriage ☐3 Abortion ☐4	Birth ☐1 Still birth ☐2 Miscarriage ☐3 Abortion ☐4	Birth ☐1 Still birth ☐2 Miscarriage ☐3 Abortion ☐4	Birth ☐1 Still birth ☐2 Miscarriage ☐3 Abortion ☐4	Birth ☐1 Still birth ☐2 Miscarriage ☐3 Abortion ☐4
Duration of pregnancy (weeks)	☐☐	☐☐	☐☐	☐☐	☐☐
Breast-fed	Yes ☐1 No ☐2 Not applicable ☐7 Do not know ☐9	Yes ☐1 No ☐2 Not applicable ☐7 Do not know ☐9	Yes ☐1 No ☐2 Not applicable ☐7 Do not know ☐9	Yes ☐1 No ☐2 Not applicable ☐7 Do not know ☐9	Yes ☐1 No ☐2 Not applicable ☐7 Do not know ☐9

Method of administration

The questionnaire can be either self-administered or interviewer-administered. In general, self-administered questionnaires must be simpler and much more carefully designed than those intended for use by interviewers.

Recording and coding of responses

Most questionnaires will be prepared to allow numerical coding of all responses for processing by computer. Every possible answer on the form is assigned a code (as in Examples A2.1.2 to A2.1.4). Numerical data (e.g., number of pregnancies) do not require coding, as the exact number can be entered. But even with such pre-coded questionnaires, some coding of data collection will still be required for some open-ended questions or for the 'Other: please specify' category of closed-ended questions (as in Example A2.1.2).

Coding of questionnaires may be a complex task and it may be necessary to develop a coding manual with specific coding rules. Various classification systems have been developed and published which can be used to code cancers by their topography (e.g., *International Classification of Diseases,* WHO, 1992) and by their morphology and behaviour (e.g., *International Classification of Diseases for Oncology*, Percy *et al.*, 1990) (see Appendix 2.2), occupations (e.g., *Classification of Occupations*, OPCS, 1970), and many other variables.

A2.1.3 Evaluation of a questionnaire

Questionnaires should be subject to two forms of evaluation: pre-testing and assessment of validity.

Pre-testing

All questionnaires should be pre-tested. This involves testing the draft questionnaire on samples of subjects similar to those who will ultimately be studied. Its purpose is to identify questions that are poorly understood, ambiguous, or evoke hostile or other undesirable responses. Pre-tests should be carried out using the same procedures that will finally be used in administering the questionnaire. Interviewers and study subjects should be asked to provide feedback and the questions revised in the light of their comments. Several rounds of pre-testing will usually be necessary before the final form of a questionnaire is developed.

Assessment of validity

The validity of the questionnaire as a measure of the variables of interest should always be determined in a sample of subjects before the main study is undertaken. This requires comparison of the results obtained using the questionnaire with those obtained using a gold standard test (see Section 2.6). For instance, questions on past hospitalizations and surgical interventions may be validated against hospital records. Validation is usually difficult, often expensive, and may sometimes be impossible, when no appropriate gold standard is available.

A2.1.4 Use of standard questionnaires

If a standard questionnaire for measurement of a particular exposure is available, it may be best to use this, rather than spending time and effort designing a new one. Moreover, the standard questionnaire will have been used extensively and proved satisfactory, and may even have been validated (although validity in one population may not ensure validity in another). Use of a standard questionnaire will also allow comparison of the data gathered with those collected in other studies.

Some changes in the format of a standard questionnaire may be needed to make it suitable for a particular study population. Be aware that such changes may affect the validity of the questionnaire; however, any modification can be tested for validity against the original questionnaire.

A full discussion of questionnaire design is given by Armstrong *et al.* (1992).

Appendix 2.2
Classification of diseases

Neoplasms can be classified in many ways, but the most important classifications for the epidemiologist are those based on:

(1) Topography—the site in the body where the tumour is located.
(2) Morphology (or histology)—the microscopic characteristics of the tumour.
(3) Behaviour—the tendency to invade other tissues (malignant, benign, *in situ,* and uncertain).

Uniform definitions and uniform systems of classification are fundamental to the quantitative study of diseases. Without a standard classification tool that remains fixed for periods of time and is applied uniformly, meaningful comparative analyses of morbidity and mortality data would be impossible. The *International Classification of Diseases* (ICD), published by the World Health Organization, is such a standard classification tool. It is revised every ten years or so (Table A2.2.1); the 10th revision (ICD-10) (WHO, 1992) is currently in use. An historical review of disease classification from the first revision, the Bertillon Classification of Causes of Death, until 1947 can be found in the introduction to ICD-7 (WHO, 1957), and an account of classification in the years 1948–1985 is given by Muir and Percy (1991).

Table A2.2.1.
Revisions of the International Classification of Diseases.

Revision	Publication year	Publisher
1st (ICD-1)	1900	French Government
2nd (ICD-2)	1910	
3rd (ICD-3)	1920	
4th (ICD-4)	1929	Health Organization of the League of Nations
5th (ICD-5)	1938	
6th (ICD-6)	1948	World Health Organization
7th (ICD-7)	1957	
8th (ICD-8)	1967	
9th (ICD-9)	1977	
10th (ICD-10)	1992	

Although retaining the traditional structure of ICD-9, the 10th revision of the ICD uses an alphanumeric coding scheme—the first character of the category is a letter—replacing the numeric codes of ICD-9 and previous revisions. This change provides a larger coding frame and leaves scope for future inclusion of new disease entities without disrupting the numbering system.

ICD-10 has three volumes. Volume 1 deals with the tabular list of classification at the level of three and four characters, special tabulations of morbidity and mortality, and definitions and nomenclature regulations. Volume 2 is essentially an instruction manual. Volume 3 contains an alphabetical index.

The ICD chapter that deals with neoplasms presents a primarily topographic classification arranged according to the anatomical site of the tumour, with the exception of a few histological types such as lymphomas and leukaemias (Table A2.2.2). Organs are ordered according to organ systems. Neoplasms with a given behaviour are grouped as malignant, benign, *in situ* and of uncertain behaviour.

Table A2.2.2.

Classification of neoplasms according to ICD-10 (WHO, 1992).

C00-C75	Malignant neoplasms, stated or presumed to be primary, of specified sites, except of lymphoid, haematopoietic and related tissue	
	C00-C14	Lip, oral cavity and pharynx
	C15-C26	Digestive organs
	C30-C39	Respiratory and intrathoracic organs
	C40-C41	Bone and articular cartilage
	C43-C44	Skin
	C45-C49	Mesothelium and soft tissue
	C50	Breast
	C51-C58	Female genital organs
	C60-C63	Male genital organs
	C64-C68	Urinary tract
	C69-C72	Eye, brain and other parts of central nervous system
	C73-C75	Thyroid and other endocrine glands
C76-C80	Malignant neoplasms of ill-defined, secondary and unspecified sites	
C81-C96	Malignant neoplasms, stated or presumed to be primary, of lymphoid, haematopoietic and related tissue	
C97	Malignant neoplasms of independent (primary) multiple sites	
D00-D09	*In situ* neoplasms	
D10-D36	Benign neoplasms	
D37-D48	Neoplasms of uncertain or unknown behaviour	

The first morphological classification was developed in 1951 and many others have since emerged (Table A2.2.3). The *Manual of Tumor Nomenclature and Coding* (MOTNAC) (American Cancer Society, 1951; Percy *et al.*, 1968) and, more recently, the *International Classification of Diseases for Oncology* (ICD-O) (WHO, 1976; Percy *et al.*, 1990) have been the most widely used. They provide not only morphology and behaviour codes, but also topography codes that are directly related to the ICD codes. A full discussion of the merits and drawbacks of each of these classifications is given by Muir and Percy (1991).

Publication year	Morphological code manual	Publisher	Main characteristics
1951	*Manual of Tumour Nomenclature and Coding (MOTNAC)* 1st edition	American Cancer Society	Morphology codes Behaviour codes
1956	*Statistical code for Human Tumours (STAT CODE)*	World Health Organization	Topography codes from ICD-7 Morphology codes from MOTNAC Behaviour codes from MOTNAC
1965	*Systematized Nomenclature of Pathology (SNOP)* *(Section 8,9 – neoplasms)*	College of American Pathologists	Topography codes unrelated to ICD Morphology codes
1968	*Manual of Tumor Nomenclature and Coding (MOTNAC)* 2nd edition	American Cancer Society	Topography codes from ICD-8 Morphology codes from SNOP
1976	*ICD-O*, 1st edition	World Health Organization	Topography codes from ICD-9 Morphology codes from MOTNAC (with one-digit extension) Behaviour codes from MOTNAC
1977	*Systematized Nomenclature of Medicine (SNOMED)* *(Section 8,9 – neoplasms)*	College of American Pathologists	Review of SNOP Topography codes unrelated to ICD Morphology codes from ICD-O
1990	*ICD-O*, 2nd edition	World Health Organization	Topography codes from ICD-10 Morphology codes from ICD-O, 1st edition Behaviour codes from ICD-O, 1st edition

Table A2.2.3.
Morphology and behaviour classifications of neoplasms.

The major advantage of ICD is that it is truly international, being used by all WHO Member States for tabulating the causes of death and for most health statistics. The main disadvantage is that, for the majority of sites, no separation on the basis of morphology is possible. As a result, it is generally recommended that agencies interested in identifying both the site and morphology of tumours, like cancer registries and pathology laboratories, use ICD-O, which is a dual-axis classification providing independent coding systems for topography and morphology.

As new classifications and new revisions of ICD and ICD-O have come into use, data coded by previous classifications must be converted to the new codes. The National Cancer Institute of the USA has produced a series of conversion tables for neoplasms (e.g., Percy, 1980, 1981, 1983; Percy & van Holten, 1979). Summary tables of equivalence between various revisions of the ICD have also been published in certain volumes of *Cancer*

Incidence in Five Continents (e.g., Waterhouse *et al.*, 1976; Muir *et al.*, 1987). Programs that perform conversions from ICD-O (1st edition) to ICD-O (2nd edition) and vice versa, from ICD-O (1st and 2nd editions) to ICD-9, and from ICD-O (2nd edition) to ICD-10 have been developed by the International Agency for Research on Cancer (IARC) and are available on diskette for use on microcomputers (Ferlay, 1994).

Chapter 3
Describing and presenting data

All epidemiological studies involve the collection of data on the exposures and outcomes of interest. In a well planned study, the raw observations that constitute the data contain the information that satisfies the objectives of the study. The aim of data analysis is to extract the pertinent information from these raw observations in a concise way.

The first stage in data analysis is the preparation of an appropriate form in which the relevant data can be collected and coded in a format suitable for entry into a computer; this stage is referred to as data processing. The second stage is to review the recorded data, checking for accuracy, consistency and completeness; this process is often referred to as data editing. Next, the investigator summarizes the data in a concise form to allow subsequent analysis—this is generally done by presenting the distribution of the observations according to key characteristics in tables, graphs and summary measures. This stage is known as data reduction. Only after data processing, editing and reduction should more elaborate statistical manipulation of the data be pursued.

3.1 Data processing

All the various steps of data processing should be planned when the study is designed, before any data are collected. All forms used for recording data should be carefully designed and tested to ensure that the data can easily be extracted for processing. This general principle applies to all data-collection forms: questionnaires, as well as forms for recording results from laboratory assays, data extraction forms from hospital notes, etc.

Most epidemiological studies involve the collection of large amounts of data that are not easy to process by hand. Fortunately, microcomputers are now available at reasonable prices (see Chapter 18). Before data collected on a form can be entered into a computer file, they must first be coded. For instance, sex may be coded as 1 for male, or 2 for female; only the number 1 or 2 will be entered in the computer file. Numerical data (e.g., number of children) do not require coding, as the exact number can be entered. Most data-collection forms are designed so that every possible answer is assigned a code. However, even when such 'pre-coded' forms are used, further data coding will still be required for the answers to 'open-ended' questions or to the 'other' category of 'closed-ended' questions. For a more detailed discussion of these issues, see Appendix 2.1 and Section 18.3.6.

For each type of data-collection form, a computer file will be created to enter the data. Data-entry programs can be designed so that the computer screen resembles the layout of the data-collection form. This helps to minimize errors made during data entry.

3.2   Data editing

Basic editing of the data involves checking each variable for illogical or unusual values. For example, sex may be coded 1 for male or 2 for female. Another code, perhaps 9, is used to designate an unknown value. It is preferable to assign specific codes to unknown or missing information than to leave these values blank, as it is impossible to tell whether a blank field corresponds to data that are truly missing or to data that have been omitted in error. A code of zero should, however, be avoided, because missing information may be interpreted by some computers or programs as zero. The range and distribution of each variable should be examined, and any inadmissible values should be checked against the original data forms.

In addition to checking for incorrect or unusual values, the distribution of each variable should be examined to see if it appears reasonable. Such an evaluation may reveal important problems that might not otherwise come to light. It is also necessary to cross-check the consistency of codes for related variables. For instance, males should not have been admitted to hospital for hysterectomy or females for prostatectomy. Careful editing will involve many such consistency checks and is best accomplished by computer programs designed to flag such errors.

Most data-entry programs can check and edit data interactively as they are entered. The computer can be programmed to display an error message on the screen and give an audible warning, allowing inadmissible values to be rejected and corrected immediately. A sophisticated data-entry program can also check for consistency between variables and can eliminate some potential inconsistencies by providing appropriate codes automatically. For example, if a subject is male, the program can automatically supply the correct code for 'Have you ever been pregnant?'. Nevertheless, even with the most sophisticated editing during data entry, it remains essential to edit the data before analysis, to check on their completeness, and to examine the distribution of each variable, as data-entry programs cannot perform these functions (see Section 18.3.6).

To minimize error during the handling of data, three basic precautions are recommended. First, avoid any unnecessary copying of data from one form to another. Second, use a verification procedure during data entry. Data should always be entered twice, preferably by two people; the two data-sets can then be compared and any inconsistencies resolved. Third, check all calculations carefully, either by repeating them or, for example, by checking that subtotals add to the correct overall total. All computer procedures should be tested initially on a small subset of the data and the results checked by hand.

3.3   Data reduction

After the data are edited, they should be examined by means of simple tabulations, graphs and basic summary measures. Different types of data must be presented and summarized in different ways: the correct choice of methods used therefore depends on the type of data collected. The remainder of this chapter describes ways of presenting and summarizing two main types of data: quantitative and categorical (or qualitative) variables.

3.3.1   Quantitative data

Quantitative variables can either have a numerical value along a continuous scale (e.g., age, weight, height), or can be whole numbers representing counts of a particular event (e.g., number of children, number of sexual partners).

Presentation of quantitative data

The frequencies with which the different possible values of a variable occur in a group of subjects is called the frequency distribution of the variable in the group. For example, we may wish to present the distribution of height (in cm) of a sample of 1250 women who were examined in a certain breast-screening clinic. As height is measured on a continuous scale, it can have a large number of distinct values; it is therefore more useful to group the values before presenting the distribution (Table 3.1).

Height (cm)	Number of women	Percentage
145–149	75	6.0
150–154	153	12.2
155–159	261	20.9
160–164	323	25.8
165–169	201	16.1
170–174	144	11.5
175–179	91	7.3
180–184	2	0.2
Total	**1250**	**100.0**

Table 3.1.
Distribution of height in a sample of 1250 women attending a certain breast-screening clinic: hypothetical data.

The percentage frequency distribution shown in the final column allows one to make comparison with distributions in other groups of women. There is no need to calculate the percentages precisely: for example, 56 out of 1250 can often be expressed 4.5%, rather than 4.48%. When percentage frequency distributions are reported on their own, the total number of subjects on which the distribution is based should always be given (in this example, 1250). For instance, it might be misleading to report that 20% of women were between 155 and 159 cm tall if only five women had been measured in total.

There are no universal rules on how the data should be grouped. As a rough guide, the number of groups should be 5–20, depending on the number of observations involved. If the interval chosen is wide, too much detail will be lost; if it is narrow, the table may be difficult to interpret. All intervals should have the same width, although the categories at either extreme may be open-ended (e.g., ≥180 cm). There should be no gaps between the groups. The table should be labelled to show clearly how observations that fall on the boundaries are classified.

A frequency distribution can be displayed graphically as a *histogram*, as shown in Figure 3.1. In this type of graph, the number (or percentage) of observations is plotted for different values, or groups of values, of the variable being studied (in this example, height). In a histogram, it is the *area* of the rectangle, not its height, that represents the frequency—the vertical scale is measured in frequency per unit of value and the horizontal scale in units of value. The larger the sample measured, the narrower the grouping interval that can be chosen, so that the histogram becomes smoother and more closely resembles the distribution of the total population. At the limit, when the width of the intervals is so narrow that they practically correspond to a single unit, the resulting diagram would be a smooth curve.

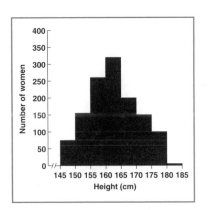

Figure 3.1.
Histogram showing the distribution of height in 1250 women who attended a breast-screening clinic (data shown in Table 3.1).

Summarizing quantitative data

Tabular and graphical methods are an important way of examining the data. But it is also useful to summarize the data numerically. The two most important features of a distribution are usually the central value and the spread about this value.

Measures of central value

(1) The most commonly used measure of the central value of a distribution is the *arithmetic mean*. This is the sum of the observations divided by n, the number of observations. For example, if the weights (in kg) of eight healthy women are

45.3, 49.8, 50.5, 60.7, 65.2, 69.4, 73.2, 75.9,

the arithmetic mean of the weights of these women is

$(45.3 + 49.8 + 50.5 + 60.7 + 65.2 + 69.4 + 73.2 + 75.9)/8 = 490/8 = 61.25 = 61.3$ kg

(2) The *median* is another commonly used measure of central value. It is the value that divides the distribution in half when the observations are ranked in order. Thus, the median is the middle observation. For an even number of observations, the median is calculated as the mean of the two middle values. A general expression for finding the median is:

Median = $(n+1)/2$ th value of the ordered observations,

where n is the total number of observations.

In this example, the value of the median is the 4.5th value, i.e., the average of the fourth and fifth values, (60.7 + 65.2) / 2 = 63.0 kg.

The choice of measure used will depend on the nature of the data and the purpose of the analysis. The mean is often the preferred measure of central value because it takes into account every observation and it is easy to use in the most common types of statistical analysis. Its major disadvantage is that it can be affected by *outliers*—single observations that are extreme in comparison with most observations and whose inclusion or exclusion changes the mean markedly.

The median is a useful descriptive measure when outliers make the mean unrepresentative of the majority of the data. It is also particularly useful when certain observations are not recorded precisely because they are above or below a certain level; in these circumstances, the mean cannot be calculated, but the median can determined so long as definite values are known for more than one half of all subjects. For instance, the mean survival time of a group of cancer patients can be calculated only when all the patients have died; however, the median survival time can be calculated while almost half the patients are alive. The main disadvantage of this measure is that it ranks the data, but does not make use of their individual values.

When the shape of a distribution is roughly symmetric about a central axis, the mean and the median are approximately equal (as is the case for the data on weight given in the example above).

Measures of variation

In addition to a measure of the central value of a distribution, it is also useful to have an idea of the variation or spread of values around this central value. Several measures of variation are used:

(1) The *range* is the interval between the largest and smallest values. The major advantage of this measure is that it is very simple to calculate. The main disadvantage is that it is based only on two extreme observations and gives no indication of how other observations are distributed in between.

(2) The three values that divide a distribution into quarters are called the *quartiles*. Of the total number of observations, 25% lie below the lower quartile, 50% below the middle quartile and 75% below the upper quartile. The middle quartile is the median. The distance between the lower quartile and the upper quartile is called the *inter-quartile range* and is sometimes used to describe variability. The inter-quartile range contains 50% of the observations.

Similarly, *percentiles* are values that divide the distribution into percentages. The 50th percentile corresponds to the median, while the 25th and the 75th percentiles correspond to the lower and upper quartiles, respectively.

A simple but useful semi-graphical way of summarizing data using percentiles is the box-and-whisker plot. Figure 3.2 shows a box-and-whisker

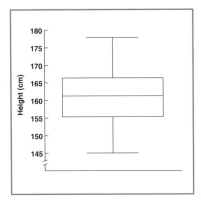

Figure 3.2.
Box-and-whisker plot of the heights of a sample of 1250 women (data shown in Table 3.1).

plot for the data given in Table 3.1. The box indicates the lower and upper quartiles, while the central line is the median. The points at the ends of the 'whiskers' are the 2.5th and the 97.5th percentile values.

(3) The *standard deviation* is the most commonly used measure of the average spread of values about the mean. If the values of a variable do not vary greatly within a population, observations will lie closely around the mean, whereas if there is substantial variation, the observations will be scattered widely about the mean.

This variability or *variance* can be measured in terms of how much, on average, observations differ from the mean: in other words how far, on average, each observation *deviates* from the mean. Figure 3.3 illustrates this for the weights of the eight healthy women given in the example above. The deviations from the mean are shown by the lines d_1, d_2, ... d_8. First, the sum of the these deviations is calculated; however, the sum of the deviations from the arithmetic mean is, by definition, zero, since negative deviations cancel out positive deviations. In calculating the dispersion of values around the arithmetic mean, it is irrelevant whether the deviations are positive or negative: only their absolute numerical magnitude is of interest. Hence, to avoid getting zero when the deviations are added together, the individual deviations are first squared, eliminating negative values. The average of these squared deviations is called the *variance*.

$$\text{Variance} = (d_1^2 + d_2^2 + ... + d_8^2)/n$$

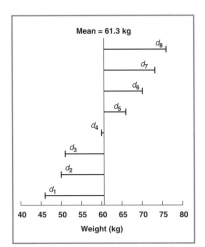

Figure 3.3.
Deviations from the mean of the weights of eight women: hypothetical data.

The variance is a very useful mathematical measure of the average spread of values around the mean, but is difficult to interpret because it is expressed as the square of the units measured. In our example, the variance of weight will be expressed as kg^2. As it is usually more convenient to express the variation in terms of the original, unsquared units, the *square root of the variance* is usually used. This is known as the *standard deviation* (SD). In this example, the SD is equal to 10.8 kg.

A small standard deviation indicates that most values are very close to the mean, whereas a large one indicates that many lie far from the mean: i.e., the more the values in a population vary, the bigger the standard deviation.

As a general rule, provided a distribution is roughly symmetrical and has a bell-like shape, with a dome of central values and two tails at the extremes (characteristic of what statisticians call a 'normal distribution'), the mean is the central value and the standard deviation is a measure of spread such that one standard deviation either side of the mean includes roughly 70% of the observations, and two standard deviations include roughly 95% (Figure 3.4).

3.3.2 Categorical data

The values of categorical (also called qualitative) variables represent attributes, rather than actual measurements of some quantity. The following are examples of categorical variables: sex (male/female), marital status (single/married/divorced/widowed), oral contraceptive use (ever-users/never-users), country of birth (Colombia, Spain, etc.).

There are various types of categorical variable. If the variable can only have two different values, the categorical variable is called binary (e.g., sex). Sometimes the different categories of a variable can be ordered on some scale (e.g., the severity of pain could be categorized as mild, moderate or severe). In this case, the variable is called an ordered categorical variable.

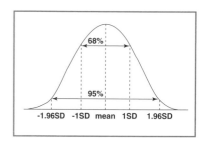

Figure 3.4.
A normal distribution. SD = standard deviation.

Presentation of categorical data

As with quantitative variables, we can present the frequency distribution of a categorical variable as the number of times each value (category) occurs in the group of subjects being studied. Consider Example 3.1:

> **Example 3.1.** *A study was conducted in Spain and Colombia to assess the relationship between cervical cancer and exposure to human papillomavirus (HPV), selected aspects of sexual and reproductive behaviour, use of oral contraceptives, screening practices and smoking. The study included 436 cases of histologically confirmed squamous-cell carcinoma and 387 controls randomly selected from the general population that generated the cases. Each participant responded to a structured questionnaire which collected data on a large number of variables: age, number of sexual partners, educational level, smoking, etc. (Bosch et al., 1992). Table 3.2 shows the distribution of the cervical cancer cases by educational status and oral contraceptive use.*

Baseline characteristics	Number of cases	Percentage
Education (schooling)		
Ever	317	72.7
Never	119	27.3
Total	**436**	**100.0**
Oral contraceptive use		
Ever	141	32.4
Never	291	66.7
Unknown	4	0.9
Total	**436**	**100.0**

[a] Data from Bosch *et al.* (1992).

Table 3.2.
Distribution of cervical cancer cases by educational status and oral contraceptive use.[a]

Bar charts are often used to present the distribution of categorical variables (Figure 3.5). In this type of graph, the value of the quantity of interest is represented by the length of the bar.

Figure 3.5.
Distribution of cervical cancer cases by oral contraceptive use (data from Bosch *et al.*, 1992).

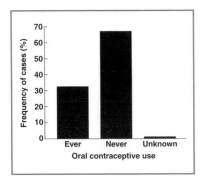

Summarizing categorical data

For categorical data, percentages are the only summary measures that can be calculated (as in Table 3.2). They are particularly useful when making comparisons between different groups.

3.3.3 Two variables—quantitative or categorical

So far, we have considered the frequency distribution of a variable within a single group of subjects. Often, we need to compare frequency distributions between two or more groups defined by another variable; for example, the distribution of oral contraceptive use among Colombian and Spanish cases of cervical cancer. Thus, we wish to examine the association between two categorical variables: oral contraceptive use and country of residence. One way to do this is to tabulate the data as in Table 3.3.

Table 3.3.
Distribution of cervical cancer cases by oral contraceptive use (rows) according to country of residence (columns).[a]

| Oral contraceptive use | Country of residence (number (%)) | |
	Colombia	Spain
Ever	77 (41.4)	64 (25.6)
Never	109 (58.6)	182 (72.8)
Unknown	0 (0)	4 (1.6)
Total	**186 (100.0)**	**250 (100.0)**

[a] Data from Bosch *et al.* (1992)

When considering two variables simultaneously, it is useful to classify them according to their purpose in the investigation, as either *explanatory* or *response* variables. Explanatory variables are characteristics of the subjects (exposures) that will be used to explain some of the variability in the response, which is the outcome of interest.

Table 3.3 shows the distribution of the response variable (oral contraceptive use) according to each category of the explanatory variable (country of residence). In this example, it is appropriate to calculate column percentages to show the distribution of the response variable.

These data may also be presented as in Table 3.4. In this case, it is appropriate to calculate row percentages.

The distribution of oral contraceptive use among cervical cancer cases in the two countries can be illustrated in a two-bar chart arranged as in Figure 3.6.

Table 3.4.
Distribution of cervical cancer cases by oral contraceptive use (columns) according to country of residence (rows).[a]

| Country of residence | Oral contraceptive use (number (%)) | | | |
	Ever	Never	Unknown	Total
Colombia	77 (41.4)	109 (58.6)	0 (0)	**186 (100.0)**
Spain	64 (25.6)	182 (72.8)	4 (1.6)	**250 (100.0)**

[a] Data from Bosch *et al.* (1992)

Quantitative variables (such as age) can also be tabulated by grouping the values of the variable. Table 3.5 shows the age distribution of cervical cancer cases at the time of their enrollment into the study in each country. The distribution of the response variable (age) is shown according to each category of the explanatory variable (country).

Tabulations are useful for showing the association between categorical variables; they are not suitable for illustrating the association between quantitative variables (unless they are grouped into categorical variables as in Table 3.5). This is discussed in more detail in Section 11.2.1; here, only graphical representation of the association between two quantitative variables is considered. As an example, we can plot data on vitamin C intake and levels in the plasma in a sample of 25 individuals on a *scattergram* (Figure 3.7). The values of each variable are represented on an axis. A symbol (often a dot or a cross) is used to represent each individual.

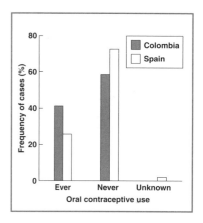

Figure 3.6.
Distribution of cervical cancer cases by oral contraceptive use according to country of residence (data from Bosch *et al.*, 1992).

Age group (years)	Country of residence (number (%))	
	Colombia	**Spain**
<30	15 (8.1)	7 (2.8)
30–39	48 (25.8)	41 (16.4)
40–44	27 (14.5)	30 (12.0)
45–54	50 (26.9)	61 (24.4)
≥55	46 (24.7)	111 (44.4)
Total	**186 (100.0)**	**250 (100.0)**

[a] Data from Bosch *et al.* (1992).

Table 3.5.
Age distribution of cervical cancer cases according to country of residence.[a]

3.4   Final remarks

Data analyses should always begin by using basic tables, graphical techniques and summary statistics to explore the data. Tables, graphs and summaries should, however, be presented in a sensible way, and must not be misleading.

General rules for designing tables

(1) A table should have a title that gives a clear indication of its contents. The reader should be able to determine without difficulty precisely what is tabulated.

(2) Column and row headings should be brief but self-explanatory.

(3) The source of the data should be included, so that original sources can be checked.

(4) Units of measurement should be clearly indicated.

(5) Totals should be given. These are helpful in indicating the quantity of data in the table and to allow comparison with data presented elsewhere.

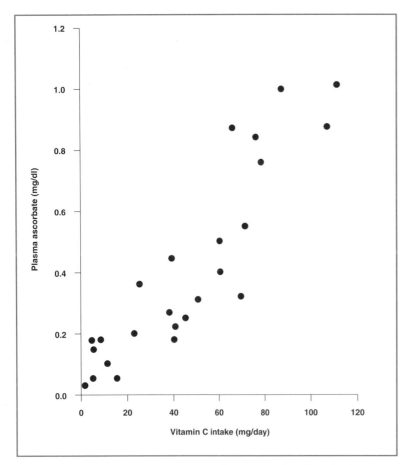

(6) If percentages are given, the base for the percentage should be clearly indicated. In a complex table displaying percentages without indication of their base, the reader is uncertain how or in which way the percentages total 100%. Such a table can easily be misinterpreted. A glance at the location of the 100% value almost always informs the reader immediately how the percentages in the table were derived.

(7) Approximations and omissions can be explained in footnotes. If some observations are excluded from the table, their number should be indicated clearly.

(8) Tables are used to present results in a more concise and clear way than would be possible in the text. Often, a certain degree of complexity is necessary to save space. However, avoid compressing too much information into a single table. Two or three simple tables may be better than a single large and complex one.

Figure 3.7.
Plasma ascorbate levels in 25 study subjects in relation to their vitamin C intake: hypothetical data.

General rules for designing graphs

(1) A graph should have a self-explanatory legend.

(2) A graph should help the reader to understand the data. It should not be cluttered with too much detail.

(3) Axes should be clearly labelled and units of measurement indicated. It is important for the reader to be able to tell precisely what is being illustrated and in which units.

(4) Scales are extremely important. Whenever feasible, they should start at zero; otherwise, this should be clearly indicated by a break in the axis.

(5) Graphs are generally more easily interpreted if the explanatory (exposure) variable is displayed along the horizontal axis and the response (outcome) variable along the vertical axis.

(6) Avoid graphs that give a three-dimensional impression, as they may be misleading (people visualize less easily in three dimensions).

(7) Choose the type of graph that uses as little ink as possible without loss of information. Figure 3.8 presents the same data in two different ways. In graph (*a*) the data are difficult to interpret because of the three-dimensional columns, multiple outcome scales, grid-lines and hatching. Most ink was used to present features that can be

omitted without any loss of information. The same data are shown in a much simpler and clearer manner in graph (*b*).

General rules for reporting summary measures

(1) Always report the number of observations on which the summary is based. For binary responses (A or B), report the percentage of A or B, but not both.

(2) If the median is used as a measure of the central value of a quantitative distribution, give the lower and upper quartiles (or the range) as well.

(3) If the mean is used as a measure of the central value of a quantitative distribution, give the standard deviation as well.

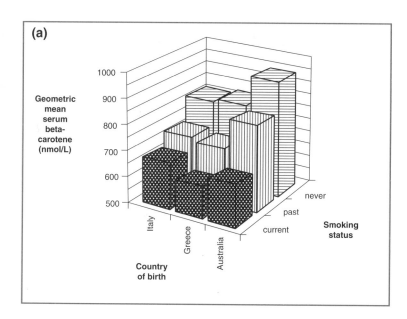

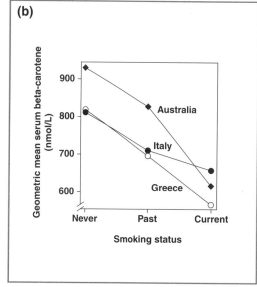

Figure 3.8.
Two graphical presentations of data from 750 subjects on their country of birth, smoking status and serum concentrations of beta-carotene: (*a*) 'business' graph; (*b*) 'scientific' graph (reproduced, with permission, from Jolley, 1993. © by The Lancet Ltd, 1993).

Further reading

* Further details of ways of presenting and summarizing data are given by Altman (1991) and Bland (1987).

* An excellent book on graphical methods is that by Tufte (1983).

* A critical view of the use (and misuse) of graphs in epidemiology is given by Jolley (1993).

Box 3.1. Key issues

- After the data have been edited, they should be examined using simple tabulations, graphs and summary measures.

- The choice of the correct methods to present and summarize the data depends on the type of data collected: *quantitative* or *categorical*.

- The frequency distribution of a *quantitative* variable can be presented in tables, or graphically, in histograms. It can be summarized by reporting a measure of central value and a measure of spread of the distribution (i.e., arithmetic mean with standard deviation, or median with inter-quartile range).

- The frequency distribution of a *categorical* variable can be presented in tables, or graphically, in bar charts. Percentages of individual values in each category are the only summary measures that can be calculated for this type of variable.

- Tables and bar charts can be used to examine the relationship between two categorical variables, and scattergrams to examine the association between two quantitative variables. It is important, however, to first decide which variable is the explanatory variable and which is the response variable.

- Tables, graphs and summary measures should be intelligently designed so as to ensure accurate representation of the data.

Chapter 4
Measures of occurrence of disease and other health-related events

4.1 Introduction

Epidemiological research is based on the ability to quantify the occurrence of disease (or any other health-related event) in populations. To do this, the following must be clearly defined:

(1) What is meant by a case, i.e., an individual in a population who has the disease, or undergoes the event of interest (e.g., death).
(2) The population from which the cases originate.
(3) The period over which the data were collected.

4.1.1 Defining a case—the numerator

In epidemiology, it is seldom easy to define what is meant by a 'case', even for a well known condition. The epidemiological definition of a case is not necessarily the same as the clinical definition, and epidemiologists are often forced to rely on diagnostic tests that are less invasive and cheaper than those normally used by clinicians. Nevertheless, for study purposes, it is important to standardize the case definition. For instance, should 'cancer cases' comprise only those that were confirmed histologically? Should *in situ* lesions be included? For cancers of paired organs (e.g., breast, testis, kidney), should the number of cases counted reflect the number of individuals who develop the cancer or the number of organs affected? Cancer epidemiologists are also interested in measuring the frequency of other health-related event, so, for example, someone who smokes, uses oral contraceptives or uses a certain health service might be counted as a case.

Another important consideration when dealing with recurrent non-fatal conditions (e.g., the common cold) is to decide whether, for a given individual, each episode or occurrence should be counted as a case, or only the first attack. In this chapter, we assume that individuals can only suffer from one episode of the condition of interest; however, the measures of occurrence presented can be modified to cover recurrent episodes.

Cases may be identified through disease registries, notification systems, death certificates, abstracts of clinical records, surveys of the general population, etc. It is important, however, to ensure that the numerator both includes all cases occurring in the study population, and excludes cases from elsewhere. For instance, when measuring the occurrence of a disease in a particular town, all cases that occurred among its residents should be included in the numerator, even those diagnosed elsewhere. In contrast, cases diagnosed in people who are normally resident elsewhere should be excluded.

4.1.2   Defining the population at risk—the denominator

Knowing the number of cases in a particular population is on its own of little use to the epidemiologist. For example, knowing that 100 cases of lung cancer occurred in city A and 50 cases in city B does not allow the conclusion that lung cancer is more frequent in city A than in city B: to compare the frequency of lung cancer in these two populations, we must know the size of the populations from which the cases originated (i.e., the denominator).

The population at risk must be defined clearly, whether it be the residents of one particular town, the population of a whole country or the catchment population of a hospital. The definition must exclude all those who are not usually resident in that area. If possible, it should also exclude all those who are not at risk of the event under investigation. For instance, in quantifying the occurrence of cervical cancer in a population, women who have undergone hysterectomy should ideally be excluded, as they cannot develop this cancer. However, as the data necessary to exclude such women are seldom available, all women are usually included in the denominator.

4.1.3   Time period

As most health-related events do not occur constantly through time, any measure of occurrence is impossible to interpret without a clear statement of the period during which the population was at risk and the cases were counted. The occurrence of lung cancer in most western countries illustrates this point: incidence of this disease was much lower in the early years of this century than today.

4.2   Measures of occurrence

There are two principal measures of occurrence: prevalence and incidence.

4.2.1   Prevalence

Point prevalence is the proportion of existing cases (old and new) in a population at a single point in time.

$$\text{Point prevalence} = \frac{\text{No. of existing cases in a defined population at one point in time}}{\text{No. of people in the defined population at the same point in time}}$$

This measure is called point prevalence[a] because it refers to a single point in time. It is often referred to simply as prevalence.

[a] Period prevalence is a variation that represents the number of people who were counted as cases at any time during a specified (short) period, divided by the total number of people in that population during that time. This measure is used when the condition is recurrent and non-fatal, and so is seldom used in cancer epidemiology. An example of period prevalence would be the proportion of women who have used oral contraceptives at any time during the 12-month period preceding the day of the survey.

Example 4.1. Each line in Figure 4.1 represents an individual (subject) in a particular population. Some subjects developed the condition of interest and either recovered or died from it. Others left the population and went to live elsewhere. Because of these dynamic changes, the magnitude of the prevalence varies from one point in time to another.

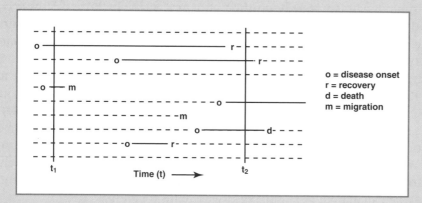

o = disease onset
r = recovery
d = death
m = migration

Figure 4.1.
Changes in the disease status and migration of members of a population over time, and how these changes affect the prevalence of the disease in the population.

Prevalence at time $t_1 = {}^2/_{10} = 0.20 = 20\%$
Prevalence at time $t_2 = {}^3/_8 = 0.38 = 38\%$

Although as with any proportion, prevalence has no time units, the point in time to which it refers must always be specified (Examples 4.1 and 4.2). The term 'prevalence rate' is often wrongly used instead of 'prevalence': this is incorrect, as prevalence is, by definition, a proportion not a rate (see Section 4.2.2).

Example 4.2. In 1985, a study was carried out in a small town to determine the prevalence of oral contraceptive use among women aged 15–44 years. All women between these ages resident in the town were interviewed and asked about their current use of oral contraceptives. The prevalence of oral contraceptive use in that town in 1985 among women aged 15–44 years was 0.5 (50%).

It may be difficult to define a prevalent cancer case. Cancer registries generally assume that once diagnosed with cancer, an individual represents a prevalent case until death (see Section 17.6.1). However, this assumption is not always correct, as people diagnosed with cancer may survive for a long period without any recurrence of the disease and may die from another cause.

Prevalence is the only measure of disease occurrence that can be obtained from cross-sectional surveys (see Chapter 10). It measures the burden of disease in a population. Such information is useful to public-health professionals and administrators who wish to plan the allocation of health-care resources in accordance with the population's needs.

4.2.2 Incidence

The number of cases of a condition present in a population at a point in time depends not only on the frequency with which new cases occur and are identified, but also on the average duration of the condition (i.e., time to either recovery or death). As a consequence, prevalence may vary from one population to another solely because of variations in duration of the condition.

Prevalence is therefore not the most useful measure when attempting to establish and quantify the determinants of disease; for this purpose, a measurement of the flow of new cases arising from the population is more informative. Measurements of incidence quantify the number of new cases of disease that develop in a population of individuals at risk during a specified time interval. Three distinct measures of incidence may be calculated: risk, odds of disease, and incidence rate.

Risk

Risk is the proportion of people in a population that is initially free of disease who develop the disease within a specified time interval.

$$\text{Risk} = \frac{\text{No. of new cases of disease arising in a defined population over a given period of time}}{\text{No. of disease free people in that population at the beginning of that time period}}$$

Both numerator and denominator include only those individuals who are free from the disease at the beginning of the given period and are therefore at risk of developing it. This measure of incidence can be interpreted as the average probability, or risk, that an individual will develop a disease during a specified period of time.

Often, other terms are used in the epidemiological literature to designate risk, for example, incidence risk and incidence proportion.

Like any proportion, risk has no time units. However, as its value increases with the duration of follow-up, the time period to which it relates must always be clearly specified, as in Example 4.3.

Example 4.3. A group of 5000 healthy women aged 45–75 years was identified at the beginning of 1981 and followed up for five years. During this period, 20 new cases of breast cancer were detected. Hence, the risk of developing breast cancer in this population during this five-year period was 20/5000 = 0.4%.

Example 4.4. *A total of 13 264 lung cancer cases in males were diagnosed in a certain population in 1971. These cases were followed up for five years. At the end of this follow-up period, only 472 cases were still alive. The probability of surviving during this five-year period was 472/13 264 = 3.6%. Thus, the probability of dying during the period was 100% – 3.6% = 96.4%. These measures are risks, as they represent the proportion of lung cancer cases who were still alive (or who died) at the end of the follow-up period out of all cases diagnosed at the beginning of the study. These calculations assume that all individuals were followed up for the entire five-year period (or until death if it occurred earlier).*

Risk is a measure commonly used to quantify the survival experience of a group of subjects, as in Example 4.4.

The measures in Example 4.4 are often called survival and fatality 'rates'; this is incorrect as, by definition, they are proportions (see later in this section). These two measures are discussed further in Chapter 12.

Odds of disease

Another measure of incidence is odds of disease, which is the total number of cases divided by the total number of persons who remained disease-free over the study period.

$$\text{Odds of disease} = \frac{\text{No. of new cases of disease arising in a defined population over a given period of time}}{\text{No. of people in that population who remain disease-free during that period}}$$

Example 4.5. *One hundred disease-free individuals were followed up for a certain period of time. By the end of this period, ten had developed the disease of interest (Figure 4.2).*

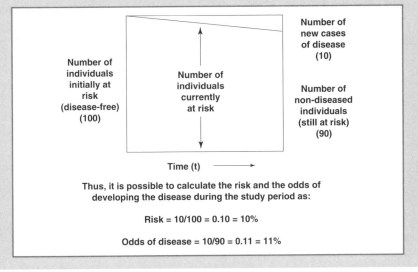

Thus, it is possible to calculate the risk and the odds of developing the disease during the study period as:

Risk = 10/100 = 0.10 = 10%

Odds of disease = 10/90 = 0.11 = 11%

Figure 4.2.
Follow-up of the 100 disease-free individuals described in Example 4.5.

This measure is a *ratio* of the probability of getting the disease to the probability of not getting the disease during a given time period. Thus, it can also be expressed as:

Odds of disease = risk/(1 – risk)

Risk and odds of disease use the same numerator (number of new cases) but different denominators. In the calculation of risk, the denominator is the total number of disease-free individuals at the beginning of the study period, whereas when calculating the odds of disease, it is the number of individuals who remained disease-free at the end of the period (Example 4.5).

Incidence rate

Calculations of risk and odds of disease assume that the entire population at risk at the beginning of the study period has been followed up during the specified time period. Often, however, some participants enter the study some time after it begins, and some are lost during the follow-up; i.e., the population is dynamic. In these instances, not all participants will have been followed up for the same length of time. Moreover, neither of these two measures of incidence takes account of the time of disease onset in affected individuals.

To account for varying lengths of follow-up, the denominator can be calculated so as to represent the sum of the times for which each individual is at risk, i.e., the sum of the time that each person remained under observation and was at risk of becoming a case. This is known as person-time at risk, with time being expressed in appropriate units of measurement, such as person-years (often abbreviated as pyrs).

> **Example 4.6.** *Consider a hypothetical group of nine persons who were followed up from the beginning of 1980 to the end of 1984. Subjects joined the study at different points, as shown in Figure 4.3. Three subjects, (2), (6) and (7), developed the disease of interest during the study period and one, (4), was last contacted at the end of 1983.*

Figure 4.3.
Calculation of an individual's time at risk and total person-time at risk for the nine study subjects described in Example 4.6.

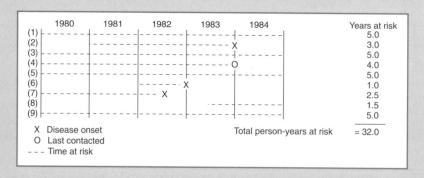

Example 4.6 illustrates the calculation of person-time at risk using a hypothetical group of nine persons. Subject (1) joined the study at the beginning of 1980 and was followed up throughout the study period. Therefore, (1) was at risk of becoming a case for the entire five years of the study. Subject (4) also joined at the beginning of the study, but was last contacted at the end of 1983; thus, (4) was at risk for only four years. Subject (6) joined the study at the beginning of 1982, and developed the disease by the end of that year; after that, (6) was no longer at risk (assuming there can be no recovery from the disease of interest). The total person-years at risk is the sum of all the individuals' time at risk.

The incidence rate accounts for differences in person-time at risk and is given by:

$$\text{Incidence rate} = \frac{\text{No. of new cases of disease arising in a defined population over a given time period}}{\text{Total person–time at risk during that period}}$$

This measure of disease frequency is also called incidence density or force of morbidity (or mortality). Like risk and odds, the numerator of the incidence rate is the number of new cases in the population. The denominator, however, is the sum of each individual's time at risk. In the above example, the incidence rate will be equal to:

3/32 = 0.094 per person-year or 9.4 per 100 person-years

When presenting an incidence rate, the time units must be specified; that is, whether the rate measures the number of cases per person-day, person-month, person-year, etc. Although the above definitions of risk, odds and rate are now widely accepted, the terms risk and rate are used interchangeably in much of the literature, and especially in older publications.

4.2.3 The relationship between prevalence, rate and risk

As stated in Section 4.2.2, prevalence depends on both the incidence and the duration of the disease. When both incidence and duration are stable and the prevalence of the disease is low (as with cancer), this association may be expressed as follows:

Prevalence = incidence rate × average duration of disease

Example 4.7 provides an illustration of the relationship between prevalence, incidence and duration of the disease.

Example 4.7. *A total of 50 new cases of a particular cancer are diagnosed every year in a population of 100 000 people. The average duration of (i.e., survival from) this cancer is four years. Thus, the prevalence of the cancer in that population is:*

Prevalence = 0.0005 per person-year × 4 years = 0.2%

Risk depends both on the incidence rate and on the duration of the at-risk period. It is also affected by mortality from diseases other than the disease of interest; some of those who died from other diseases would have been expected to develop the disease of interest had they survived. If mortality from other diseases is disregarded, and if the incidence rate is constant throughout the period at risk, the following relationship applies:

Risk = 1 – exp (– incidence rate × duration of the period at risk)

The symbol exp indicates that the mathematical constant e = 2.72 should be raised to the power of the expression in parentheses. For diseases that have a low incidence rate or when the period at risk is short, the following approximation may be used:

Risk = incidence rate × duration of the period at risk.

This is clearly illustrated in Example 4.8.

Example 4.8. The incidence rate of a particular condition in a population is 50 per 100 000 person-years. The risk for an individual in this population of developing this condition during a five-year period (assuming no other causes of death) is given by:

Five-year risk = 1 – exp (– 0.0005 per person-year × 5 years) = 0.0025 = 0.25%.

The same value can be obtained using the simplified formula:

Five-year risk = 0.0005 per person-year × 5 years = 0.0025 = 0.25%

Consider now a common condition with an incidence rate of 300 per 1000 person-years:

Five-year risk = 1 – exp (– 0.3 per person-year × 5 years) = 0.78 = 78%

In this instance, the simplified formula yields a meaningless result:

Five-year risk = 0.3 per person-year × 5 years = 1.5 = 150%

(As risk is a proportion, it can never have a value above 1, or 100%.)

4.3 Using routine data to measure disease occurrence

Rates can be estimated from routinely collected data (e.g., vital statistics data, cancer registration data), even though direct measures of the person-time at risk are not available (Example 4.9). An estimate of the person-time at risk during a given period can be made as follows:

> Population at the mid-point of the calendar period of interest × length of the period (in suitable units of time, usually years).

Provided that the population remains stable throughout this period, this method yields adequate estimates of person-time at risk.

Example 4.9. Suppose that we wish to estimate the incidence of stomach cancer in men living in Cali, Colombia. Volume VI of Cancer Incidence in Five Continents *(Parkin et al., 1992) provides data on the total number of stomach cancer cases that occurred in Cali during the years 1982–86 and on the total male population in 1984. The incidence rate of stomach cancer can be calculated from these data as shown below:*

No. of male stomach cancer cases, Cali, 1982–86 = 655
Total male population, Cali, 1984 = 622 922
Total person-years at risk, 1982–86 = 5 (years) × 622 922 = 3 114 610 pyrs
Mean annual incidence rate, Cali, 1982–86 = 655/3 114 610 = 21.03 per 100 000 pyrs

Thus the mean annual incidence rate of stomach cancer in men living in Cali during the years 1982–86 was 21 per 100 000 pyrs.

This method of estimating person-time at risk is appropriate for rare conditions such as cancer. However, common conditions demand more sophisticated approaches that exclude from the denominator those who have the disease and are therefore no longer at risk.

In most developed countries and many developing countries, a population census is taken, usually once every ten years. This provides the baseline count of the total population. As a source of denominator data, censuses are somewhat limited: they are relatively incomplete for some population subgroups (e.g., homeless and nomadic people) and can rapidly become out of date. Most census offices provide estimates of the population size between censuses (for intercensal years), which are based on population birth, death and migration rates. When available, these annual population estimates can be taken as the best estimates of the person-time at risk in each calendar year. Thus in the above example, the sum of the annual population estimates for the years 1982–86 could have been used to provide an estimate of the total person-years at risk for the entire study period.

4.3.1 Crude and stratum-specific measures

The measures of disease occurrence discussed in Section 4.2 may be calculated for a whole population—so-called crude measures—or separately for specific sub-groups (strata) of the population—called stratum-specific measures. For example:

$$\text{Crude incidence rate per 100 000 pyrs} = \frac{\text{No. of new cases arising in a defined population in a specific period of time}}{\text{Total person - years at risk in that population during that period of time}} \times 100\ 000$$

Crude rates are widely used, in part because they are summary measures and so are easily interpreted, and in part because their calculation requires relatively little information. Crude rates may obscure the fact that subgroups of the population have marked differences in incidence; for instance, people in different age groups have a different risk of death. This should be borne in mind when comparing crude rates from various populations, as disparities might reflect differences in their population structure rather than in disease incidence (see Section 4.3.3).

To gain an understanding of certain epidemiological aspects of a disease, more detailed rates, specific for sex and other demographic characteristics such as age, are needed. For example, age-specific rates can be calculated as follows:

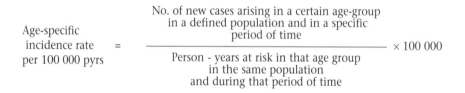

$$\text{Age-specific incidence rate per 100 000 pyrs} = \frac{\text{No. of new cases arising in a certain age-group in a defined population and in a specific period of time}}{\text{Person - years at risk in that age group in the same population and during that period of time}} \times 100\ 000$$

Person-time at risk is calculated separately for each age group. Plotting these age-specific rates against age yields an age–incidence curve, which can reveal important clues to the epidemiology of a disease (see Figure 4.5a). Note that cancer rates are usually sex-specific, i.e., calculated separately for males and females, because cancer incidence for most sites differs markedly between the sexes.

4.3.2 Changes in disease incidence with time

The risk of getting a disease also changes with calendar time, and this should be taken into account during follow-up. This is illustrated in Example 4.10

Example 4.10. Consider a group of people (cohort) aged from 30 to 54 years who were followed up from 1950 to the end of 1969. Study subjects contributed person–time at risk from the time they joined the cohort to the end of the study in 1969 (or until their 55th birthday if it occurred earlier). The experience of one study subject is shown in Figure 4.4; this subject joined the cohort on 1 October 1952, on his 30th birthday, and was 47 years and 3 months old when the study ended on 31 December 1969.

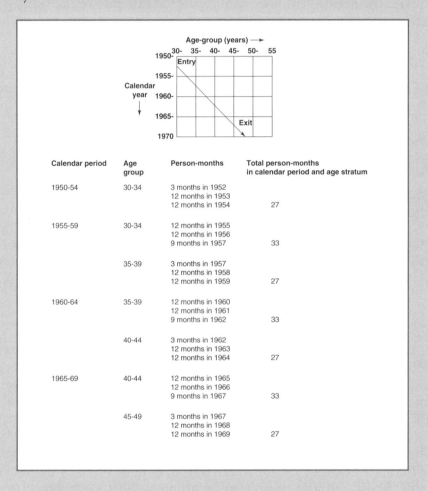

Figure 4.4.
Lexis diagram showing the follow-up of the study subject described in Example 4.10 and the calculation of his person-months contribution to each calendar period and age stratum.

Calendar period	Age group	Person-months	Total person-months in calendar period and age stratum
1950-54	30-34	3 months in 1952 12 months in 1953 12 months in 1954	27
1955-59	30-34	12 months in 1955 12 months in 1956 9 months in 1957	33
	35-39	3 months in 1957 12 months in 1958 12 months in 1959	27
1960-64	35-39	12 months in 1960 12 months in 1961 9 months in 1962	33
	40-44	3 months in 1962 12 months in 1963 12 months in 1964	27
1965-69	40-44	12 months in 1965 12 months in 1966 9 months in 1967	33
	45-49	3 months in 1967 12 months in 1968 12 months in 1969	27

The experience of a whole cohort can be represented in a *Lexis diagram*, which consists of age and calendar time cells or strata (see Figure 4.4). This diagram can be used to assess individual follow-up simultaneously in relation to two different time-scales: age and calendar period. Once a subject enters the cohort, he moves diagonally through the Lexis diagram as he ages, contributing person-time at risk to various strata as he moves through them. Stratum-specific rates can be calculated by dividing the total number of cases arising in each age and calendar period stratum by the corresponding total person-time at risk.

Even when data on date of birth are not available, the Lexis diagram can be used with routine data to describe the incidence of a disease in successive generations. Mortality rates from cancer of the lung in men in England and Wales during 1941–78 are shown in Table 4.1: columns show changes in the incidence rates with age, and rows show changes in the age-specific rates over calendar time. In any age × calendar-period two-way table, diagonal lines represent successive birth cohorts, although the earliest and the most recent birth cohorts (in the extremes of the table) will have very few data points.

Table 4.1.
Mortality (per million person-years) from cancer of the lung, in males in England and Wales, 1941–78, by age group and calendar period; the central year of birth is indicated on the diagonals.[a]

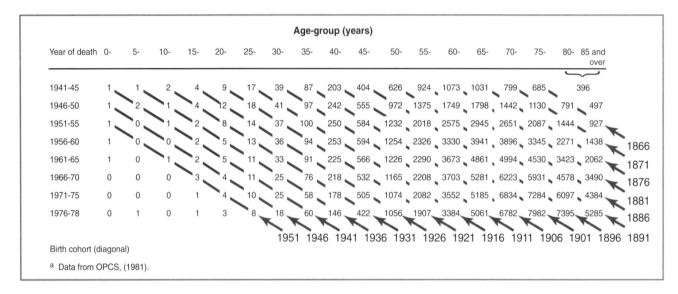

Age-group (years)																		
Year of death	0-	5-	10-	15-	20-	25-	30-	35-	40-	45-	50-	55-	60-	65-	70-	75-	80-	85 and over
1941-45	1	1	2	4	9	17	39	87	203	404	626	924	1073	1031	799	685	396	
1946-50	1	2	1	4	12	18	41	97	242	555	972	1375	1749	1798	1442	1130	791	497
1951-55	1	0	1	2	8	14	37	100	250	584	1232	2018	2575	2945	2651	2087	1444	927
1956-60	1	0	0	2	5	13	36	94	253	594	1254	2326	3330	3941	3896	3345	2271	1438
1961-65	1	0	1	2	5	11	33	91	225	566	1226	2290	3673	4861	4994	4530	3423	2062
1966-70	0	0	0	3	4	11	25	76	218	532	1165	2208	3703	5281	6223	5931	4578	3490
1971-75	0	0	0	1	4	10	25	58	178	505	1074	2082	3552	5185	6834	7284	6097	4384
1976-78	0	1	0	1	3	8	18	60	146	422	1056	1907	3384	5061	6782	7982	7395	5285

Birth cohort (diagonal): 1866, 1871, 1876, 1881, 1886

1951 1946 1941 1936 1931 1926 1921 1916 1911 1906 1901 1896 1891

a Data from OPCS, (1981).

The diagonals of Table 4.1 (from upper left to lower right), for instance, define the lung cancer mortality experience for successive generations of men who were born together and hence aged together. For example, a man aged 40–44 years in 1941–45, was aged 45–49 in 1946–50, 50–54 in 1951–55, etc. To be 40–44 in 1941–45, he could have been born at any time between January 1896 (44 in 1941) and December 1905 (40 in 1945). These so-called birth cohorts are typically identified by their central year of birth; for example, the 1901 birth cohort, or more precisely the 1900/1 birth cohort, contains those men born during the 10-year period from 1896 to 1905. The diagonal just above this one shows the rates pertaining to the 1896 cohort, i.e., those men born between 1891 and 1900. As the years of birth for each cohort are estimated from the age and calendar period data, adjacent cohorts inevitably overlap, i.e., they have years of birth in common. When data on exact year of birth are available, these estimates need not be made, and so successive birth cohorts do not overlap.

Analyses by birth cohort thus use the same age-specific rates as in calendar time period analyses, but these rates are arranged in a different way. Comparison of rates in successive birth cohorts allows us to assess how incidence may have changed from one generation to another.

The data in Table 4.1 can be plotted in different ways to illustrate changes in age-specific rates over calendar time—*secular trends*—or changes from generation to generation—*cohort trends*.

Figure 4.5 clearly illustrates that secular trends in lung cancer mortality differ by age. In older age-groups, rates increased over the study period, while in younger groups, they declined. When rates are presented by year of birth (Figure 4.6), it becomes apparent that while rates for successive generations of men born until the turn of the century increased, they declined for generations born since then. These trends closely parallel trends in cigarette smoking (not shown).

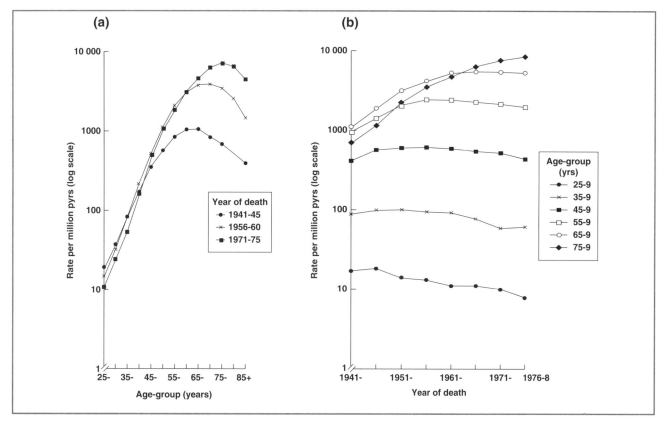

In certain situations, cohort analysis gives the most accurate picture of changes in the patterns of disease over time, for example, if exposure to a potential risk factor occurs very early in life and influences the lifetime risk of a particular disease, or if the habits of adults are adopted by successive generations (as with cigarette smoking and lung cancer, and exposure to sunlight and malignant melanoma of skin). In other situations, secular analysis might be more appropriate: for example, if exposure to the risk factor affects all age groups simultaneously (as with the introduction of a new medical treatment). However, in most situations, it is not clear which analysis is most appropriate to describe temporal trends, and the results of both should be examined.

Figure 4.5.
Mortality from lung cancer in men in England and Wales, 1941-78. (*a*) Rates presented to show differences in age-specific curves between three selected calendar periods; (*b*) rates presented to show secular (calendar) trends in age-specific rates. For clarity, only rates for alternate age-groups are shown; the first five age-groups are omitted because of the small number of deaths (data from Table 4.1).

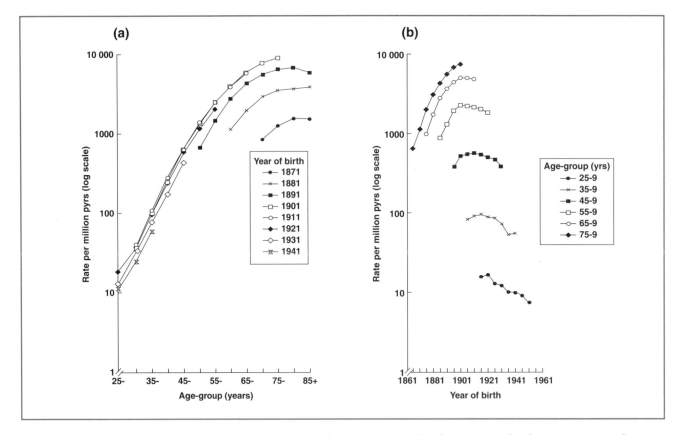

Figure 4.6.
Mortality from lung cancer in men in England and Wales, 1941–78. (*a*) Rates presented to show differences in age-specific curves for successive birth cohorts; (*b*) rates presented to show cohort trends in age-specific rates. For clarity, only rates for alternate age-groups or cohorts are shown; the first five age-groups are omitted because of the small number of deaths (data from Table 4.1).

Descriptive analyses by age, calendar time and cohort are a popular epidemiological tool for examining temporal changes in the incidence of a disease. These analyses are based on the inspection of tables and graphs, in much the same way as described here, although statistical models can also be used to assess whether there is a statistically significant trend in rates over calendar time, or between birth cohorts (Clayton & Schifflers, 1987a,b).

4.3.3 Controlling for age

For comparison of incidence between populations, crude rates may be misleading. As an example, let us compare stomach cancer incidence among men living in Cali, Colombia and Birmingham, England. The data are extracted from *Cancer Incidence in Five Continents* (Parkin *et al.*, 1992).

Table 4.2 shows that the crude incidence rate (the rate for all ages combined) for Birmingham was much higher than that for Cali. However, before concluding that the incidence of male stomach cancer in Birmingham (1983–86) was higher than in Cali (1982–86), the age-specific rates for the two must be compared. Surprisingly, age-specific rates were higher for Cali in all age-groups. The discrepancy between crude and age-specific rates is because these two populations had markedly different age-structures (Table 4.3), with Birmingham having a much older population than Cali.

Age (years)[b]	Cali			Birmingham		
	No. of cancers (1982–86)	Male population (1984)	Mean annual rate[c] (1982–86)	No. of cancers (1983–86)	Male population (1985)	Mean annual rate[c] (1983–86)
0–44	39	524 220	1.5	79	1 683 600	1.2
45–64	266	76 304	69.7	1037	581 500	44.6
65+	315	22 398	281.3	2352	291 100	202.0
All ages	620	622 922	19.9[d]	3468	2 556 200	33.9

[a] Data from Parkin *et al.* (1992)
[b] For simplicity, only three broad age-groups are used throughout this example.
[c] Rate per 100 000 person-years.
[d] This crude rate is slightly lower than in Example 4.9 (21.03 per 100 000 person-years) because cases of unknown age (35 in total) were excluded here. The exclusion of two cases of unknown age in Birmingham did not affect the value of the crude rate calculated here.

The lower crude rate for Cali is thus explained by its male population being younger than that of Birmingham, and the fact that younger people have a much lower incidence of stomach cancer than older people (Figure 4.7). In this situation, age is a confounding variable, i.e., age is related to exposure (locality) and it is itself a risk factor for the outcome of interest, stomach cancer (see also Chapter 13).

Table 4.2.
Incidence of stomach cancer in males by age group in Cali, 1982–86, and Birmingham, 1983–86.[a]

Age (years)	Percentage of total male population	
	Cali (1984)	Birmingham (1985)
0–44	84	66
45–64	12	23
65+	4	11
All ages	100	100

[a] Data from Parkin *et al.* (1992).

Table 4.3.
Age distribution of the male population in Cali, 1984, and Birmingham, 1985.[a]

Figure 4.7.
Age-incidence curve of stomach cancer in males in Cali, 1982-86, and Birmingham, 1983-86 (data from Parkin *et al.*, 1992).

As incidence rates for stomach cancer change considerably with age, differences in the age distribution of populations need to be considered before attempting to compare incidence. One approach is to compare age-specific rates, as in the example above; however, this can become cumbersome when comparing several populations each with many age-groups. The ideal would be to have a summary measure for each population, which has been controlled, or adjusted, for differences in the age structure. Several statistical methods can be used to control for the effects of confounding variables, such as age (see also Chapters 13 and 14). Here, only one such method, *standardization*, is discussed.

Standardization is by far the most common method used when working with routine data. Although this method is usually employed to adjust

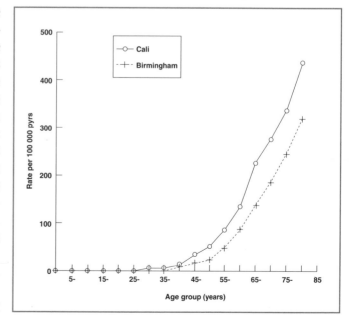

for the effect of age, it can equally be used to control for any other confounding variable such as social class, area of residence, etc. There are two methods of standardization: direct and indirect.

Direct method of standardization

Let us take a hypothetical population, and call it our standard population, the age-structure of which is shown in Table 4.4. How many cases of stomach cancer would we expect in males in Cali if its male population had the same age distribution as this standard population?

As shown in Figure 4.8, this is relatively easy to calculate. Each age-specific rate for Cali is simply multiplied by the standard population figures in the corresponding age-group; the sum over all age categories will give the total number of male stomach cancer cases expected in Cali if its male population had the same age distribution as the standard.

It is also possible to determine how many male stomach cancer cases would be expected in Birmingham if its male population had the same age distribution as the standard population; the calculations are similar to those described for Cali, but are based on the age-specific rates for Birmingham (Figure 4.8).

Summary incidence rates for Cali and Birmingham, assuming the age-structure of the standard population, can be obtained by dividing the total expected cases by the total person-years at risk in the standard population. These rates are called mean annual age-adjusted or age-standardized incidence rates; they can be seen as the crude incidence rates that these populations would have if their age distributions were shifted from their actual values in the mid-1980s to the age distribution of the standard population. These standardized rates are a fiction: they are not the stomach cancer incidence rates that actually existed, but rather those that these two populations would have had if, while retaining their own age-specific rates, they had a hypothetical (standard) population. The fiction is useful, however, because it enables the epidemiologist to make summary comparisons between populations from different areas, or during different time periods, which are free from the distortion that arises from age differences in the actual populations.

Age (years)	Population
0–44	74 000
45–64	19 000
65+	7 000
All ages	100 000

Table 4.4.
A standard population.

Figure 4.8.
The direct method of standardization.

Mean annual age-specific rates in Cali, 1982-86 (per 100 000 pyrs)			Mean annual age-specific rates in Birmingham, 1983-86 (per 100 000 pyrs)	
Age	Rate		Age	Rate
0–44	1.5		0–44	1.2
45–64	69.7		45–64	44.6
65+	281.3		65+	202.0

Standard Population

Age	Population
0–44	74 000
45–64	19 000
65+	7 000

No. of male stomach cancer cases expected if the male population of Cali and Birmingham had the same age distribution as the standard population

a) Cali

Age	Expected cases	
0–44	$0.000015 \times 74\ 000 =$	1.11
45–64	$0.000697 \times 19\ 000 =$	13.24
65+	$0.002813 \times 7\ 000 =$	19.69
Total expected		**= 34.04**

Mean annual age-adjusted rate for Cali, 1982-86 =
= 34.04/100 000 =
= 34.0 per 100 000 pyrs

b) Birmingham

Age	Expected cases	
0–44	$0.000012 \times 74\ 000 =$	0.89
45–64	$0.000446 \times 19\ 000 =$	8.47
65+	$0.002020 \times 7\ 000 =$	14.14
Total expected		**= 23.50**

Mean annual age-adjusted rate for Birmingham, 1983-86 =
= 23.5/100 000 =
= 23.5 per 100 000 pyrs

The age-standardized rate can be seen as a weighted average of the age-specific rates, the weights being taken from the standard population. Age-adjusted rates can be compared directly, provided that they refer to the same standard population, i.e., that the weights given to the age-specific rates are the same. In the example above, the mean annual age-standardized incidence rate for Cali is higher than that for Birmingham; this is in agreement with the age-specific rates. An age-standardized rate ratio can be calculated by dividing the rate for Cali by that for Birmingham, to yield a rate ratio:

34.0 per 100 000 pyrs/23.5 per 100 000 pyrs = 1.45

This measure is called the *standardized rate ratio (SRR)* or *comparative morbidity (or mortality) figure (CMF)*. In this example, it reveals that the estimated incidence of stomach cancer was 45% higher in Cali than in Birmingham in the mid-1980s, and that this excess is independent of age differences between these two populations.

This method of adjusting for age is called the direct method of standardization. It requires knowledge of the age-specific rates (or the data to calculate them) for all the populations being studied, and also the definition of a standard population. The standard population can be any population: one of those being compared or any other. However, the standard population used must always be specified, as its choice may affect the comparison. Conventional standard populations, such as the world standard and the European standard populations, have been defined and are widely used so as to allow rates to be compared directly (see Appendix 4.1). The standard population given in Table 4.4 is in fact a summary of the world standard population.

For simplicity, we use only three broad age-groups in the example given in this section. However, this does not provide an adequate age-adjustment, and narrower age groups should be used. Five-year age-groups are usually employed, as they are the most common grouping in publications on site-specific cancer data. When five-year age-groups are used for age-adjustment of the data on stomach cancer presented in the example above (Figure 4.8), the age-adjusted rates per 100 000 person-years are 36.3 for Cali and 21.2 for Birmingham; the rate ratio is now 1.71. When rates change dramatically with age, narrower age groups (e.g., one-year groups) may be required to obtain an adequate age-adjustment.

It is important to remember that an age-standardized rate is not an actual rate but rather an artificial one, which permits the incidence of a disease in one population to be compared with that in another, controlling for differences in their age composition. Therefore, age-standardized rates should not be used when what is needed is an accurate measurement of disease occurrence in a population, rather than a comparison.

Indirect method of standardization

Suppose that the total number of stomach cancers in Cali in 1982–86 is known, but their distribution by age is not available (Table 4.5). In this case, the direct method of standardization cannot be used.

Table 4.5.
Incidence of stomach cancer in Cali, 1982–86, and Birmingham, 1983–86.[a]

Age (years)[b]	Cali				Birmingham		
	No. of cancers (1982–86)	Male population (1984)	Mean annual rate[b] (1982–86)		No. of cancers (1983–86)	Male population (1985)	Mean annual rate[b] (1983–86)
0–44	NA	524 220	–		79	1 683 600	1.2
45–64	NA	76 304	–		1037	581 500	44.6
65+	NA	22 398	–		2352	291 100	202.0
All ages	620	622 922	19.9		3468	2 556 200	33.9

NA, data assumed to be not available (see Table 4.2).
[a] Data from Parkin *et al.*, 1992.
[b] Rate per 100 000 person-years.

It is, however, possible to calculate how many male cases of stomach cancer would be expected in Cali if males in both Cali and Birmingham had the same age-specific incidence rates. In other words, the Birmingham age-specific rates can be treated as a set of standard rates. The calculations are shown in Figure 4.9. The expected number of cancer cases in Cali is calculated by multiplying the mean annual age-specific rates for Birmingham by the person-years at risk in the corresponding age-group in Cali; the sum over all age categories will give the total number of male cancer cases that would be expected in Cali if its male population had the same age-specific incidence rates for stomach cancer as that of Birmingham. Evidently, the number of expected cases in Birmingham is equal to the number observed.

Note that these expected stomach cancer cases relate to what would happen if Cali and Birmingham had the same age-specific incidence rates for stomach cancer rather than the same population structure. So it would be meaningless to calculate summary rates for each locality by dividing the total number of expected cases by the corresponding total person-years at risk. However, for

Figure 4.9.
The indirect method of standardization.

Mean annual age-specific rates in Birmingham, 1983-86 (per 100 000 pyrs)

Age	Rate
0–44	1.2
45–64	44.6
65+	202.0

Total person-years at risk in Cali, 1982-86

Age	Person-years
0–44	524 220 × 5 = 2 621 100
45–64	76 304 × 5 = 381 520
65+	22 398 × 5 = 111 990
All ages	= 3 114 610

Total person-years at risk in Birmingham, 1983-86

Age	Person-years
0–44	1 683 600 × 4 = 6 734 400
45–64	581 500 × 4 = 2 326 000
65+	291 100 × 4 = 1 164 400
All ages	= 10 224 800

No. of expected male stomach cancer cases if the populations have the same stomach cancer age-specific incidence rates as Birmingham

a) Cali

Age	Expected cases	
0–44	0.000012 × 2 621 100 =	31.45
45–64	0.000446 × 381 520 =	170.15
65+	0.002020 × 111 990 =	226.22
Total expected (E), 1982-86		427.82
Total observed (O), 1982-86		620
O/E (%) =		145

b) Birmingham

Age	Expected cases	
0–44		
45–64		
65+		
Total expected (E), 1983-86 =		3 468
Total observed (O), 1983-86 =		3 468
O/E (%) =		100

each locality, the numbers of cases observed and expected can be compared, because both refer to the same population. The ratio of the observed number of cases to that expected is called the standardized incidence ratio (SIR) or the standardized mortality ratio (SMR) if a case is defined as death. These ratios are usually expressed as a percentage.

In the example above, the SIR (%) for Birmingham is 100; by definition, the number of observed cases of stomach cancer is equal to the number of expected cases when using the age-specific stomach cancer incidence rates for Birmingham as the standard rates. The SIR (%) for Cali is 145, meaning that the number of cases observed was 45% higher than that expected if Cali had the same incidence of stomach cancer as Birmingham. This result is similar to that obtained using the direct method of standardization.

This method is called the indirect method of standardization. As with the direct method, the results depend in part upon the standard chosen. However, the indirect method of standardization is less sensitive to the choice of standard than the direct one.

Which method is the best?

In comparisons of incidence of disease between two or more populations, direct and indirect standardization tend to give broadly similar results in practice. However, the choice of method might be affected by several considerations:

(1) The direct method requires that stratum-specific rates (e.g., age-specific rates) are available for all populations studied. The indirect method requires only the total number of cases that occurred in each study population. If stratum-specific rates are not available for all study populations, the indirect method may be the only possible approach.

(2) Indirect standardization is preferable to the direct method when age-specific rates are based on small numbers of subjects. Rates used in direct adjustment would thus be open to substantial sampling variation (see Section 6.1.4). With the indirect method, the most stable rates can be chosen as the standard, so as to ensure that the summary rates are as precise as possible.

(3) In general, when comparing incidence in two or more populations, direct standardization is open to less bias than indirect standardization. The reasons for this are subtle and are beyond the scope of this text.

For a more detailed discussion of the advantages and disadvantages of each method of standardization, see pp. 72–76 in Breslow & Day (1987).

Is the use of adjusted summary measures always appropriate?

Although age-adjusted measures provide a convenient summary of age-specific rates, the age-specific rates themselves give the most infor-

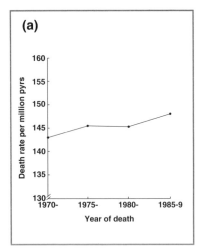

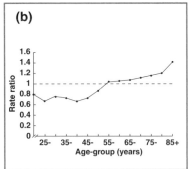

Figure 4.10.
Ovarian cancer mortality in England and Wales, 1970–89. (a) Rates are age-standardized to the 1981 female population of England and Wales; (b) age-specific mortality rate ratios, 1970–74 and 1985–89 (rates in 1970–74 taken as the baseline).

mation. It must be emphasized that, under certain circumstances, it may not be appropriate to summarize disease rates in a single summary measure. Consider this example. We wish to monitor trends in mortality from ovarian cancer in England and Wales. The age-adjusted death rates for this cancer in England and Wales increased slightly from 1970–74 to 1985–89, as shown in Figure 4.10a. However, trends in the age-specific rates for this period reveal that they did not increase across all age-groups. Figure 4.10b shows the rate ratio of the 1985–89 to the 1970–74 age-specific rates. It becomes apparent that while death rates were increasing at older ages (rate ratios above 1), there was no increase in women below age 55 years (rate ratios below 1). If age-standardized death rates for all ages are calculated, this information is lost, because mortality rates from this cancer at younger ages were so low that they were dominated by the much higher mortality rates in the older age-groups. So in this case, the age-adjusted summary measure is misleading.

Before age-adjusted summary measures are calculated, the age-specific rate ratios should always be examined to determine whether this approach is appropriate. If these ratios vary systematically with age, this information would inevitably be lost in the summary age-adjusted measure.

4.3.4 Cumulative rate

The cumulative rate is another measure of disease occurrence that is increasingly used in cancer epidemiology. This measure has been included in recent editions of *Cancer Incidence in Five Continents* (see, for example, Parkin *et al.*, 1992).

A cumulative rate is the sum of the age-specific incidence rates over a certain age range. The age range over which the rate is accumulated must be specified, and depends on the comparison being made. Thus for childhood tumours, this might be age 0–14 years. In general, however, the most appropriate measure is calculated over the whole life span, usually taken as 0–74 years.

The cumulative rate can be calculated by the sum of the age-specific incidence rates (provided they are expressed in the same person-time units, e.g., 100 000 pyrs), multiplied by the width of the age-group. Thus for five-year age-groups, the cumulative rate would be five times the sum of the age-specific incidence rates over the relevant age range (Figure 4.11). If the age-groups are of different width, each age-specific rate should be first multiplied by the width of the corresponding age-group; the sum over all age-categories yields the cumulative rate. This measure is usually expressed as a percentage.

The cumulative rate can be interpreted as a form of direct age-standardization with the same population size (i.e., denominator) in each age-group. Thus, it avoids the arbitrary choice of a standard population.

Another advantage of the cumulative rate is that it provides an estimate of cumulative risk, i.e., the risk an individual would have of devel-

Age-group (years)	Mean annual age-specific incidence rate (per 100 000 pyrs)
0–4	0
5–9	0
10–14	0
15–19	0
20–24	0.1
25–29	0.1
30–34	0.9
35–39	3.5
40–44	6.7
45–49	14.5
50–54	26.8
55–59	52.6
60–64	87.2
65–69	141.7
70–74	190.8
Total	**524.9**
Total x 5	**2624.5**

Cumulative rate = 100 x (2624.5/100 000) = 2.6%
Cumulative risk = 100 x {1–exp(–cumulative rate/100)} = 2.6%

Figure 4.11.
Calculation of cumulative rate and cumulative risk over the age range 0–74 years for male stomach cancer in Birmingham, 1983-86 (data from Parkin *et al.*, 1992).

oping a particular cancer over a defined life span in the absence of any other cause of death. The cumulative risk can be calculated as follows:

$$\text{Cumulative risk} = 100 \times \{1-\exp(-\text{cumulative rate}/100)\}$$

However, if the cumulative rate is lower than 10%, its value is practically equal to that of the cumulative risk. Thus, in Figure 4.11, the estimated risk for a Birmingham male of developing stomach cancer between the ages of 0–74 years is 2.6% (assuming no other cause of death). This is equal to the cumulative rate.

Table 4.6 shows the crude rates, five-year age-standardized rates and cumulative rates for male stomach cancer in Cali and Birmingham. In contrast to the crude rates, both age-standardized rates and cumulative rates give an accurate picture of the relative incidence of stomach cancer in the two populations.

4.3.5 Lack of proper denominators

Sometimes, no suitable denominator is available to permit calculation of one of the measures of incidence discussed so far. This may be because there are no data on denominators (e.g., no census has been carried out), because a catchment population cannot be defined (e.g., for a hospital-based registry), or because case-finding has been so incomplete that denominators derived from other sources (e.g., the census) are not comparable with the numerator data. In these circumstances, it is traditional

Table 4.6.
Mean annual crude incidence rates,
mean annual age-standardized rates
and cumulative rates for male stomach
cancer, Cali, 1982–86, and Birmingham,
1983–86.

	Cali, 1982–86	Birmingham, 1983–86	Rate ratio
Crude rates (per 100 000 pyrs)	19.9	33.9	0.59
Age-standardized rate[a] (per 100 000 pyrs)	36.3	21.2	1.71
Cumulative rate, 0–74 years (%)	4.6	2.6	1.77

[a] Standardized to the world standard population. These age-standardized rates differ slightly from those in Figure 4.8, being age-adjusted within five-year age-groups.

to calculate proportional measures; that is, to express the number of cases of a particular condition as a proportion of the total number of cases of all conditions:

$$\text{Proportional incidence (\%)} = \frac{\text{No. of cases of the disease of interest in a specified time period}}{\text{Total number of cases of all conditions in the same time period}} \times 100$$

Comparisons of incidence between populations can then be made by calculating proportional incidence ratios (PIRs); likewise, mortality can be compared by using mortality data to calculate proportional mortality ratios (PMRs). These ratios are calculated as follows:

$$\text{PIR (\%)} = \frac{\text{Proportion of cases from a specific cause in population A}}{\text{Proportion of cases from the same cause in population B}} \times 100$$

As with rates, these proportions can be standardize for age (or any other potential confounding factor).

Note that a proportional measure is not equivalent to a rate, as the denominator is derived from the total number of cases, and not from the population at risk. While proportional measures reveal the proportion of cases (or deaths) that can be attributed to a particular disease, a cause-specific rate reflects the risk of developing (or dying from) a particular disease for members of a specific population.

Proportional measures can be misleading because their denominator is the total number of cases (or deaths), a measure that depends on the number of cases (or deaths) from all causes, not just that being studied. For example, although the proportion of deaths due to cancer is greater in middle-aged women than in elderly women, death rates from cancer are actually higher among the elderly (Figure 4.12). This is because the total number of deaths from other causes, particularly from cardiovascular disease, is also considerably higher in the elderly. Thus, although the total number of deaths from cancer is greater in the elderly, they constitute a smaller proportion of all deaths than at younger ages.

These measures (and the use of odds ratios as an alternative) are discussed further in Chapter 11.

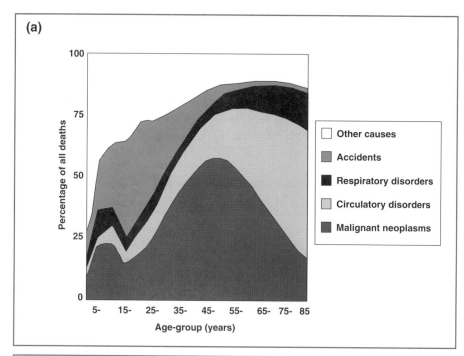

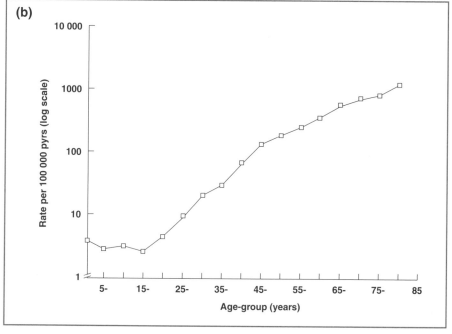

Figure 4.12.
Female deaths in England and Wales, 1993. (a) Proportion of deaths due to cancer and other causes by age; (b) cancer mortality rates by age (data from OPCS, 1995).

Further reading

* Most of the measures of disease occurrence discussed here are dealt with in more detail in Breslow & Day (1987) and Estève *et al.* (1994).

* A more elaborate discussion of age, calendar time and cohort effects can be found in Clayton & Schifflers (1987a,b).

Box 4.1. Key issues

- Quantification of the occurrence of disease and other health-related events in populations requires a clear definition of the cases (numerator), the population at risk (denominator), and the time frame to which these refer.

- There are two major measures of disease occurrence: *prevalence* and *incidence*. Prevalence refers to the total number of existing (new and old) cases of a condition in a population at a specific point in time. Incidence refers to the occurrence of new cases in a population over a specific time period.

- Incidence can be measured as either *risk, odds of disease*, or *rate*. The calculation of risk and odds requires complete follow-up of all study subjects for the entire study period. In contrast, the calculation of rates takes into account individual differences in length of follow-up.

- Measures of disease occurrence can be calculated for the whole population, as *crude* measures; or separately for certain subgroups of the population, as *stratum-specific* measures.

- Incidence of a disease varies with time. These changes occur simultaneously according to three different time scales: age, calendar period (*secular trends*) and date of birth (*cohort trends*), but can be examined separately in an age-by-calendar period two-way Lexis diagram. The diagonals in this diagram represent successive birth cohorts.

- Crude rates can be misleading when comparing incidence from different populations because they do not take into account differences in population age-structure. *Age-standardization*, either direct or indirect, can be used to obtain summary measures that are adjusted for differences in age structure. Alternatively, *cumulative rates* may be calculated.

- Proportional measures, such as *proportional incidence ratios*, can be calculated when no suitable denominators are available. These ratios should be interpreted cautiously, as their denominator is the total number of cases, not the population at risk.

Appendix 4.1
Conventional standard populations

The choice of the standard population to be used in the direct method of standardization is, to a certain extent, arbitrary. For example, if the aim is to compare disease occurrence in several groups in England and Wales, an appropriate standard might be the adult population of England and Wales. On the other hand, this may not be an appropriate standard when making comparisons between countries.

For international comparisons, various conventional standard populations have been used (Table A4.1). These standard populations range from an African population with a low proportion of old people, through an intermediate world population, to a European population with a high proportion of old people. In the earliest volumes of *Cancer Incidence in Five Continents*, rates were standardized to these three populations; however, the European and African standards were dropped in Volume IV (Waterhouse *et al.*, 1982) and replaced by cumulative rates over the age ranges 0–64 and 0–74 years.

The truncated population is derived from the world population but comprises only the middle age-groups. This truncated population was often used in the past, because data for older age-groups were likely to be less reliable than those for the middle age-groups, and because for most forms of cancer, virtually no cases arise in groups under 35 years.

Table A4.1.
Conventional standard populations
used for international comparisons.

Age group (years)	African	World	European	Truncated
0	2 000	2 400	1 600	–
1–4	8 000	9 600	6 400	–
5–9	10 000	10 000	7 000	–
10–14	10 000	9 000	7 000	–
15–19	10 000	9 000	7 000	–
20–24	10 000	8 000	7 000	–
25–29	10 000	8 000	7 000	–
30–34	10 000	6 000	7 000	–
35–39	10 000	6 000	7 000	6 000
40–44	5 000	6 000	7 000	6 000
45–49	5 000	6 000	7 000	6 000
50–54	3 000	5 000	7 000	5 000
55–59	2 000	4 000	6 000	4 000
60–64	2 000	4 000	5 000	4 000
65–69	1 000	3 000	4 000	–
70–74	1 000	2 000	3 000	–
75–79	500	1 000	2 000	–
80–84	300	500	1 000	–
85+	200	500	1 000	–
Total	100 000	100 000	100 000	31 000

Chapter 5
Overview of study designs

In epidemiology, measuring the occurrence of disease or other health-related events in a population is only a beginning. Epidemiologists are also interested in assessing whether an exposure is associated with a particular disease (or other outcome of interest). For instance, researchers may be interested in obtaining answers to the following questions:

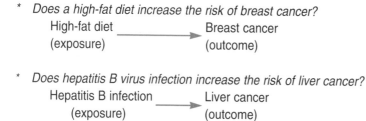

The first step in an epidemiological study is to define the hypothesis to be tested. This should include a precise definition of the exposure(s) and outcome(s) under study. The next step is to decide which study design will be the most appropriate to test that specific study hypothesis.

5.1   Types of study design

There are two basic approaches to assessing whether an exposure is associated with a particular outcome: experimental and observational. The *experimental* approach is perhaps more familiar to clinicians, since it corresponds to the approach used for investigations in laboratory-based research. In an experiment, investigators study the impact of varying some factor which they can control. For example, the investigators may take a litter of rats, and randomly select half of them to be exposed to a supposedly carcinogenic agent, then record the frequency with which cancer develops in each group. The equivalent of this animal experiment in human beings would entail selecting a group of individuals, randomly allocating half of them to exposure to a hypothesized disease-producing factor, and then comparing the occurrence of disease in subjects who were exposed with that in subjects who were not. For ethical reasons, it would be impossible to conduct such a study in human subjects. It is, however, possible to conduct a trial to test whether removal of such an exposure will decrease subsequent incidence and mortality. Thus, experimental studies in epidemiology are limited to interventions that are believed to be of potential benefit.

Since epidemiologists can rarely conduct experiments, their role is usually limited to observing the occurrence of disease in people who are already segregated into groups. For instance, we can follow up people who happen to be or not be infected with the hepatitis B virus, to see whether their risks of liver cancer are different. These studies are *observational*, because the role of the investigator is merely to observe what happens, noting who is exposed or unexposed and who has or has not developed the outcome of interest.

A major problem with observational studies is that the observed groups may differ in many other characteristics, in addition to the one under study. Thus, people in various occupations may differ not only in exposure to occupational hazards but also in other lifestyle characteristics such as socioeconomic background, health status, fitness for the job, smoking and alcohol habits and many other factors. Because of these *confounding* and often unmeasurable factors, the role of a specific exposure under investigation is more difficult to establish than in experimental studies.

Epidemiological studies can thus generally be classified as *intervention* or *observational* studies. Within each of these two broad categories, studies can be further organized as in Figure 5.1

Figure 5.1.
Main types of epidemiological study design.

```
Intervention (experimental) studies
        Clinical trials
        Field trials
                individual level
                aggregated level (community trials)
Observational (non-experimental) studies
        Cohort studies
        Case–control studies
        Cross-sectional surveys
        Routine-data-based studies
                individual level
                aggregated level (ecological studies)
```

The classification scheme shown in Figure 5.1 should be taken as just a simple way of presenting and discussing the different study designs. There are, of course, many other ways in which epidemiological study designs may be classified. Also, in reality, many studies have mixed features.

5.1.1 Intervention studies

Intervention studies are characterized by the fact that the study subjects are allocated by the investigator to the different study groups through the use of *randomization* (Figure 5.2). This ensures that the assignment of subjects to the various groups is determined by chance alone and is not subjectively influenced by the investigators or the participants (see Section 7.9.1). There are two main types of intervention study: clinical trials and field trials.

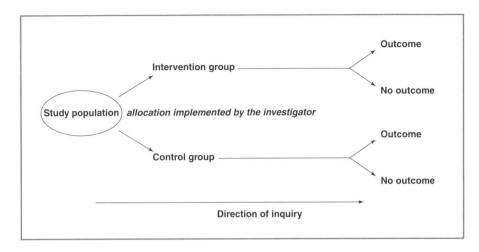

Figure 5.2.
Outline of an intervention trial.

The objective of a *clinical trial* is to evaluate new forms of treatment of a disease or condition. Thus clinical trials are usually carried out in hospitals or clinics among people who have already developed the disease.

Example 5.1. *The Women's Intervention Nutrition Study was set up to assess whether a low-fat diet will reduce cancer recurrence and improve survival of women who have surgery for early and moderate stage breast cancer. A total of 2000 postmenopausal women with resected breast cancer are being recruited and randomized to receive standard treatment plus a low-fat dietary intervention or standard treatment alone. The standard treatment consists of tamoxifen, and radiotherapy and/or chemotherapy as appropriate. The study will last for five years (Chlebowski & Grosvenor, 1994; Henderson, 1995).*

In Example 5.1, women who had already developed breast cancer (and had surgery) were randomized to standard treatment accompanied by a low-fat dietary regimen ('intervention group') or standard treatment alone ('control group') to assess whether a low-fat diet reduces recurrence of the tumour and increases survival.

Example 5.2. *The Women's Health Initiative is a randomized trial taking place in the USA to determine whether a sustained low-fat diet will reduce the incidence of breast cancer. A total of 48 000 postmenopausal women with no prior history of breast or colon cancer are being randomized to the intervention or control group. The dietary intervention is designed to reduce fat intake to 20% of total kilocalories and to increase intake of fruits and vegetables. The trial will last 11 years (Chlebowski & Grosvenor, 1994; Henderson, 1995).*

In contrast to clinical trials, *field trials* deal with subjects who are disease-free and, therefore they generally have to be conducted in the 'field' rather than in hospitals or clinics. Their main objective is to evaluate whether an agent or procedure reduces the risk of developing disease among those free from the condition at enrolment.

In Example 5.2, women are being randomized to receive ('intervention group') or not receive ('control group') the dietary intervention programme.

Whereas complications from breast cancer are quite common among women who already suffer from the disease, the risk of healthy women developing breast cancer is very small, even in high-risk populations. As a result, the field trial in Example 5.2 involves a much larger number of subjects followed for a much longer period than the clinical trial in Example 5.1

> **Example 5.3.** *The Gambia Hepatitis Intervention Study is a large-scale hepatitis B vaccination project initiated in The Gambia in July 1986. In this trial, 60 000 infants received a course of hepatitis B vaccine and a similar number did not. A national surveillance system will detect all new cases of hepatocellular carcinoma (and other chronic liver diseases) over a period of 30 to 40 years (Gambia Hepatitis Study Group, 1987).*

In Example 5.3, half the infants participating in the trial received a course of hepatitis B vaccine ('intervention group') and the other half did not ('control group'). This study has a remarkably long follow-up period (it will not be able to answer the main research question before the year 2020!). This is because the intervention had to be given to infants before they were infected with hepatitis B, whereas most cases of hepatocellular carcinoma are expected in adulthood.

These last two examples clearly illustrate the complexities involved in the design and implementation of field trials when cancer is the outcome of interest. Because cancer is a relatively rare condition, they require the enrolment of large numbers of subjects who have to be followed up for relatively long periods of time. One advantage of such trials is that it is possible to assess the impact of the intervention on several outcomes. For instance, the effect of a low-fat diet on the incidence of colon cancer (Example 5.2) and of hepatitis B vaccination on the incidence of other chronic liver diseases (Example 5.3) are also being assessed in the trials described.

In field trials, the unit of allocation to the intervention may be the *individual* (as in Example 5.2) or, alternatively, a *group* of people. The group may be a household, a school or a whole community. If the unit of allocation is a community (as in Example 5.4) the study is called a community trial.

Intervention trials are very powerful for testing hypotheses. Despite this, they are not the most commonly used study design in epidemiology, mainly because of ethical constraints.

Example 5.4. *The Community Intervention Trial for Smoking Cessation is an on-going trial designed to evaluate a community-wide smoking cessation programme in the USA. Eleven pairs of communities were selected and one member of each pair was randomly assigned to receive a smoking cessation programme, while the other acted as a control. The intervention was designed to promote smoking cessation by using a wide range of community resources to affect community attitudes and policies towards smoking (COMMIT Research Group, 1991).*

5.1.2 Cohort studies

Cohort studies are observational studies in which the starting point is the selection of a study population, or cohort. Information is obtained to determine which members of this cohort are exposed to the factor of interest. The entire population is then followed up over time and the incidence of the disease in the exposed individuals is compared with the incidence in those not exposed (Figure 5.3). This type of observational study is the one that most closely resembles intervention studies, except that allocation of subjects to the exposure is *not* controlled by the investigator.

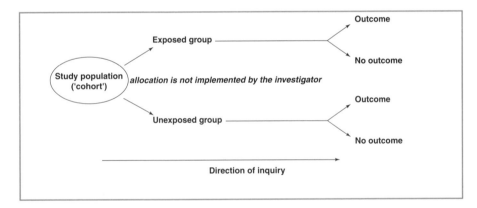

Figure 5.3.
Outline of a cohort study.

Example 5.5. *In 1980, 89 538 registered nurses in the USA, aged 34 to 59 years and with no past history of cancer, completed a previously validated dietary questionnaire designed to measure individual consumption of total fat, saturated fat, linoleic acid and cholesterol, as well as other nutrients. The nurses were then classified in five groups of similar size according to their levels of fat intake, followed up in time and the incidence of breast cancer in each of these groups measured and compared (Willett et al., 1987).*

Cohort studies take individuals and classify them according to their exposure status. Sometimes they can be simply classified as exposed/unexposed. More usually, various degrees of exposure can be identified. In Example 5.5, the US nurses (the 'cohort') were classified into five groups (quintiles) according to their levels of fat intake. The incidence of breast cancer ('outcome') was then measured and compared across these quintiles.

> ***Example 5.6.*** *A cohort study of Chinese male government employees in Taiwan was set up to investigate the association between hepatitis B virus infection and the development of primary hepatocellular carcinoma. All participants completed a health questionnaire and provided a blood sample at their entry into the study. A total of 22 707 men were enrolled into the study: 3454 were positive for hepatitis B surface antigen (HBsAg) and 19 253 were negative. These men were then followed up and the incidence of hepatocellular carcinoma among HBsAg carriers was compared with the incidence among non-carriers (Beasley et al., 1981).*

In Example 5.6, the cohort consisted of Chinese male government employees in Taiwan. Subjects were classified as HBsAg carriers ('exposed') or non-carriers ('unexposed') at the time of their enrolment into the study and were followed up to assess whether the risk of hepatocellular carcinoma ('outcome') was higher in those exposed than in those unexposed.

In cohort studies, it is important that the groups being compared are as similar as possible with respect to all other factors that may be related to the disease. Since the investigator has no control over who is or is not exposed, it is likely that the exposure groups will differ in relation to factors other than the one being investigated, so that special techniques have to be used in the analysis to ensure that these uneven distributions are taken into account (see Chapters 8, 13 and 14).

5.1.3. Case–control studies

Case–control studies are observational studies in which the starting point is the identification of 'cases' of the disease (or condition) of interest, and of suitable 'controls' without that disease (or condition). Cases and controls are then compared to assess whether there were any differences in their past exposure to putative risk factors (Figure 5.4).

Figure 5.4.
Outline of a case–control study.

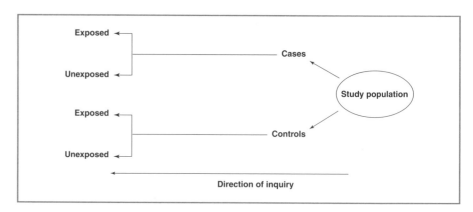

Example 5.7. *A case–control study was conducted in Singapore to investigate the role of diet in breast cancer. Two hundred Chinese women with histologically confirmed breast cancer and 420 controls without this disease participated in the study. A dietary questionnaire was used to measure past dietary intake. Cases and controls were then compared to assess whether there were any differences in their past intake of selected foods and nutrients (Lee et al., 1991).*

In Example 5.7, women with ('cases') and without ('controls') breast cancer were identified and their past diet ('exposure') compared.

Example 5.8. *A case–control study was carried out in Taiwan to assess whether hepatitis B infection played a role in the etiology of primary hepatocellular carcinoma. A total of 128 histologically or cytologically confirmed cases of hepatocellular carcinoma and 384 controls without the disease were included in the study. Of the cases, 77% were carriers of the hepatitis B surface antigen (HbsAg) compared with only 28% of the controls (Chuang et al., 1992).*

In Example 5.8, subjects with ('cases') and without ('controls') hepatocellular carcinoma were identified and the frequencies of the HBsAg carrier status ('exposure') in the two groups were compared.

The major difference between cohort and case–control methods is in the selection of study subjects. In a cohort study, subjects are selected who are initially free of disease and are then followed over time. In contrast, in the case–control approach, subjects are selected on the basis of the presence or absence of the disease (or any other outcome) under study.

Case–control studies are particularly suitable for investigating rare diseases such as cancer. A cohort study would require the follow-up of a large number of individuals for a long period of time in order to accrue enough cases of a rare disease. Case–control methods are also more appropriate for studying diseases with a long induction period. This is because the case–control study starts with subjects who have already developed the condition of interest, so there is no need to wait for time to elapse between an exposure and the manifestation of disease as in cohort studies.

The number of subjects necessary for a case–control study is much smaller than the number required for cohort studies. Examples 5.5 and 5.6 involved large numbers of subjects followed up for relatively long periods of time. The same questions were addressed in Examples 5.7 and 5.8 using much smaller numbers of subjects. Thus, case–control studies are relatively inexpensive to carry out, at least compared with cohort studies.

Results from case–control studies are, however, more difficult to interpret. First, controls should represent the same study population from which the cases were drawn. If not, the results will be distorted by *selection bias* (see Chapter 9). Secondly, one cannot be sure that the exposure did precede the disease (except when the exposure is a fixed attribute such as blood type that does not change over time). In Example 5.7, it is conceivable that the reported diet may be a *consequence* rather than a *cause* of breast cancer.

5.1.4 Cross-sectional surveys

In a cross-sectional survey, a sample of individuals is selected from a previously defined population and contacted at a particular point in time to obtain simultaneously information on both the exposure(s) and outcome(s) of interest.

> **Example 5.9.** *To assess whether there is an association between* Helicobacter pylori *infection and chronic atrophic gastritis, a relatively common condition and an established precursor of gastric cancer, a cross-sectional survey was performed among 1815 randomly selected healthy blood donors in four prefectures of Japan. Blood samples were taken from all study subjects and measurements made of serum* H. pylori *IgG antibodies and serum pepsinogen I and II (markers of chronic atrophic gastritis). The prevalence of antibodies against the bacterium among subjects with chronic atrophic gastritis was then compared with the prevalence among individuals without chronic atrophic gastritis (Fukao et al., 1993).*

In Example 5.9, a sample of 1815 study subjects was selected from a well defined population (healthy blood donors in certain prefectures of Japan) and a blood sample taken from each of them at a particular point in time to measure both the levels of *H. pylori* antibodies ('exposure') and the levels of pepsinogen I and II ('outcome').

In this type of study, it is crucial to ensure that the sample of subjects who participate in the study is representative of the whole population to whom the results will be extrapolated. Otherwise, the results will be distorted by *selection bias*. The best way to safeguard against selection bias is to use *random sampling* methods. These methods ensure that chance alone determines who will and who will not be included in the sample (see Chapter 10).

Cross-sectional surveys are generally used to estimate the prevalence of common conditions of reasonably long duration. Thus this design is not appropriate for studying diseases such as cancer, since it would be necessary to survey a very large population to identify enough cases to be able to draw any conclusions. Moreover, prevalent cancer cases are a biased sample of all cases, in which those with long survival tend to be over-represented.

The main use of cross-sectional surveys in cancer epidemiology has been to examine the distribution and determinants of common conditions, such as human papillomavirus infection or skin naevi, which are known (or suspected) to be associated with cancer. This type of study has also been used to investigate the distribution and determinants of known (or potential) high-risk behaviours, such as being a smoker or being a regular sunbed user.

These studies are relatively simple to conduct and take only a short time because they do not require follow-up of the study subjects. Their main disadvantage is that, as with case–control studies, it is not possible to know whether the outcome followed the exposure in time or the exposure resulted from the outcome, since information on both exposure and outcome is collected at the same single point in time. In Example 5.9, it is not possible to establish whether *H. pylori* infection preceded or followed chronic atrophic gastritis. This is obviously not a problem for exposures that do not change over time such as gender, ethnicity or genetically determined traits. For exposures that are likely to change over time, cross-sectional surveys may include questions about past as well as current exposures. For example, in a health survey of workers in a particular industry, workers may be asked details about their current job and any other jobs they have had in the past.

5.1.5. Routine-data-based studies

The distinguishing feature of this type of study is that the data on the exposure(s) and outcome(s) of interest are obtained from routine data-collection systems, without the researcher contacting any of the study subjects. Routine-data-based studies can be carried out at an *individual* or at an *aggregated* level.

Individual level

Many routine data-collection systems collect data on personal attributes such as age, sex, place of birth, place of residence, occupation, etc. Cancer occurrence can then be examined in relation to these variables. The objective is to search for patterns that might suggest or confirm specific etiological hypotheses.

In Example 5.10, data on place of birth, place of residence and age at migration ('exposures') and on breast cancer ('outcome') were available from population censuses, social security records and cancer registries for each of the study individuals.

The key feature of this type of study is that data on both the exposure and the outcome(s) of interest are obtained for each of the study subjects from routine data-collection systems. In terms of their analysis and interpretation, they can be regarded as being similar to cohort or case–control studies. For instance, Example 5.10 can be regarded as a cohort of women who were classified into four different exposure categories according to their place of birth, residence and age at migration. These women were then followed up in time and the occurrence of breast cancer in each group was measured and compared.

The main advantage of routine-data-based studies in relation to other observational studies is that they can be carried out relatively quickly and cheaply because the data have already been collected and there is no need to contact the individuals. A major limitation, however, is that few vari-

Example 5.10. The risk of female breast cancer was studied in four population groups: (1) Japanese women born and resident in Japan (homeland); (2) Japanese women who migrated later in life to the USA; (3) Japanese women who migrated early in life to the USA; and (4) women born in the USA. The main results are shown in Figure 5.5. They suggest that environmental factors (e.g. diet) in early life may be important in the development of breast cancer (Shimizu et al., 1991).

Figure 5.5.
Age-adjusted incidence rates of female breast cancer for USA residents (1972–85) by birthplace and age at migration, and for Japan (1973–81) (reproduced, by permission of Churchill Livingston, from Shimizu *et al.*, 1991).

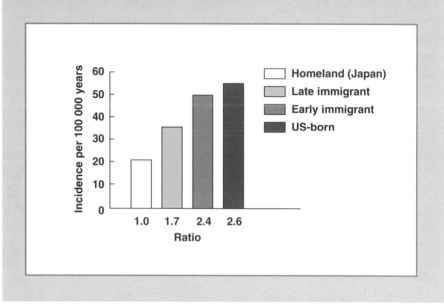

ables are usually available and they have not been collected with the specific needs of the study in mind. In Example 5.10, the variables 'country of birth' and 'country of residence' are only proxy measures for more biologically relevant exposures, such as reproductive factors, diet and other lifestyle characteristics, for which no data were available in the routine data-sets.

Aggregated level (ecological studies)

Studies which involve investigating the frequency of disease (or any other outcome of interest) in relation to the level of exposure in several groups of people (or in the same group over different periods of time) are called ecological studies. In this type of study, it is not possible to link the exposure of a particular individual to his or her outcome. Thus, the *group* rather than the individual is the unit of observation and analysis. The groups may be defined in a large number of ways, such as according to place of residence, place of birth, socioeconomic status, occupation, etc.

Most ecological studies in cancer epidemiology make use of routinely collected data. Data on the average (or frequency of) exposure in different population groups may be available from government or private sources that routinely collect data on demographic, environmental and lifestyle variables. Disease rates may be available from surveillance programmes, cancer registries or death certification systems.

In Example 5.11, it is not possible to link the breast cancer experience of any individual woman with her diet because the only two pieces of information available for each of the countries were their breast cancer incidence rate and an estimate of their average *per caput* consumption of fat.

Example 5.11. *Breast cancer incidence data and average* per caput *daily consumption of a wide range of foods for 24 countries were extracted from routinely collected data sources (Armstrong & Mann, 1985). The relationship between fat consumption and breast cancer is illustrated in Figure 5.6.*

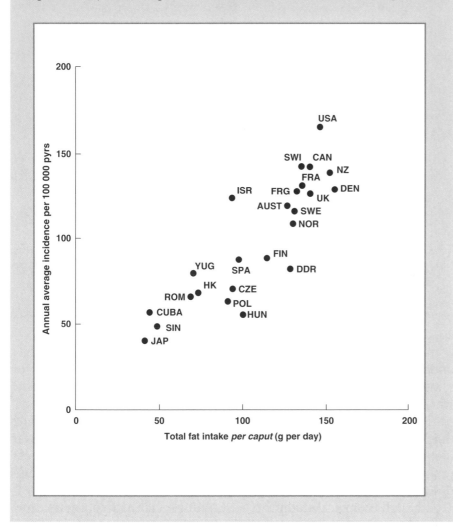

Figure 5.6.
Estimated daily consumption of fat *per caput* in 1964-66 and age-adjusted breast cancer incidence rates in women aged 35-64 years in 1972-77 in 24 countries (reproduced, by permission of Oxford Univesity Press, from Armstrong & Mann, 1985).

Sometimes data on the exposure(s) or outcome(s) of interest may not be available from routine data-collection systems but may be obtained from previously conducted surveys (as in Example 5.12).

Figure 5.7.
Prevalence of *H. pylori* IgG antibodies and gastric cancer mortality in 46 rural Chinese counties; each county is represented by a dot in the graph (reproduced by permission of Wiley-Liss, Inc., a subsidiary of John Wiley & Sons, Inc., from Forman *et al.*, 1990).

Example 5.12. A study was carried out to examine the association between prevalence of Helicobacter pylori *infection and mortality from gastric cancer in 46 rural counties of the People's Republic of China. The results are plotted in Figure 5.7 (Forman* et al., *1990).*

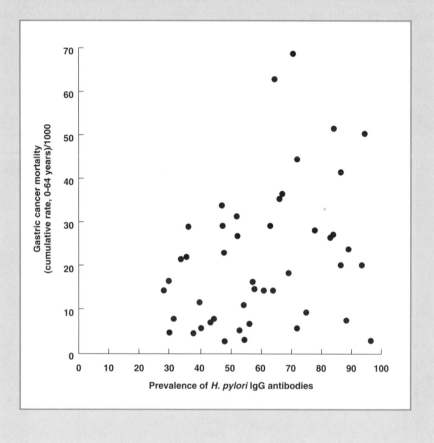

In Example 5.12, information on the average prevalence of *H. pylori* IgG antibodies ('exposure') and on gastric cancer mortality ('outcome') for samples of individuals in each of 46 rural counties (the groups of interest) was obtained from surveys previously conducted in China.

The main advantage of ecological studies is that they can be done quickly and inexpensively. For instance, the question 'does a high-fat diet increase the risk of breast cancer' can be addressed in a much quicker and cheaper way in an ecological study than using any other study design (Examples 5.2, 5.5 and 5.7).

Although ecological studies are useful for generating hypotheses, they are of limited value in assessing whether there is a true exposure–outcome relationship at an individual level, since their results refer to *groups* of people and cannot be extrapolated to individuals. Attempts to infer associations at the individual level from those observed at the group level are subject to the *'ecological fallacy'* (see Section 11.2). For instance, in Example 5.11, we do not know whether the women who developed breast cancer in each country were those who actually consumed a high-fat diet.

Despite these limitations, ecological studies may be the best approach to study exposures that are easier to measure at a group rather than at an individual level, such as air pollution and water quality. They are also useful for monitoring the effectiveness of population interventions such as health education campaigns and mass screening programmes (see Chapter 16).

5.2   Measures of exposure effect

The basic aim of an epidemiological study is to quantify the association between the exposure and the outcome of interest. To achieve this, the incidence of disease in a group of individuals exposed to the putative risk factor must be compared with the incidence in a group of persons not exposed. This comparison can be summarized by calculating either the ratio of the measures of disease occurrence for the two groups, which indicates the likelihood of developing the disease in the exposed individuals *relative* to those unexposed, or the difference between the two, which provides information about the *absolute* effect of the exposure in those exposed compared with those unexposed.

5.2.1   Relative measures of exposure effect

These measures estimate the magnitude of the association between exposure and disease, indicating how much more likely the exposed group is to develop the disease than the unexposed group. Three types of relative measure can be calculated:

$$\text{Risk ratio} \ = \ \frac{\text{Risk in the exposed group}}{\text{Risk in the unexposed group}}$$

$$\text{Rate ratio} \ = \ \frac{\text{Incidence rate in the exposed group}}{\text{Incidence rate in the unexposed group}}$$

$$\text{Odds ratio (of disease)} = \frac{\text{Odds of disease in the exposed group}}{\text{Odds of disease in the unexposed group}}$$

These measures are often collectively called measures of *relative risk*.

The *relative risk* is used as a measure of *etiological strength*. A value of 1.0 indicates that the incidence of disease in the exposed and unexposed

Table 5.1.
Hypothetical data from a cohort of 20 000 individuals followed up for a period of two years.

Example 5.13. *Suppose that 20 000 workers were recruited into a cohort study. At the time of their entry into the study, individuals were classified as exposed or unexposed to a particular chemical substance on the basis of the type of job they had at that time. The whole cohort was then followed up for a period of two years to establish whether those exposed had an increased risk of dying from cancer. The results are presented in Table 5.1.*

	Exposure	
	Yes	No
No. initially at risk	4000	16 000
Deaths	30	60
Person-years at risk[a]	7970	31 940

Risk ratio $= \dfrac{30/4000}{60/16\,000} = \dfrac{7.5 \text{ per } 1000}{3.75 \text{ per } 1000} = 2.0000$

Rate ratio $= \dfrac{30/7970 \text{ pyrs}}{60/31\,940 \text{ pyrs}} = \dfrac{3.76 \text{ per } 1000 \text{ pyrs}}{1.88 \text{ per } 1000 \text{ pyrs}} = 2.0038$

Disease odds ratio $= \dfrac{30/(4000-30)}{60/(16\,000-60)} = \dfrac{0.00756}{0.00376} = 2.0076$

[a] Assuming that on average all deaths occurred in the middle of the follow-up period.

groups is identical and thus that there is no observed association between the exposure and the disease. A value greater than 1.0 indicates a positive association, or an increased risk among those exposed. Similarly, a relative risk less than 1.0 means that there is an observed inverse association or a decreased risk among those exposed. In Example 5.13, workers exposed to the particular occupational hazard were twice as likely to die from cancer as those who were not exposed.

Note that in the above example the three measures of effect give similar estimates of relative risk. Death from cancer is a rare occurrence and therefore the number at risk remains practically constant throughout the study, since the cases represent a negligible fraction of the population. In practice, the three measures of effect will yield similar estimates of relative risk only for rare conditions (e.g., cancer). The estimates obtained by these three measures may differ considerably when a common disease (e.g., most infectious diseases) is examined or when a moderately rare disease is studied over a long period of time (e.g., coronary heart disease in women followed over 20 years).

5.2.2 Absolute measures of exposure effect

Information on the relative risk alone does not provide the full picture of the association between exposure and disease. Table 5.2 shows relative risks, calculated as rate ratios, of diseases A and B among those exposed to a certain risk factor. Although the rate ratio is higher for disease A, the incidence rate for disease A is increased by only 15 cases per 100 000 person-years at risk, whereas the incidence rate for disease B is increased by 40 cases per 100 000 person-years at risk. Clearly, the absolute impact of the exposure, measured by the rate difference, is quite different for these two diseases.

The *excess risk* (also called *attributable risk*) is an absolute measure of exposure effect. It indicates how many extra cases the exposure is respon-

	Disease A	Disease B
Incidence rate in the exposed group[a]	20	80
Incidence rate in the unexposed group[a]	5	40
Rate ratio	4.0	2.0
Rate difference[a]	15	40
[a] Rates per 100 000 pyrs.		

Table 5.2.
Incidence of disease A and B among persons exposed and persons unexposed to a particular risk factor, rate ratios and rate differences: hypothetical data.

sible for, *assuming that the relationship between exposure and disease is causal*. It can be calculated either as the difference of risk (*risk difference*) or of rates (*rate difference*).

Excess risk is equal to:

Risk difference = risk in the exposed – risk in the unexposed

or

Rate difference = rate in the exposed – rate in the unexposed

The excess risk is especially useful in evaluating the impact of introduction or removal of a risk factor and its value can be translated into the number of cases of the disease among the exposed that could be prevented if the exposure were completely eliminated. In the above example, the importance of the exposure as an etiological factor was given by the rate ratio and it was greater for disease A than for disease B, but, from a public health viewpoint, the exposure is much more important for disease B because more cases of disease B than of disease A would be avoided if the exposure were removed (assuming that the public health costs of a case of disease A are similar to those of disease B). Thus, relative risk measures the *strength* of the association between the exposure and the outcome of interest, whereas the excess risk measures the *impact* of the association in public health terms. In contrast to the relative risk, however, the magnitude of the excess risk cannot be generalized to other populations because it depends on the baseline incidence in the unexposed group, which tends to vary between populations.

It is useful to express the excess risk in relation to the risk (or rate) in the exposed group. This measure is called the *excess fraction* (also known as the *excess risk percentage* or *attributable risk percentage*) and can be calculated as

Excess fraction (%) = 100 × (excess risk/risk (or rate) in the exposed)

In the above example, the excess fraction for diseases A and B would be

Excess fraction (%) for disease A = 100 × (15 per 100 000 pyrs/20 per 100 000 pyrs) = 75%

Excess fraction (%) for disease B = 100 × (40 per 100 000 pyrs/80 per 100 000 pyrs) = 50%

This excess fraction represents the proportion of cases among the exposed that can be attributed to the exposure (assuming causality). In other words, it represents the proportion of cases among the exposed that could have been prevented if they had never been exposed. Thus, 75% of the cases of disease A and 50% of the cases of disease B could have been prevented among the exposed if they had never been exposed.

Example 5.14. *A total of 34 439 British male doctors were followed up for 40 years and their mortality in relation to smoking habits was assessed (Doll et al., 1994a). Mortality from certain diseases is shown in Table 5.3.*

Table 5.3.
Mortality by smoking habits from selected causes among male British doctors.[a]

Underlying cause of death	Never smoked regularly Rate[b] (1)	Current cigarette smoker Rate[b] (2)	Rate ratio (2)/(1)	Rate difference[b] (2)–(1)	Excess fraction (%) (2)–(1)/(2) × 100
Cancer					
All sites	305	656	2.2	351	54
Lung	14	209	14.9	195	93
Oesophagus	4	30	7.5	26	87
Bladder	13	30	2.3	17	57
Respiratory diseases (except cancer)	107	313	2.9	206	66
Vascular diseases	1037	1643	1.6	606	37
All causes	1706	3038	1.8	1332	44

[a] Data from Doll et al., 1994a.
[b] Age-adjusted rates per 100 000 pyrs.

Example 5.14 shows that 44% of the deaths that occurred among male British doctors who smoked could be attributed to smoking (assuming causality). The proportion of deaths that could be attributed to smoking varied by disease. For those diseases shown in Table 5.3, this proportion was highest for lung cancer (93%) and lowest for vascular diseases (37%). However, if smokers had never smoked, the total number of deaths prevented would have been much greater for vascular diseases (606 per 100 000 pyrs) than for lung cancer (195 per 100 000 pyrs).

Similar absolute measures of effect can be calculated when those exposed have a lower risk of developing the disease than those unexposed. In these circumstances, we would have

Risk reduction = risk (or rate) in the unexposed – risk (or rate) in the exposed

Prevented fraction (%) = 100 × (risk reduction/risk (or rate) in the unexposed)

Example 5.15. *Suppose that a group of oral contraceptive users and a group of never users were followed up in time and their ovarian cancer incidence was measured and compared. The results from this hypothetical study are shown in Table 5.4.*

	Oral contraceptive use	
	Ever	Never
Ovarian cancer cases	29	45
Person-years at risk	345 000	321 429
Rate per 100 000 pyrs	8.4	14.0

Rate ratio = 8.4 per 100 000 pyrs/14.0 per 100 000 pyrs = 0.60
Risk reduction = 14.0 per 100 000 pyrs – 8.4 per 100 000 pyrs = 5.6 per 100 000 pyrs.
Prevented fraction (%) = 100 × (5.6 per 100 000 pyrs / 14.0 per 100 000 pyrs) = 40%.

Table 5.4.
Distribution of ovarian cancer cases and person-years at risk by oral contraceptive use: hypothetical data.

In Example 5.15, 40% of ovarian cancer cases could have been prevented among never-users if they had used oral contraceptives.

5.3 Conclusions

Before implementing a study, careful consideration must be given to the appropriateness of the proposed study design, especially in terms of practical feasibility, information to be obtained, expected duration of the study and total costs. The advantages and disadvantages of each of these study designs are covered in more detail in subsequent chapters (7–11).

Further reading

* References to books and papers dealing with each study design are given in the relevant chapters.

All the measures of effect discussed in this chapter can be directly calculated from intervention and cohort studies, since the incidence of disease in those exposed and in those unexposed is known. This is not the case in other study designs, where these measures of effect can be estimated only indirectly. For instance, in case–control studies, the subjects are selected on the basis of their disease status (sample of subjects with ('cases') and without ('controls') a particular disease), not on the basis of their exposure status. Therefore, it is not possible to calculate the incidence in exposed and unexposed individuals. It is, however, possible to calculate the odds of exposure among cases and the odds of exposure among controls and obtain an odds ratio of exposure (see Chapter 9). It can be shown that, depending on the sampling scheme used to select controls, this measure provides an unbiased estimate of one of the three relative measures of effect considered in Section 5.2.1. This is discussed in detail in later chapters (9-11, 16).

Box 5.1. Key issues

- There are two main types of epidemiological study: intervention (experimental) and observational.

- In *intervention studies*, the allocation of the study subjects to the different study groups is implemented by the investigator. Thus, if conducted properly, the intervention and the control groups would be similar in all respects apart from the exposure under study. There are two types of intervention study:

  Clinical trials, where the main aim is to assess the value of new forms of treatment.

  Field trials, where the objective is to evaluate whether an intervention decreases the risk of disease among disease-free people. Field trials can be conducted at an individual level, if the unit of allocation is the individual, or at an aggregated level, if the unit is a group of people. Community trials are an example of trials carried out at an aggregated level, where whole communities are the unit of allocation.

- In *observational studies*, the researchers limit themselves to observing the occurrence of disease in people who are already segregated into different exposure groups. There are various types of observational study:

  Cohort studies, in which a study population (or 'cohort') is selected and the exposure status of its members assessed. The cohort is followed up in time and the occurrence of disease in the different exposure groups is measured and compared.

  Case—control studies, in which a group of patients with a particular disease or condition ('cases') and a suitable group of subjects without that disease or condition ('controls') are selected and their past exposure to putative risk factors is ascertained and compared

Box 5.1. Key issues (Contd)

Cross-sectional surveys, in which a sample of subjects from a defined population is selected and information on the exposure(s) and outcome(s) of interest is collected simultaneously at a single point in time.

Routine-data-based studies, in which the data are derived from routine data-collection systems (e.g., cancer registration or death certification). They may be carried out at an individual level if information on the exposure(s) and outcome(s) of interest is available for each of the study subjects or at an aggregated level (ecological studies) if the group rather than the individual is the unit of study.

• Once the data from a particular study have been collected, the association between the exposure and the outcome of interest can be quantified by calculating an appropriate *measure of effect*. This may be expressed as either the ratio of the measure of disease occurrence in the exposed relative to that in the unexposed (*relative* measure) or as the difference between the two (*absolute* measure). The first type of measure is particularly important when assessing etiology, whereas the second type is more useful for evaluations of the public health impact of the association.

• Each study design has its own limitations and strengths. These are considered in detail in subsequent chapters of this book (Chapters 7–13).

Chapter 6
Evaluating the role of chance

6.1 Populations and samples

Suppose that as part of a general health cross-sectional survey, we wish to determine the proportion of men in a particular town who currently smoke cigarettes. For practical and financial reasons, it is impossible to interview every single man in this town, so we decide to select a random sample of 30 men. In this sample, the proportion of current smokers is 7/30 = 23%.

Usually it is impossible to examine every single individual of a population of interest, and we are limited to examining a sample (or subset) of individuals drawn from this population in the hope that it is representative of the whole population[a].

If we do not have information about the whole population, we cannot know the true proportion of the population. However, the proportion computed from a random sample can be used as an estimate of the proportion in the entire population from which the sample was drawn. In the above example, the sample proportion (23%) is our best guess of the true but unknown proportion of current smokers in the whole town.

6.1.1 How reliable is our sample proportion?

There is nothing special about the particular random sample we have used, and different random samples will yield slightly different estimates of the true population proportion. This implies that our sample estimate is subject to *sampling error*. The proportion of current smokers in the whole town is unlikely to be exactly the 23% found in our sample, due to sampling error. The question is, how far from 23% is it likely to be?

To try to answer this question, we first recognize that the sample we picked was only one of a very large number of possible samples of 30 individuals. Suppose we were able to look at 100 000 samples. For each sample, we interview 30 individuals and calculate the sample proportion of current smokers p. The value of p will vary from sample to sample. If we plot all values of p, we would see a distribution like the one shown in Figure 6.1.

This distribution is called the sampling distribution of p. It shows that although most sample estimates are likely to be concentrated around the true (population) proportion π, some will be a long way from this true value. The amount of spread tells us how precise our sample proportion p is likely to be, as an estimate of the true proportion π. If the distribution is wide, there is a lot of sampling error and our p may be a long way from

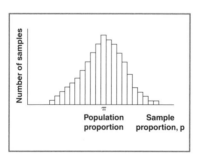

Figure 6.1.
Sampling distribution of p for 100 000 repeated samples of size 30.

[a] To ensure representativeness, the sample of individuals should be *randomly selected* from the population of interest. That is, every individual in the population should have an equal chance of being included in the sample. The different ways in which a random sample can be drawn from a specific population are dealt with in Chapter 10.

the true value π. If it is narrow, there is little sampling error, and our p is likely to be very close to π.

We have already seen in Section 3.3.1 that the spread of a distribution can be measured by a quantity called the standard deviation. It can be shown that the standard deviation of a sampling distribution of p is given by

$$\text{SE}(p) = \sqrt{\frac{\pi(1-\pi)}{n}}$$

where n represents the size of the sample. SE stands for *standard error*, which is the term we generally use for the standard deviation of a sampling distribution. The standard error is a measure of the precision with which our sample value p estimates the true value π. Notice that if we increase the sample size, n, we decrease the standard error and the sampling distribution will become narrower. This is just what we would expect, as larger samples should provide more reliable estimates of π.

When we actually do our survey, of course, we do not know the value of π (otherwise we would not need to do the survey!), and so we cannot actually use the above formula to calculate the $\text{SE}(p)$. We can make a close estimation of it by replacing π in the formula with our sample estimate p, giving

$$\text{SE}(p) = \sqrt{\frac{p(1-p)}{n}}$$

which can be rearranged as

$$\text{SE}(p) = \sqrt{\frac{p^2(1-p)}{a}}$$

where a is the numerator of the proportion $p = a/n$ (in our sample $a = 7$, the observed number of current smokers). This last formula is particularly useful because it shows that the standard error is inversely related to the observed number of cases. It is the number of cases in the numerator of p that mainly determines the magnitude of the standard error, and not the sample size in itself.

It is possible to show mathematically that, in sufficiently large samples, approximately 95% of all the sample estimates will fall within 1.96 standard errors of the true value π; 2.5% of the sample estimates (one sample in 40) will be more than 1.96 SEs below the true value, and 2.5% (one in 40) will be more than 1.96 SEs above the true value (Figure 6.2).

Now what can we say about π from our single sample of 30 individuals? Our sample may have come from any part of the distribution shown in Figure 6.2. However, before drawing the sample, there was a 95% chance that the observed sample proportion p would lie within two standard errors (more precisely $1.96 \times$ SE) of the true value π. As a logical consequence, intervals from samples of similar size but centred on each sample proportion p will include π if p is within two standard errors of π. Hence, an interval bounded by the following lower and upper limits

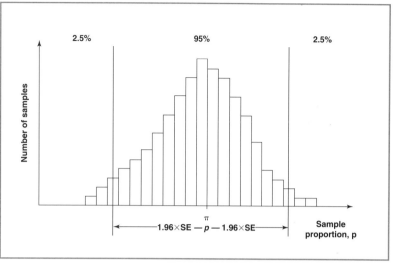

Figure 6.2.
Sampling distribution of p with 95% confidence limits.

$$p - 1.96 \times \text{SE} \quad \text{and} \quad p + 1.96 \times \text{SE}$$

(usually written $p \pm 1.96 \times \text{SE}(p)$) will include the true proportion π with probability 95%. These limits, calculated from the sample data, are called *lower* and *upper confidence limits*, respectively, and the interval between them is called a *95% confidence interval* of the unknown population proportion π.

In our example for estimating the proportion of men currently smoking,

$$n = 30, a = 7 \text{ and } p = 0.23$$

We estimate standard error of p to be

$$\text{SE}(p) = \sqrt{\frac{0.23^2(1-0.23)}{7}} = 0.076$$

A 95% confidence interval for the true proportion of men who currently smoke in the whole town is therefore given by

$$0.23 \pm 1.96 \times 0.076 = 0.081 \text{ to } 0.379$$

So our best estimate of the proportion of current smokers in the whole town is 23%, but the true value could easily be anywhere between 8% and 38%.

In strict terms, the confidence interval is a range of values that is likely to cover the true population value but we are still not certain that it will.

In reality, a confidence interval from a particular study may or may not include the actual population value. The confidence interval is based on the concept of repetition of the study under consideration. Thus if the study were to be repeated 100 times, we would expect 95 of the 100 resulting 95% confidence intervals to include the true population value.

If we want to be even more confident that our interval includes the true population value, we can calculate a *99% confidence interval*. This is done simply by replacing 1.96 with 2.58 in the above formula. That is, we use

$$p \pm 2.58 \times \sqrt{\frac{p^2(1-p)}{a}}$$

In our example, the corresponding 99% confidence interval for the proportion of current smokers in the whole town is 0.034 to 0.426, or roughly 3% to 43%.

Similarly, we can calculate a *90% confidence interval* by replacing 1.96 with 1.64 in the formula:

$$p \pm 1.64 \times \sqrt{\frac{p^2(1-p)}{a}}$$

In our example, the corresponding 90% confidence interval for the proportion of current smokers in the whole town is 0.105 to 0.355, or 11% to 36%.

6.1.2   How good are other sample estimates?

This useful way of describing sampling error is not limited to the sample proportion. We can obtain confidence intervals for any other sample estimates such as means, risks, rates, rate ratios, rate differences, etc. The underlying concept is similar to the one illustrated above for proportions. In all these cases, the confidence intervals provide an indication of how close our sample estimate is likely to be to the true population value.

Suppose that, as part of the same general health survey, we wished to determine the mean height of the men in the same town. We measured the 30 individuals from our sample and obtained a sample mean height of 165 cm. Again, the mean height of the male adult population in the whole town is unlikely to be exactly 165 cm. However, if a very large number of samples of 30 individuals were drawn from this population and for each one the mean height were calculated and plotted, a sampling distribution of the mean would be obtained. This sampling distribution will have a shape similar to that of the sampling distribution of a proportion (Figure 6.1), i.e., the distribution would be bell-shaped, with most sample estimates centred around the true population mean.

We can, therefore, obtain a 95% confidence interval in a similar way to that used for proportions:

Sample mean ± 1.96 × SE of the mean[b]

The *standard error of a mean* can be estimated by

SE (mean) = SD/√ n

where SD represents the standard deviation described in Section 3.3.1. Suppose that, in the above example, the standard deviation was found to be 7.1 cm. The standard error of the mean will be given by

SE (mean) = 7.1/√ 30 = 1.3 cm

A 95% confidence interval for this sample mean will be equal to

165 cm ± 1.96 × 1.3 cm = 162 cm to 168 cm

How do we interpret this confidence interval? If the study were done 100 times, of the 100 resulting 95% confidence intervals, we would expect 95 of them to include the true population value. Thus, the confidence interval from this particular sample of 30 men provides a range of values that is likely to include the true population mean, although we cannot be sure that it does.

As long as the sampling distribution of a particular estimate is approximately bell-shaped (i.e., it is what statisticians call a 'Normal distribution'), as it will always be if the sample size is sufficiently large, we can summarize the calculation of a 95% confidence interval as follows:

Sample estimate ± 1.96 × SE(sample estimate)

(To obtain a 90% or a 99% confidence interval, all we need to do is to replace 1.96 in the formula with, respectively, 1.64 or 2.58.)

In Example 6.1, men employed for 10 or more years were estimated to have an excess of 92 cancer deaths per 10 000 pyrs compared with those employed for less than 1 year, with a 95% confidence interval ranging from 61 to 122 deaths per 10 000 pyrs. This confidence interval was calculated using the above general formula as follows:

Rate difference ± 1.96 × SE(rate difference)

where the SE of the rate difference was about 15 deaths per 10 000 pyrs.

[b] The precise value to be used in this formula varies with the size of the sample and it is given in tables of the *t*-distribution. However, for large sample sizes (≥30) this factor is close to 1.96.

Example 6.1. In a cohort study of 15 326 men employed in a particular factory, their cancer mortality was assessed in relation to duration of their employment (Table 6.1).

Table 6.1.

Age-adjusted mortality rate ratios and rate differences of cancer (all sites combined) by duration of employment: hypothetical data.

Duration of employment (years)	No. of cases	Person -years	Rate[a]	Rate ratio (95% CI)[b]	Rate difference[a] (95% CI)[b]
<1[c]	44	40 056	11	1.0	0
1.0-1.9	67	21 165	32	2.9 (1.9–4.3)	21 (12–29)
2.0-4.9	19	3 105	61	5.6 (3.1–9.7)	50 (23–78)
5.0-9.9	48	5 067	95	8.6 (5.6–13.3)	84 (57–111)
≥10	43	4 192	103	9.3 (6.0–14.6)	92 (61–122)

[a] Rates per 10 000 person-years.

[b] CI = confidence interval.

[c] Baseline category.

The corresponding rate ratio was 9.3 with a 95% confidence interval ranging from 6.0 to 14.6. Thus, our best guess is that men employed for 10 or more years were nine times more likely to die from cancer than those employed for less than one year, but the true rate ratio might lie somewhere between 6.0 and 14.6 (and is unlikely to lie outside this range).

You might have noticed in this example that, whereas the confidence limits of a rate difference are equidistant from the sample estimate, this is not the case for the confidence limits of a rate ratio. This can be seen clearly in Figures 6.3 and 6.4(a). In contrast to the rate difference, the sampling distribution of a rate ratio is not symmetric, since the minimum possible value it can take is zero, whereas the maximum is infinity. To obtain a more symmetric distribution, a logarithmic transformation of the data was used. As a consequence of this transformation, the confidence limits are equidistant from the sample estimate of the rate ratio on the logarithmic scale (Figure 6.4(b)) but asymmetric when converted back to the original scale (Figure 6.4(a)) (see Appendix 6.1, at the end of this chapter, which provides formulae to calculate confidence intervals for difference and ratio measures).

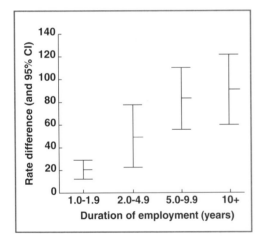

Figure 6.3.

Graphical display of rate differences (indicated by the middle horizontal lines) and their 95% confidence intervals (vertical lines) on an arithmetic scale (data from Table 6.1).

6.1.3 Display of confidence intervals

If we have two or more groups, we can display the sample estimates and their 95% confidence intervals in a graph. For instance, the rate ratios and rate differences from Table 6.1 and their respective confidence intervals are displayed in Figures 6.3 and 6.4.

The middle horizontal lines show the observed rate differences and rate ratios, while the vertical lines indicate the 95% confidence intervals. Note how the confidence interval is much narrower when the number of cases is large (e.g., category 1–1.9 years (based on 67 cases)). It is the number of cases in the numerator of rates and proportions which determines the size of the standard error and, therefore, the width of the confidence interval.

6.1.4 Further comments

Statistical inference is a process by which we draw conclusions about a population from the results observed in a sample. The above statistical methods assume that the sample of individuals studied has been randomly selected from the population of interest, which was properly defined beforehand. That is, every individual in the population has an equal chance of being in the selected sample. Quite often in epidemiology, getting a truly random sample is impossible and thus we have to be concerned about *selection bias* (see Chapter 13). Confidence intervals convey only the effects of sampling variation on the precision of the sample estimates and cannot control for non-sampling errors such as bias in the selection of the study subjects or in the measurement of the variables of interest. For instance, if the smoking survey only included men who visited their doctors because of respiratory problems, the sample would be unrepresentative of the whole male population in the community. The statistical techniques described above assume that no such bias is present.

The other issue that needs to be kept in mind in epidemiological studies is that even when whole populations are studied, questions of random variability still need to be addressed. Death rates may be computed from national vital statistics, or incidence rates determined from cancer registries that cover whole populations, but there will still be random variation in the number of cases from one year to another.

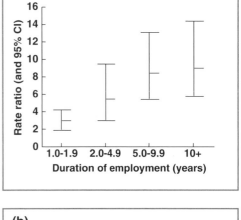

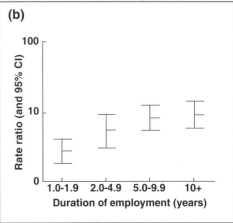

Figure 6.4.
Graphical display of rate ratios and their 95% confidence intervals: (*a*) on an arithmetic scale and (*b*) on a logarithmic scale (data from Table 6.1).

Example 6.2. Table 6.2 shows that there is considerable random fluctuation in the number of female lip cancer cases registered from year to year in England and Wales.

Table 6.2.
Number of incident cases of lip cancer by year of registration, females, England and Wales, 1979-89.[a]

Year of registration										
1979	1980	1981	1982	1983	1984	1985	1986	1987	1988	1989
58	57	60	46	57	64	53	47	51	58	62

[a] Data from OPCS (1983a to 1994b).

Even though the whole population of the country was studied to produce the data in Example 6.2, there was still random variability in the number of lip cancer cases from year to year, which cannot be explained in terms of changes in underlying risk. In these situations, we are sampling 'in time', that is the population in any particular year can be viewed as a 'sample'. The methods discussed above should still be used to assess the degree of precision of the observed rates. Of course, not all of the variation from year to year may be random and there may, for example, be an underlying trend, upwards or downwards, over a particular time period (see Section 4.3.2).

When the rates are based on small numbers of cases, so that the confidence intervals are very wide, it may be useful to reduce the random variation by pooling data over five or even ten adjacent calendar years and calculating the average annual incidence (or mortality) rates.

6.2 Testing statistical hypotheses

An investigator collecting data generally has two aims: (*a*) to draw conclusions about the true population value, on the basis of the information provided by the sample, and (*b*) to test hypotheses about the population value.

Example 6.3. In a clinical trial on metastatic cervical cancer, 218 patients were randomly assigned to a new treatment regimen or to the standard treatment. All patients were followed up for one year after their entry into the trial (or until death if it occurred earlier). The numbers of women still alive at the end of this follow-up period are shown in Table 6.3.

Table 6.3.
Number of patients still alive one year after entry into the trial by type of treatment administered: hypothetical data.

		Type of treatment	
		New	**Standard**
Alive at the end	**Yes**	68	45
of the first year	**No**	40	65
	Total	108	110

The data in Example 6.3 show that 63.0% (68 out of 108) patients administered the new treatment were still alive compared with 40.9% (45 out of 110) of those given the standard treatment. From these results the new treatment appears superior but how strong is the evidence that this is the case?

In general, when comparing the effects of two levels of an exposure or of two treatments, two groups are sampled, the 'exposed' and the 'unexposed', and their respective summary statistics are calculated. We might wish to compare the two samples and ask: 'Could they both come from the same population?' That is, does the fact that some subjects were exposed and others were not influence the outcome we are observing? If there is no strong evidence from the data that the exposure influences the outcome, we might assume that both samples came from the same population with respect to the particular outcome under consideration.

Statistical significance testing is a method for quantification of the chance of obtaining the observed results if there is no true difference between the groups being examined in the whole population.

6.2.1 The null hypothesis

An investigator usually has some general (or theoretical) hypothesis about the phenomenon of interest before embarking on a study. Thus, in Example 6.3, it is thought that the new treatment is likely to be better than the standard one in the management of metastatic cervical cancer patients. This hypothesis is known as the *study hypothesis*. However, it is impossible to prove most hypotheses conclusively. For instance, one might hold a theory that all Chinese children have black hair. Unfortunately, if one had observed one million Chinese children and found that they all had black hair, this would not have proved the hypothesis. On the other hand, if just one fair-haired Chinese child were seen, the theory would be disproved. Thus there is often a simpler logical setting for disproving hypotheses than for proving them. Obviously, the situation is much more complex in epidemiology. The observation that both the new and the standard treatments had similar effects in one single patient would not be enough to 'disprove' the study hypothesis that the two treatments were different in effect.

Consider again the cervical cancer clinical trial (Example 6.3). In addition to the study hypothesis that the new treatment is better than the standard one, we consider the *null hypothesis* that the two treatments are equally effective. If the null hypothesis were true, then for the population of all metastatic cervical cancer patients, the one-year survival experience would be similar for both groups of patients, regardless of the type of treatment they received. The formulation of such a null hypothesis, i.e., a statement that there is no true statistical association, is the first step in any statistical test of significance.

6.2.2 Significance test

After specifying the null hypothesis, the main question is:

If the null hypothesis were true, what are the chances of getting a difference at least as large as that observed?

For example, in the cervical cancer trial, what is the probability of getting a treatment difference at least as large as the observed 63.0% − 40.9% = 22.1%? This probability, commonly denoted by P (capital P rather than the small p we used earlier for the sample proportion), is determined by applying an appropriate statistical test.

A simple example

To understand the basis for a statistical significance test, let us look first at an example that uses numbers small enough to allow easy calculations. Suppose that an investigator has a theory that predicts there will be an excess of male births among babies resulting from *in-vitro* fertilization (IVF) and he therefore wants to study the question 'Are there more boys than girls among IVF babies?'

The investigator formulates a null hypothesis that there is an equal proportion (0.5 or 50%) of males and females in the population of IVF babies. Next, he samples five records from one IVF clinic and finds that they are all males in this sample of births. We can now calculate the probability of obtaining five males and no females if the null hypothesis of equal numbers of males and females were true.

Probability that the first sampled is a male	= 0.5	
Probability that the first and the second sampled are males	= 0.5 x 0.5	= 0.25
Probability that the first, second and third sampled are males	= 0.5 x 0.5 x 0.5	= 0.125
Probability that the first, second, third and fourth sampled are males	= 0.5 x 0.5 x 0.5 0.5	= 0.0625
Probability that all five sampled are males	= 0.5 x 0.5 x 0.5 x 0.5 x 0.5	= 0.03125

Thus, there is a 3.125% chance of obtaining five males in a row even if the true proportions of males and females born in the whole population were equal. We have just done a statistical significance test! It yields the probability (P) of producing a result as large as or larger than the observed one if no true difference actually existed between the proportion of males and females in the whole population of IVF babies.

What can we conclude from this probability? This P-value can be thought of as a measure of the consistency of the observed result with the null hypothesis. The smaller the P-value is, the stronger is the evidence provided by the data against the null hypothesis. In this example, the probability of obtaining five boys in a row if the null hypothesis were really true was fairly small. Hence, our data provide moderate evidence that the number of boys is greater than the number of girls among IVF babies.

However, in spite of this small probability, the null hypothesis may well be true. Our final interpretation and conclusions depend very much on our previous knowledge of the phenomenon we are examining. (The situation can be compared to tossing a coin. Even after getting five tails in a series of five tosses, most people would still believe in the null hypothesis of an unbiased coin. However, if the first 20 tosses were all tails the investigators would be very suspicious of bias, since the probability of this happening by chance is only $(0.5)^{20} = 0.00000095$.)

Comparing two proportions

In the cervical cancer treatment trial (Example 6.3), if the null hypothesis of no difference in survival between the two treatments is true, what is the probability of finding a sample difference as large as or larger than the observed 22.1% (= 63.0% – 40.9%)? If the null hypothesis were true, the only reason for the observed difference to be greater than zero is sampling error. In other words, even if the true population difference in proportions were zero, we would not expect our particular sample difference to be exactly zero because of sampling error. In these circumstances how far, on average, can we reasonably expect the observed difference in the two proportions to differ from zero?

We have already seen in this chapter that the standard error of a proportion gives an indication of how precisely the population value can be estimated from a sample. We can define the standard error of the difference between two proportions in a similar fashion. Theoretically, if we were to repeat the above cervical cancer trial over and over again, each time using the same number of patients in each group, we would obtain a sampling distribution of differences in proportions of a shape similar to that shown in Figure 6.1. The spread of this sampling distribution could be summarized by using a special formula to calculate the standard error. Its application to the cervical cancer trial data yields a standard error equal to 6.6%. The essence of the statistical test we apply to this situation is to calculate how many standard errors away from zero the observed difference in proportions lies. This is obtained as follows:

$$\text{Value of the test statistic} = \frac{\text{observed difference in proportions} - 0}{\text{standard error of difference}}$$

In the cervical cancer trial, the test statistic has a value of

$$\frac{0.221 - 0}{0.066} = 3.35$$

The observed difference between the two treatments (22.1%) is 3.35 standard errors from the null hypothesis value of zero. A value as high as this is very unlikely to arise by chance, since we already know that 95% of observations sampled from a bell-shaped distribution (i.e., a Normal distribution) will be within 1.96 standard errors of its centre.

The larger the test value, the smaller the probability P of obtaining the observed difference if the null hypothesis is true. We can refer to tables which convert particular statistical test values into corresponding values for P. An extract from one such table, based on the Normal (bell-shaped) distribution, is shown on the next page.

In the cervical cancer example, the value of the test statistic is 3.35, even larger than the highest value shown in the extract on the next page (3.291), and so the probability P is less than 0.001. That is, if the new and the standard treatments were really equally effective, the

test statistic exceeds in absolute value[a]	0.674	with probability	0.5	(50%)
"	1.282	"	0.2	(20%)
"	1.645	"	0.1	(10%)
"	1.960	"	0.05	(5%)
"	2.576	"	0.01	(1%)
"	3.291	"	0.001	(0.1%)

[a] Absolute value means that the plus or minus signs should be ignored; for example, −1 and +1 have the same absolute value of 1.

chances of getting so great a difference in survival would be less than one in a thousand. According to conventional use of statistical terminology, we would say that the difference in percentages is *statistically significant at the 0.1% level*. Hence, there is strong evidence that the new treatment is associated with a better one-year survival than is the standard treatment.

6.2.3 Interpretation of *P*-values

Cox & Snell (1981) give the following rough guidelines for interpreting *P*-values:

If $P > 0.1$, the results are reasonably consistent with the null hypothesis.

If $P \approx 0.05$, there is moderate evidence against the null hypothesis.

If $P \leq 0.01$, there is strong evidence against the null hypothesis.

It is common to consider $P<0.05$ as indicating that there is substantial evidence that the null hypothesis is untrue. (The null hypothesis is rejected and the results of the study are declared to be statistically significant at the 5% level.) However, *this emphasis on P<0.05 should be discouraged*, since 0.05 is an arbitrary cut-off value for deciding whether the results from a study are statistically significant or non-significant. It is much better to report the actual *P*-value rather than whether *P* falls below or above certain arbitrary limiting values.

When *P* is large, investigators often report a 'non-statistically significant' result and proceed as if they had proved that there was no effect. All they really did was fail to demonstrate that there was a statistically significant one. The distinction between demonstrating that there is no effect and failing to demonstrate that there is an effect is subtle but very important, since the magnitude of the *P*-value depends on both the extent of the observed effect and the number of observations made. Therefore, a small number of observations may lead to a large *P*-value despite the fact that the real effect is large. Conversely, with a large number of observations, small effects, so small as to be clinically and epidemiologically irrelevant, may achieve statistical significance. These issues are of great importance to clinical and epidemiological researchers and are considered in detail in later chapters (13 and 15).

6.2.4   Comparing other sample estimates

Although we have introduced significance testing for one particular problem (comparing two proportions), the same procedure can be applied to all types of comparative study. For instance, it can be used to compare other sample estimates (e.g., means, rates) or to assess more generally associations between variables.

Example 6.4. *In a case–control study to investigate the association between past history of infertility and the risk of developing benign ovarian tumours, the data shown in Table 6.4 were obtained.*

	Past history of infertility	
	Yes ('exposed')	**No ('unexposed')**
Women with benign ovarian tumours ('cases')	16	42
Healthy women ('controls')	9	120

$$\text{Odds ratio} = \frac{\text{odds of infertility among the cases}}{\text{odds of infertility among the controls}} = \frac{16/42}{9/120} = 5.08$$

(The calculation of odds ratios from case–control studies is discussed in detail in Chapter 9.)

Table 6.4.
Distribution of benign ovarian tumour cases and controls according to past history of infertility: hypothetical data.

In Example 6.4, the null hypothesis assumes that the two groups of women have a similar risk of getting benign ovarian tumours, i.e., the true odds ratio in the population is equal to one. After using an appropriate statistical test, as described in Appendix 6.1, the researchers obtained a P-value of 0.0003, i.e., if the null hypothesis were true, the probability of getting an odds ratio as large as, or larger than, 5.08 would be very small (less than 1 in 1000). Thus, the data from this study provide strong evidence against the null hypothesis.

6.3   Confidence intervals and hypothesis testing

Statistical significance testing is designed to help in deciding whether or not a set of observations is compatible with some hypothesis, but does not provide information on the size of the association (or difference of effects). It is more informative not only to think in terms of statistical significance testing, but also to estimate the size of the effect together with some measure of the uncertainty in that estimate.

This approach is not new; we used it in Section 6.1 when we introduced confidence intervals. We stated that a 95% confidence interval for a sample estimate could be calculated as

Sample estimate ± 1.96 × standard error of a sample estimate

A 95% confidence interval for the difference in two proportions can be calculated in a similar way:

Observed difference ± 1.96 × standard error of the difference

(The calculation of the standard error of a difference between proportions is illustrated in the Appendix, Section A6.1.2).

In the cervical cancer trial (Example 6.3), this 95% confidence interval is

$$0.221 \pm 1.96 \times 0.066 = 0.092 \text{ to } 0.350 = 9.2\% \text{ to } 35.0\%$$

Thus, it is plausible to consider that the real difference in one-year survival between the new treatment and the standard treatment lies somewhere between 9% and 35%.

This confidence interval is consistent with the result of the statistical test we performed earlier (Section 6.2.2). The value of the test for the null hypothesis of no difference between the two treatments was 3.35, which corresponded to $P < 0.001$.

Note that if the 95% confidence interval for a difference *does not include the null hypothesis value of zero*, then P is lower than 0.05. Conversely, if this confidence interval includes the value 0, i.e. one limit is positive and the other is negative, then P is greater than 0.05.

This example shows that there is a close link between significance testing and confidence intervals. This is not surprising, since these two approaches make use of the same ingredient, the standard error. A statistical test is based on how many standard errors the observed sample estimate lies away from the value specified in the null hypothesis. Confidence intervals are calculated from the standard error and indicate a range of values that is likely to include the true but unknown population parameter; this range may or may not include the value specified in the null hypothesis and this is reflected by the value of the test statistic.

In Example 6.5, the P-values are large, indicating that the results are consistent with the null hypothesis of no difference in risk between relatives of mycosis fungoides patients and the general population of England and Wales. However, inspection of the confidence intervals reveals that the confidence interval for all malignancies is quite narrow, whereas the one for non-Hodgkin lymphoma is wide and consistent with an almost five-fold increase in risk as well as with a 50% reduction. This confidence interval is wide because it is based on only three cases.

To summarize, P-values should not be reported on their own. The confidence intervals are much more informative, since they provide an

Table 6.5.
Cancer incidence among first-degree
relatives of mycosis fungoides patients
(unpublished data).

Example 6.5. Various studies have suggested that relatives of patients who develop mycosis fungoides (a particular form of non-Hodgkin lymphoma) are at increased risk of developing cancer, particularly non-Hodgkin lymphomas. To clarify this issue, data on the number of cancer cases that occurred among first-degree relatives of mycosis fungoides patients diagnosed in one London hospital were ascertained. The observed number of cancer cases was then compared with those that would have been expected on the basis of the national rates for England and Wales. The results from this study are shown in Table 6.5.

Site	Number of cases observed (O)	Number of cases expected (E)[a]	Standardized incidence ratio (O/E)	95% confidence interval	P-value
All sites	34	36.8	0.9	0.6–1.3	0.719
Non-Hodgkin lymphomas	3	2.1	1.5	0.5–4.6	0.502

[a] Calculated using the national age-specific cancer incidence rates for England and Wales as the standard.

idea of the likely magnitude of the association (or difference of effects) and their width indicates the degree of uncertainty in the estimate of effect.

Appendix 6.1 gives formulae to calculate confidence intervals and statistical tests for the most commonly used epidemiological measures.

Further reading

* Gardner & Altman (1986) provide a simple overview of most of the concepts covered in this chapter and also give suggestions for presentation and graphical display of statistical results.

Box 6.1. Key issues

- Epidemiological studies are usually conducted in subsets or *samples* of individuals drawn from the population of interest. A sample estimate of a particular epidemiological measure is, however, unlikely to be equal to the true population value, due to *sampling error*.

- The *confidence interval* indicates how precise the sample estimate is likely to be in relation to the true population value. It provides a range of values that is likely to include the true population value (although we cannot be sure that a particular confidence interval will in fact do so).

- *Statistical significance* testing is used to test hypotheses about the population of interest. The P-value provides a measure of the extent to which the data from the study are consistent with the 'null hypothesis', i.e., the hypothesis that there is no true association between variables or difference between groups in the population. The smaller the P-value, the stronger is the evidence against the null hypothesis and, consequently, the stronger the evidence in favour of the study hypothesis.

- P-values should generally not be reported alone, since they do not provide any indication of the magnitude of the association (or difference of effects). For instance, small effects of no epidemiological relevance can become 'statistically significant' with large sample sizes, whereas important effects may be 'statistically non-significant' because the size of the sample studied was too small. In contrast, confidence intervals provide an idea of the range of values which might include the true population value.

- Confidence intervals and statistical significance testing deal only with sampling variation. It is assumed that non-sampling errors such as bias in the selection of the subjects in the sample and in the measurement of the variables of interest are absent.

Appendix 6.1
Confidence intervals and significance tests for epidemiological measures

This appendix provides formulae for the calculation of confidence intervals and statistical significance tests for the most commonly used epidemiological measures. The formulae presented here can only be applied to 'crude' measures (with the exception of the standardized mortality (or incidence) ratio). For measures that are adjusted for the effect of potential confounding factors, see Chapter 14. For measures not considered here, see Armitage and Berry (1994). Similar results may be easily obtained using computer packages such as EPI INFO, STATA or EGRET.

A6.1.1 Calculation of confidence intervals for measures of occurrence

Single proportion (prevalence or risk)

Prevalence is a *proportion* and therefore the standard error and the confidence interval can be calculated using the formula discussed in Section 6.1.1:

$$SE(p) = \sqrt{\frac{p^2(1-p)}{a}}$$

where a is the number of cases and $p = a/n$ (n being the sample size).

A 95% confidence interval can be obtained as

$$p \pm 1.96 \times SE(p)$$

For a 90% confidence interval, the value 1.96 should be replaced by 1.64 and for a 99% confidence interval by 2.58.

Risk is also a *proportion*. Thus the standard error and confidence interval can be obtained in exactly the same way, as long as all the subjects are followed up over the whole risk period of interest. If the follow-up times are unequal, life-table or survival analysis techniques must be used (see Chapter 12), including the appropriate standard error formulae.

The simple method for obtaining confidence intervals described above is based on approximating the sampling distribution to the Normal distribution. This 'approximate' method is accurate in sufficiently large samples (greater than 30).

An 'exact' method for calculating confidence intervals for proportions, based on the binomial distribution, is recommended for smaller samples. This method is, however, too complex for the calculations to be performed on a pocket calculator.

Single rate

If the number of cases that occur during the observation period is denoted by a and the quantity of person-time at risk by y, the estimated incidence rate (r) is

$$r = a/y$$

An 'approximate' standard error can be calculated as follows:

$$\text{SE}(r) = r/\sqrt{a}$$

The 95% confidence interval for the observed rate (r) can then be obtained as

$$r \pm 1.96 \times \text{SE}(r)$$

Table A6.1.1.
95% confidence limit factors for estimates of a Poisson-distributed variable.[a]

Observed number on which estimate is based	Lower limit factor	Upper limit factor	Observed number on which estimate is based	Lower limit factor	Upper limit factor	Observed number on which estimate is based	Lower limit factor	Upper limit factor
(a)	(L)	(U)	(a)	(L)	(U)	(a)	(L)	(U)
1	0.025	5.57	21	0.619	1.53	120	0.833	1.200
2	0.121	3.61	22	0.627	1.51	140	0.844	1.184
3	0.206	2.92	23	0.634	1.50	160	0.854	1.171
4	0.272	2.56	24	0.641	1.48	180	0.862	1.160
5	0.324	2.33	25	0.647	1.48	200	0.868	1.151
6	0.367	2.18	26	0.653	1.47	250	0.882	1.134
7	0.401	2.06	27	0.659	1.46	300	0.892	1.121
8	0.431	1.97	28	0.665	1.45	350	0.899	1.112
9	0.458	1.90	29	0.670	1.44	400	0.906	1.104
10	0.480	1.84	30	0.675	1.43	450	0.911	1.098
11	0.499	1.79	35	0.697	1.39	500	0.915	1.093
12	0.517	1.75	40	0.714	1.36	600	0.922	1.084
13	0.532	1.71	45	0.729	1.34	700	0.928	1.078
14	0.546	1.68	50	0.742	1.32	800	0.932	1.072
15	0.560	1.65	60	0.770	1.30	900	0.936	1.068
16	0.572	1.62	70	0.785	1.27	1000	0.939	1.064
17	0.583	1.60	80	0.798	1.25			
18	0.593	1.58	90	0.809	1.24			
19	0.602	1.56	100	0.818	1.22			
20	0.611	1.54						

[a] Data from Haenszel *et al.*, (1962)

These formulae are appropriate when the number of cases in the numerator of the rate, a, is greater than 30. If the number of cases is small, 'exact' confidence intervals, based on the Poisson distribution, can be obtained from Table A6.1.1. This table gives factors by which the observed rate is multiplied to obtain the lower and the upper limit of a 95% confidence interval:

Lower limit = $r \times$ lower limit factor (L)
Upper limit = $r \times$ upper limit factor (U)

Consider the following example. The total number of deaths from stomach cancer among males aged 45–54 years in Egypt during 1980 was 39 in 1 742 000 person-years (WHO, 1986). Thus, using the 'approximate' method,

r = 39/1 742 000 pyrs = 2.24 per 100 000 pyrs

SE(r) = 2.24 per 100 000 pyrs/$\sqrt{39}$ = 0.36 per 100 000 pyrs

95% CI(r) = 2.24 ± 1.96 × 0.36 = 1.53 to 2.95 per 100 000 pyrs

For the 'exact' method, the lower limit factor (L) and the upper limit factor (U) corresponding to 39 cases are obtained from the table by interpolation between the rows for 35 and 40 cases.

$$L = 0.697 + \left[(0.714 - 0.697) \times \frac{39 - 35}{40 - 35} \right] = 0.711$$

$$U = 1.39 - \left[(1.39 - 1.36) \times \frac{39 - 35}{40 - 35} \right] = 1.37$$

Thus, the limits of the 95% confidence interval are

Lower limit = 2.24 per 100 000 pyrs × 0.711 = 1.59 per 100 000 pyrs
Upper limit = 2.24 per 100 000 pyrs × 1.37 = 3.07 per 100 000 pyrs

In this example, the 'exact' and the 'approximate' confidence limits are relatively close to each other, because the rate was based on a sufficiently large number of cases. The larger the number of cases, the closer will be the confidence limits obtained by these two methods.

Let us now consider some data from Kuwait. The total number of deaths from stomach cancer among men aged 45–54 years in this country in

1980 was only 3 in 74 000 pyrs (WHO, 1983). The 'approximate' method gives

$$r = 3/74\ 000\ \text{pyrs} = 4.05\ \text{per}\ 100\ 000\ \text{pyrs}$$

$$SE(r) = 4.05\ \text{per}\ 100\ 000\ \text{pyrs}/\sqrt{3} = 2.34\ \text{per}\ 100\ 000\ \text{pyrs}$$

$$95\%\ CI(r) = 4.05 \pm 1.96 \times 2.34 = -0.54\ \text{to}\ 8.64\ \text{per}\ 100\ 000\ \text{pyrs}$$

This method gives a negative value for the lower limit, which is meaningless, as incidence and mortality rates cannot be negative. By the 'exact' method, consulting again Table A6.1.1, the limits for the 95% confidence interval are:

Lower limit = 4.05 per 100 000 pyrs × 0.206 = 0.83 per 100 000 pyrs
Upper limit = 4.05 per 100 000 pyrs × 2.92 = 11.83 per 100 000 pyrs

In this example, the 'exact and' 'approximate' confidence intervals are clearly different. When the number of cases is less than about 30, it is desirable to use the 'exact' method.

A6.1.2 Calculation of confidence intervals for measures of effect

Ratio of proportions (prevalence ratio or risk ratio)

A formula for the confidence interval around a risk ratio estimate of effect must take into account the fact that the sampling distribution of possible values for the risk ratio is highly skewed to the right. The minimum possible value a risk ratio can take is zero and the maximum is infinity. To make the distribution more symmetric, it is necessary to first convert the estimated risk ratios into their natural logarithms (denoted ln). We can then use formulae analogous to those presented in Section A6.1.1 to calculate a confidence interval around the value of the logarithm of the risk ratio rather than the risk ratio itself.

Consider the following example, in which 1000 exposed subjects and 1500 unexposed subjects were followed up for one year. The follow-up was complete for each subject. At the end of this period, 60 subjects among the exposed and 45 among the unexposed had developed the outcome of interest (Table A6.1.2).

Table A6.1.2.
Results from a cohort study in which risks were calculated as measures of occurrence of the outcome of interest in each study group: hypothetical data.

| | | Exposure | | Total |
		Yes	No	
Outcome	Yes	60 (*a*)	45 (*b*)	105 (n_1)
	No	940 (*c*)	1455 (*d*)	2395 (n_0)
Total		1000 (m_1)	1500 (m_0)	2500 (*N*)

The risk ratio (R) and its natural logarithm can be calculated as

$$R = p_1/p_0$$

$$\ln R = \ln (p_1/p_0)$$

An 'approximate' standard error of the logarithm of R can be estimated by

$$SE (\ln R) = \sqrt{\frac{1}{a} + \frac{1}{b} - \frac{1}{m_1} - \frac{1}{m_0}}$$

An 'approximate' 95% confidence interval for $\ln R$ is then given by ($\ln R$) ± 1.96 SE($\ln R$), and the 95% confidence interval for the risk ratio (R) obtained by taking antilogarithms.

Thus, in the example shown in Table A6.1.2

Risk in the exposed (p_1) = 60/1000 = 0.06

Risk in the unexposed (p_0) = 45/1500 = 0.03

Risk ratio (R) = 0.06/0.03 = 2.0

$\ln R = \ln 2.0 = 0.69$

$$SE (\ln R) = \sqrt{\frac{1}{60} + \frac{1}{45} - \frac{1}{1000} - \frac{1}{1500}} = 0.19$$

95% CI ($\ln R$) = 0.69 ± 1.96 × 0.19 = 0.318 to 1.062

The 'approximate' 95% confidence interval of the risk ratio (R) can then be obtained by taking antilogarithms:

95% CI (R) = $e^{0.318}$ to $e^{1.062}$ = 1.37 to 2.89

A similar approach can be applied when the measure of interest is a *prevalence ratio*.

'Exact' methods should be used when the risk ratio or the prevalence ratio is based on small numbers of cases, but the calculations are too complex to be shown here.

Difference of proportions (prevalence difference or risk difference)

The standard error of the difference between two proportions p_1 and p_0 can be estimated, approximately, as

$$SE\,(p_1 - p_0) = \sqrt{\frac{p_1^2(1 - p_1)}{a} + \frac{p_0^2(1 - p_0)}{b}}$$

where a and b are the numbers of cases in the two study groups. In the example shown in Table A6.1.2,

Risk difference $(p_1 - p_0) = 0.06 - 0.03 = 0.03$

$$SE\,(p_1 - p_0) = \sqrt{\frac{0.06^2\,(1 - 0.06)}{60} + \frac{0.03^2\,(1 - 0.03)}{45}} = 0.0087$$

$$
\begin{aligned}
95\%\ \mathrm{CI}\,(p_1 - p_0) &= (p_1 - p_0) \pm 1.96\ SE\,(p_1 - p_0) \\
&= 0.03 \pm 1.96 \times 0.0087 \\
&= 0.013 \text{ to } 0.047 \text{ or } 1\% \text{ to } 5\%
\end{aligned}
$$

A confidence interval for a *difference in prevalences* will be calculated in the same way.

Rate ratio

Consider the results from another hypothetical cohort study, shown in Table A6.1.3

Table A6.1.3.
Results from a cohort study in which rates were calculated as measures of occurrence of the outcome of interest in each study group: hypothetical data.

	Exposure		Total
	Yes	**No**	
Cases	60 (a)	45 (b)	105 (n)
Person-years at risk (pyrs)	4150 (y_1)	6500 (y_0)	10 650 (y)
Rate per 1000 pyrs	14.5 (r_1)	6.9 (r_0)	9.9 (r)

As with a risk ratio, a rate ratio can only take values from zero to infinity. Thus to construct a confidence interval for an estimated rate ratio (RR), its natural logarithm needs to be calculated first:

$$\ln RR = \ln\,(r_1/r_0)$$

An 'approximate' standard error of the logarithm of a rate ratio (RR) can be obtained as follows:

$$SE\,(\ln RR) = \sqrt{(1/a + 1/b)}$$

where a and b are the numbers of cases in the exposed and unexposed groups, respectively.

In this example, the incidence rate in the exposed (r_1) is equal to $60/4150 = 14.5$ per 1000 pyrs. The incidence rate in the unexposed group (r_0) is $45/6500 = 6.9$ per 1000 pyrs. Thus the rate ratio and its logarithm are:

$$RR = 14.5 \text{ per } 1000 \text{ pyrs}/6.9 \text{ per } 1000 \text{ pyrs} = 2.1$$

$$\ln RR = \ln 2.1 = 0.74$$

An 'approximate' standard error for the logarithm of a rate ratio of 2.1 based on 60 cases in the exposed group and 45 cases in the unexposed group may be calculated as follows:

$$SE (\ln RR) = \sqrt{(1/60 + 1/45)} = 0.197$$

The 'approximate' 95% confidence interval of the logarithm of the rate ratio is given by

$$
\begin{aligned}
95\% \text{ CI } (\ln RR) &= \ln RR \pm 1.96 \text{ SE } (\ln RR) \\
&= 0.74 \pm 1.96 \times 0.197 \\
&= 0.35 \text{ to } 1.13
\end{aligned}
$$

We can then obtain the 'approximate' 95% confidence interval for the rate ratio by taking the antilogarithms of these values:

$$95\% \text{ CI } (RR) = e^{0.35} \text{ to } e^{1.13} = 1.42 \text{ to } 3.10$$

There is also an 'exact' method of calculating confidence intervals for rate ratios that are based on small numbers of cases, but its discussion is beyond the scope of this chapter (see Breslow & Day, 1987, pp. 93–95).

When the rate ratio is an SMR (or SIR) (see Section 4.3.3), it is possible to calculate an 'exact' 95% confidence interval by multiplying the observed SMR (or SIR) by the appropriate lower and upper limit factors, exactly as we did for a single rate.

For instance, if the number of observed (O) leukaemia deaths in a certain town were 20 and only 15 would have been expected (E) if the town had the same age-specific rates as the whole country, the SMR would be equal to 1.33. The lower and the upper limit factors when the observed number of cases is 20 (see Table A6.1.1) are 0.611 and 1.54, respectively. Thus,

$$SMR = O/E = 20/15 = 1.33$$

$$
\begin{aligned}
95\% \text{ CI } (SMR) &= 1.33 \times 0.611 \text{ to } 1.33 \times 1.54 \\
&= 0.81 \text{ to } 2.05
\end{aligned}
$$

Rate difference

The standard error of the difference between two estimated rates (r_1 and r_0) is given by

$$SE\ (r_1 - r_0) = \sqrt{\frac{r_1^2}{a} + \frac{r_0^2}{b}}$$

where a and b refer to numbers of cases in the two groups.

The 95% confidence interval is given by

$$95\%\ CI\ (r_1 - r_0) = (r_1 - r_0) \pm 1.96\ SE(r_1 - r_0)$$

Thus in the example shown in Table A6.1.3

$$r_1 - r_0 = 14.5\ \text{per}\ 1000\ \text{pyrs} - 6.9\ \text{per}\ 1000\ \text{pyrs} = 7.6\ \text{per}\ 1000\ \text{pyrs}$$

$$SE\ (r_1 - r_0) = \sqrt{((0.0145)^2/60 + (0.0069)^2/45)} = 0.00214$$
$$= 2.14\ \text{per}\ 1000\ \text{pyrs}$$

$$95\%\ CI\ (r_1 - r_0) = 7.6 \pm 1.96 \times 2.14 = 3.41\ \text{to}\ 11.79\ \text{per}\ 1000\ \text{pyrs}$$

Odds ratio

Data from a case–control study can be presented in a 2×2 table, as shown below:

Table A6.1.4.
Results from a case–control study: hypothetical data.

	Exposure		Total
	Yes	**No**	
Cases	457 (*a*)	26 (*b*)	483 (n_1)
Controls	362 (*c*)	85 (*d*)	447 (n_0)
Total	819 (m_1)	111 (m_0)	930 (*N*)

An 'approximate' standard error of the logarithm of an odds ratio (OR) can be calculated as

$$SE\ (\ln OR) = \sqrt{(1/a + 1/b + 1/c + 1/d)}$$

In the example shown in Table A6.1.4

$$OR = \frac{\text{odds of exposure among the cases}}{\text{odds of exposure among the controls}} = \frac{457/26}{362/85} = 4.13$$

$$\ln OR = \ln 4.13 = 1.42$$

$$SE\ (\ln OR) = \sqrt{(1/457 + 1/26 + 1/362 + 1/85)} = 0.23$$

$$95\%\ CI\ (\ln OR) = 1.42 \pm 1.96 \times 0.23 = 0.97\ \text{to}\ 1.87$$

Thus an 'approximate' 95% confidence interval for the odds ratio can be obtained by taking antilogarithms:

95% CI (OR) = $e^{0.97}$ to $e^{1.87}$ = 2.64 to 6.49

It is also possible to calculate an 'exact' confidence interval for small samples, but the calculations are too complex to be carried out on a pocket calculator.

A.6.1.3 Statistical tests

Comparison of two proportions (prevalences or risks)
To test the null hypothesis that there is no true difference between two proportions (either *risks* or *prevalences*), the results from a study should first be arranged in a 2×2 table similar to Table A6.1.2. In this table, the *observed* (*O*) number of cases among exposed is *a*. We can calculate the *expected* (*E*) value in cell *a* and the *variance* (*V*), assuming that the null hypothesis of no difference between the two groups is true.

$O = a$

$E = m_1 n_1 / N$

$V = \dfrac{n_1 n_0 m_1 m_0}{N^2 (N - 1)}$

A special statistical test called the chi-squared (χ^2) test can then be applied to measure the extent to which the observed data differ from those expected if the two proportions were equal, that is, if the null hypothesis were true.

$\chi^2 = (O - E)^2 / V$

In epidemiology, this application of the χ^2 test takes the name of *Mantel–Haenszel test*.
In the example shown in Table A6.1.2

$O = 60$

$E = 1000 \times 105/2500 = 42$

$V = \dfrac{105 \times 2395 \times 1000 \times 1500}{2500^2 \times (2500 - 1)} = 24.15$

$\chi^2 = \dfrac{(60 - 42)^2}{24.15} = 13.42$

Large values of χ^2 suggest that the data are inconsistent with the null hypothesis, and therefore that there is an association between exposure and outcome. The *P*-value is obtained by comparing the calculated value of χ^2 with tables of the chi-squared distribution.

In referring the calculated χ^2 test statistics to these tables, we need to know a quantity called the 'degrees of freedom' (d.f.), which takes into consideration the number of sub-groups or 'cells' in the table which contributed to the calculation. For 2×2 tables, the number of degrees of freedom (d.f.) is one.

If the null hypothesis is true,

χ^2 test statistic (with 1 d.f.) exceeds	0.45	with probability	0.5
"	1.32	"	0.25
"	2.71	"	0.1
"	3.84	"	0.05
"	5.02	"	0.025
"	6.63	"	0.01
"	7.88	"	0.005
"	10.83	"	0.001

Thus, if the χ^2 statistic with 1 d.f. exceeds 3.84, then $P<0.05$, indicating some evidence of a real difference in the proportions. If it exceeds 6.63, then $P < 0.01$, and there is strong evidence of a difference.

In the example shown in Table A6.1.2, the value of χ^2 was 13.42, which corresponds to $P < 0.001$. There is therefore strong evidence for an association. Thus we can conclude that the observed risk ratio of 2.0 is statistically significantly different from 1, and that there is very strong evidence that the risk is higher in those who were exposed than in those who were not.

In fact, we have already performed a test for difference in two proportions in Section 6.2.2. We then used a different test statistic which gave similar results to the more general Mantel–Haenszel type of test statistic used here.

Note that the statistical test is the same regardless of the measure of effect (*risk (or prevalence) ratio* or *risk (or prevalence) difference*) that we are interested in. However, the confidence intervals are calculated in a different way (see Section A6.1.2).

Comparison of two odds

The approach discussed above for comparison of proportions can also be used to test the null hypothesis that there is no difference between the odds of exposure among the cases and the odds of exposure among the controls, that is, the odds ratio is equal to one. In the example shown in Table A6.1.4

$$O = 457$$

$$E = \frac{819 \times 483}{930} = 425.35$$

$$V = \frac{483 \times 447 \times 819 \times 111}{930^2 \times (930 - 1)} = 24.43$$

$$\chi^2 = \frac{(457 - 425.35)^2}{24.43} = 41.0$$

The χ^2 gives a measure of the extent to which the observed data differ from those expected if the two odds of exposure were equal. This χ^2 value (with one degree of freedom) corresponds to $P<0.001$. Thus, there is strong evidence against the null hypothesis.

Comparison of two rates

In cohort studies, where rates rather than risks are used as the measure of disease frequency, consideration must be given to the distribution of person-years between exposed and unexposed groups.

Consider again the example shown in Table A6.1.3. The observed number of cases among those who were exposed is $a = 60$. The expected value in cell a and the variance assuming that the null hypothesis is true (i.e., that there is no true difference in rates between the exposed and the unexposed groups) can be calculated as follows:

$$E = ny_1/y \text{ and } V = ny_1y_0/y^2$$

Then

$$\chi^2 = (O - E)^2/V$$

In the example shown in Table A6.1.3

$$O = 60$$

$$E = \frac{105 \times 4150}{10\,650} = 40.92$$

$$V = \frac{105 \times 4150 \times 6500}{(10\,650)^2} = 24.97$$

$$\chi^2 = \frac{(60 - 40.92)^2}{24.97} = 14.58$$

This χ^2 value with one degree of freedom corresponds to $P < 0.001$, providing strong evidence against the null hypothesis of no association between exposure and the incidence of the disease.

The same procedure applies when the rate ratio is an SMR. In this case, the variance is equal to the expected number of cases. Thus if the number of observed leukaemia deaths (O) in a particular town is 20 and the expected number (E) based on the national age-specific rates is 15,

$$\text{SMR} = O/E = 20/15 = 1.33$$

$$V = 15$$

$$\chi^2 = \frac{(20 - 15)^2}{15} = 1.67$$

This χ^2 value, with one degree of freedom, corresponds to $0.1 < P < 0.25$. Thus, these results are consistent with the null hypothesis of no difference in the age-specific mortality rates from leukaemia between the town and the whole country.

Note that the statistical test is the same regardless of the measure of effect (*rate ratio* or *rate difference*) we are interested in. However, the confidence intervals are calculated in a different way (see Section A6.1.2).

χ^2 test for a linear trend in proportions (prevalences or risks)

So far we have considered only situations where individuals were classified as either 'exposed' or 'unexposed'. In many circumstances, how-ever, individuals can also be classified according to levels of exposure. For instance, suppose that a survey was carried out to assess whether infection with human papillomavirus (HPV) was associated with number of sexual partners. The results from this hypothetical study are shown in Table A6.1.5.

Table A6.1.5.
Distribution of women infected and not infected with human papillomavirus (HPV) by number of lifetime sexual partners: hypothetical data.

	Lifetime number of sexual partners				Total
	1	2–3	4–5	>5	
HPV-positive	$19(a_0)$	$33(a_1)$	$51(a_2)$	$107(a_3)$	$210(n_1)$
HPV-negative	$71(b_0)$	$68(b_1)$	$42(b_2)$	$61(b_3)$	$242(n_0)$
Total	$90(m_0)$	$101(m_1)$	$93(m_2)$	$168(m_3)$	$452(N)$
Percentage of HPV positive	21.1	32.7	54.8	63.7	46.5
Score	$0(x_0)$	$1(x_1)$	$2(x_2)$	$3(x_3)$	

The results seem to support the study hypothesis of a trend for an increase in the proportion of HPV-positive women with increasing number of sexual partners. Although there is an apparent linear trend in proportions in the above table, each proportion (or percentage) is subject to sampling variability. We can use a χ^2 test for a linear trend in proportions to assess whether this trend may be due to chance.

The first step is to assign a score x to each exposure category. For example, in Table A6.1.5 '0' was assigned to those women with 1 partner, '1' to those with 2–3 partners, and so on. The second step is to use the following formulae to obtain the values of T_1, T_2 and T_3. In these formulae, the symbol Σ means sum and the subscript i stands for the subscripts 0, 1, 2, 3, etc.

$$T_1 = \Sigma a_i x_i = (19 \times 0) + (33 \times 1) + (51 \times 2) + (107 \times 3) = 456$$

$$T_2 = \Sigma m_i x_i = (90 \times 0) + (101 \times 1) + (93 \times 2) + (168 \times 3) = 791$$

$$T_3 = \Sigma m_i x_i^2 = (90 \times 0^2) + (101 \times 1^2) + (93 \times 2^2) + (168 \times 3^2) = 1985$$

The χ^2 test for trend has one degree of freedom and can be calculated as

$$\chi^2 = \frac{N\,(NT_1 - n_1 T_2)^2}{n_1 n_0\,(N\,T_3 - T_2^2)}$$

Thus, in our example

$$\chi^2 = \frac{452 \times (452 \times 456 - 210 \times 791)^2}{210 \times 242 \times (452 \times 1985 - 791^2)} = 52.41$$

A χ^2 of 52.41 with 1 d.f. corresponds to $P<0.0001$. We can therefore conclude that there is strong evidence of a linear trend for an increasing proportion of HPV-positive women as lifetime number of sexual partners increases.

χ^2 test for a linear trend in odds ratios

Consider data from a hypothetical case–control study carried out to assess whether there is a decreasing risk of developing epithelial benign ovarian tumours with increasing parity (Table A6.1.6).

The results from this study apparently support the study hypothesis. (The calculation of odds ratios from case–control studies is discussed in detail in Chapter 9.)

	Parity			Total
	0^a	1–2	≥ 3	
Benign tumour cases	30 (a_0)	23 (a_1)	7 (a_2)	60 (n_1)
Controls	46 (b_0)	48 (b_1)	35 (b_2)	129 (n_0)
Total	76 (m_0)	71 (m_1)	42 (m_2)	189 (N)
Odds ratio	1	0.73	0.31	
Score	0 (x_0)	1 (x_1)	2 (x_2)	

a Taken as the baseline category in the calculation of odds ratios.

Table A6.1.6.
Distribution of cases of benign tumours of the ovary and controls by parity: hypothetical data.

A χ^2 test for a linear trend can be used to test the hypothesis that there is a decreasing risk of ovarian benign tumours with increasing parity. The calculations are exactly the same as those used for the χ^2 test for a linear trend in proportions.

$$T_1 = \Sigma a_i x_i = (30 \times 0) + (23 \times 1) + (7 \times 2) = 37$$

$$T_2 = \Sigma m_i x_i = (76 \times 0) + (71 \times 1) + (42 \times 2) = 155$$

$$T_3 = \Sigma m_i x_i^2 = (76 \times 0^2) + (71 \times 1^2) + (42 \times 2^2) = 239$$

The χ^2 test for trend can then be calculated as:

$$\chi^2 = \frac{189 \times (189 \times 37 - 60 \times 155)^2}{60 \times 129 \times (189 \times 239 - 155^2)} = 6.15$$

This test result with 1 d.f. corresponds to $0.01 < P < 0.025$. Thus there is evidence that the risk of developing a benign ovarian tumour decreases with increasing parity.

χ^2 test for a linear trend in rates

A similar approach can be used to test for a trend in rates. Consider the following cohort study to test the hypothesis that the risk of breast cancer increases with increasing duration of oral contraceptive use.

Table A6.1.7.
Distribution of breast cancer cases and person-years at risk by duration of oral contraceptive use: hypothetical data.

	Duration of oral contraceptive use (years)			Total	
	0	1–2	≥3		
Breast cancer cases	62 (a_0)	42 (a_1)	22 (a_2)	126	(n)
Person-years at risk	31 200 (y_0)	25 100 (y_1)	11 600 (y_2)	67 900	(y)
Rate per 100 000 pyrs	198.7(r_0)	167.3(r_1)	189.7(r_2)	185.6(r)	
Score	0 (x_0)	1 (x_1)	2 (x_2)		

The observed rates by exposure level suggest, if anything, a downward trend with increasing duration of oral contraceptive use. A χ^2-test for a linear trend in rates similar to the one described above for proportions and odds ratios can be calculated as follows:

$$T_1 = \Sigma a_i x_i = (62 \times 0) + (42 \times 1) + (22 \times 2) = 86$$

$$T_2 = \Sigma y_i x_i = (31\ 200 \times 0) + (25\ 100 \times 1) + (11\ 600 \times 2) = 48\ 300$$

$$T_3 = \Sigma y_i x_i^2 = (31\ 200 \times 0^2) + (25\ 100 \times 1^2) + (11\ 600 \times 2^2) = 71\ 500$$

The χ^2 test for a linear trend in rates, which has one degree of freedom, can be calculated as follows:

$$\chi^2 = \frac{[T_1 - (n/y)T_2)]^2}{(n/y^2)\,(yT_3 - T_2{}^2)}$$

Thus, in our example,

$$\chi^2 = \frac{[86 - (126/67\ 900 \times 48\ 300)]^2}{(126/67\ 900^2) \times (67\ 900 \times 71\ 500 - 48\ 300^2)} = 0.19$$

This test value with 1 d.f. corresponds to $P > 0.5$. Hence, the results of the study provide no support for an upward or downward trend in breast cancer rates with duration of oral contraceptive use.

Validity of χ^2 tests

If in a 2×2 table the total sample size (N) is less than 40 and the expected value in any of the cells is less than 5, the χ^2 test should not be used. In these circumstances, the Fisher's exact test will be the appropriate statistical test (see Kirkwood (1988)). For larger tables, the χ^2 test is valid if no more than 20% of the expected values are less than 5, and none is less than one.

Note that the expected value (E) for a particular cell is calculated as follows:

$$E = \frac{\text{Total of the relevant row} \times \text{total of the relevant column}}{N}$$

Thus in Table A6.1.4

$$E\,(a) = n_1 m_1/N = (483 \times 819)/930 = 425.35$$

$$E\,(b) = n_1 m_0/N = (483 \times 111)/930 = 57.65$$

$$E\,(c) = n_0 m_1/N = (447 \times 819)/930 = 393.65$$

$$E\,(d) = n_0 m_0/N = (447 \times 111)/930 = 53.35$$

The χ^2 test is valid in this example since the total sample size (N) is greater than 40 and all of the expected cell values are well above 5.

Chapter 7
Intervention trials

Intervention trials are the epidemiological studies that most closely resemble the experiments conducted by scientists in the laboratory. The essential and distinguishing feature of such studies lies in the investigator's direct control over the allocation of subjects to study groups. In contrast, in observational studies, the allocation is determined by the subjects themselves and the researchers are just passive observers of what happens.

Intervention trials provide the strongest evidence with which to test hypotheses. However, they are not the most usual study design in epidemiology, mainly because of ethical constraints. It would be unacceptable to allocate people to either be or not be exposed to a substance or to be subjected to a procedure for which there is some suspicion that it may be harmful. It is, however, possible to conduct a trial to test whether removal of such an exposure will decrease subsequent incidence and mortality. Thus, intervention trials in epidemiology are limited to interventions for which there are grounds to believe that there will be a potential benefit to individuals.

7.1 Types of intervention study

Intervention trials consist of trials to prevent disease (field trials) or trials to treat established disease processes (clinical trials).

The objective of a *clinical trial* is to evaluate one or more new treatments for a disease or condition. For instance, a clinical trial may be designed to assess whether a chemotherapeutic agent can prevent recurrence of cancer, increase survival or improve quality of life (Example 7.1). Since clinical trials involve diseased people, they are often carried out in hospitals or other clinical settings where the subjects are treated and followed up for their condition.

> *Example 7.1. A total of 474 adult patients with malignant glioma (astrocytoma) grade 3 or 4 were randomized to receive 45 Gy (in 20 fractions over four weeks) or 60 Gy (in 30 fractions over six weeks) of radiotherapy postoperatively. The main objective of the study was to assess whether the higher dose would improve survival (Bleehen & Stenning, 1991).*

In contrast, *field trials* deal with subjects who are disease-free. A field trial involves evaluation of whether an agent or procedure reduces the risk of developing disease among those free from that condition at enrolment. Because these trials involve healthy rather than diseased people, they tend to be logistically more difficult to carry out than clinical trials. They generally have to be conducted in the 'field' rather than in hospitals or clinics. Moreover, whereas the adverse consequences of a given disease (e.g., disease recurrence, death) may occur with high probability during a relatively short time, typically the risk of contracting a disease among people who are initially free of it is small. This is particularly true for rare diseases such as cancer. Consequently, field trials usually require a greater number of subjects followed up for longer periods than clinical trials.

> *Example 7.2.* *A randomized trial was carried out among Whitehall (English) civil servants to measure in middle-aged men the health effects of stopping smoking. A total of 1445 male cigarette smokers aged 40–59 years who were at a high risk of developing cardiorespiratory diseases were randomly allocated to intervention (714 men) or normal care (731 men). Those in the intervention group received individual advice on the relation of smoking to health. Most then expressed their wish to stop smoking and received further support over the next 12 months. The two groups were then followed up for twenty years (Rose & Colwell, 1992).*

Field trials can be carried out among *individuals* (as in Example 7.2) or *groups of people* (as in Examples 7.3 and 7.4). In the first case, the unit of allocation to the intervention is the individual, whereas in the second, it is the group. The group may be a household, a block of houses, a school or a whole community. Field trials in which whole communities are the unit of allocation are called *community trials* (Example 7.3).

> *Example 7.3.* *The Community Intervention Trial for Smoking Cessation (COMMIT) was a multicentre project designed to evaluate a community-wide smoking cessation programme in the USA. This trial began in 1989 in 11 matched pairs of communities. One community of each pair was randomly assigned to receive the smoking cessation programme with the other acting as a control. The intervention was designed to promote smoking cessation by using a wide range of community resources to affect attitudes and policies towards smoking (COMMIT Research Group, 1991).*

> *Example 7.4.* *A randomized controlled trial was carried out to assess the effectiveness of health education leaflets in reducing the incidence of sunburn (one of the known risk factors for malignant melanoma of the skin) among British holiday-makers. The study population comprised holiday-makers travelling to warmer countries on flights from Manchester airport in the United Kingdom during August 1993. The unit of study was the flight. Flights were randomly allocated to either receive the leaflets (intervention group) or not to (control group) (Dey et al., 1995).*

There are various reasons for selecting groups rather than individuals as the study unit. Many interventions are impossible to assign at an individual level. Environmental interventions such as water fluoridation or improvement of air quality can be conducted only at a group level. Most health education interventions also fall into this category. For instance, the intervention (i.e., the smoking cessation programme) in Example 7.3 was aimed primarily at the community rather than the individual; thus, it was appropriate to choose the community as the study unit. It may also be logistically easier to conduct the trial among groups of people than among individuals. In Example 7.4, for instance, it was much easier to allocate flights to either the intervention group or the control group than it would have been to allocate individuals. By allocating flights, it was also possible to minimize the potential for 'contamination', that is, the possibility that people in the control group would end up having access to the leaflets. Such contamination would have made the two groups more alike and, consequently, would have decreased the ability of the trial to reveal any true effect that the intervention might have had (see Section 7.10).

7.2   Formulation of the study objectives

The main objectives of an intervention study should be clearly specified before its start. They should include a concise, but detailed, description of the intervention to be evaluated, the outcome(s) of interest and the population in which the study will be conducted. For example, it is not enough just to state that the objective of a trial is 'to assess whether administration of tamoxifen prevents the development of breast cancer in women'. It is necessary to define exactly the target population. For instance, does it include all women or only those at high risk of developing the disease? Which age-groups will be included? The intervention also needs to be specified in terms of dose, frequency of administration and duration. In addition, it is necessary to decide whether the comparison group will be given a placebo or nothing at all. The outcome(s) of interest and the procedures used to measure them should also be clearly stated.

It is important to decide at this stage whether the intent of the study is primarily *scientific* (explanatory) or *pragmatic* (Schwartz & Lellouch, 1967). If primarily scientific, the trial should be carried out under ideal conditions, so that it will be possible to establish the maximum benefit that the intervention can achieve. It is sensible in these circumstances to conduct the trial among special groups of people (such as volunteers) so as to ensure a high level of compliance. Pragmatic trials, by contrast, assess whether the intervention works when introduced into a public health or clinical setting, i.e., in real-life conditions. In these studies, the true effect of the intervention is likely to be diluted, among other things, by low levels of compliance.

7.3   Ethical issues

In observational studies, it is the investigator's responsibility to maintain the confidentiality of the data provided by the study subjects and to ensure that the procedures used to measure the exposures and the outcomes of interest do not involve unacceptable levels of discomfort, stress or risk for the participants.

In intervention trials, however, the situation is different. Researchers are no longer simply observing what happens to the study subjects. Since the investigator is deliberately intervening, ethical considerations are more important than in any other type of epidemiological study. Intervention trials are ethically justified only in a situation of uncertainty, when there is genuine doubt concerning the value of a new intervention in terms of its benefits and risks. The researcher must have some evidence that it may be of benefit, for instance, from laboratory and animal studies, or from observational epidemiological studies. Otherwise, there would be no justification for conducting a trial.

Unfortunately, many medical interventions have never been properly evaluated in well conducted intervention trials. For instance, radical mastectomy was used for more than a hundred years as the standard form of treatment for early breast cancer. It was not until the late 1970s, when clinical trials were finally conducted, that this form of treatment was replaced by more conservative types of breast surgery. The clinical trials revealed that there were no differences in recurrence or survival between patients who underwent radical mastectomy and other (more conservative) types of surgery (Veronesi *et al.*, 1981; Fisher *et al.*, 1985). Thus, women with early breast cancer were unnecessarily subjected to a very mutilating form of surgery for decades because clinicians were convinced that it would have been unethical to deprive women of the standard form of therapy. The lesson from this, and many other examples, is that it is best to conduct a trial when any agent or procedure is first introduced rather than after it has gained widespread acceptance and becomes considered standard practice. Failure to carry out a proper trial, when it is needed and feasible, may also be unethical.

Whether a study is considered to be ethical or unethical is a subjective judgement based on cultural norms, which vary from society to society and over time. A useful reference with proposed guidelines for research involving human subjects is that published by the Council for International Organizations of Medical Sciences (CIOMS) and the World Health Organization (WHO) (1993).

7.4 Target and experimental populations

The *target population* is the general group to whom the investigators expect the results of the trial to be applicable. A trial may concern all human beings, if it is believed that the intervention to be assessed is of potential benefit to everyone, or only certain subgroups of the population, such as women or smokers. Thus, the target population represents the scope of the public health impact of the intervention.

Once the target population has been defined, one needs to select the actual population in which the study will be carried out (Figure 7.1). The choice of this *experimental population* depends on a number of issues. First, it should not differ from the target population in such a way that generalization to the latter is impossible, although this may be sacrificed in certain circumstances. For example, intervention studies are sometimes carried out among special groups such as volunteers to ensure good compliance or to facilitate the logistics. These trials are useful to evaluate the potential effect of a new intervention, even though it may be difficult to extrapolate the results to the target population. Second, it is essential to determine whether the proposed experimental population is sufficiently large to achieve the sample size necessary for the trial (see Chapter 15). Third, it is important to choose an experimental population that will experience a sufficient number of the outcomes of interest to permit meaningful comparisons between various treatments or procedures within a reasonable period of time. Thus, most trials are carried out in populations where the risk of developing the outcome(s) of interest is high. For instance, to assess the potential benefit of a smoking cessation programme, it would make sense to select as the experimental population one with a high prevalence of tobacco use and high incidence of lung cancer.

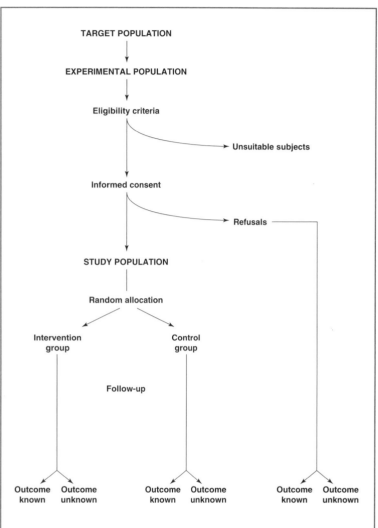

Figure 7.1.
General outline of an intervention trial.

The selection of the experimental population also depends on logistic factors. The study should be carried out in an area where it will be possible to obtain support from the local authorities or leaders of the community and where it will be possible to obtain complete and accurate follow-up information for the duration of the trial. For instance, conducting a long-term trial among a highly mobile population such as college students or nomads may result in low follow-up, which would compromise the study.

7.5   Eligibility criteria

Eligibility criteria must be clearly defined before the study begins (Figure 7.1). These should specify exactly who can be included in the study. The criteria will vary from study to study, but, in general, should be such as to eliminate subjects who may be put at greater risk by the intervention or who have an underlying condition that could interfere with the assessment. For instance, patients may be excluded if their physical and/or mental condition is inadequate to permit interview or collection of biological specimens. It is also usual to exclude pregnant women and women of childbearing age if there is any possibility, however minimal, that the intervention may be harmful to the fetus.

Once the eligibility criteria have been defined, it is possible to establish who are the eligible individuals in the experimental population. Sometimes, it may be necessary to carry out a baseline survey to identify eligible individuals, as in Example 7.5. In these circumstances, subjects must be invited to participate in the baseline survey although they may not fulfil the eligibility criteria for entry into the trial.

> *Example 7.5. An intervention study was carried out in The Gambia to determine the contribution of bedbugs to hepatitis B transmission. In order to be eligible for the trial, children had to be free from hepatitis B infection at the time of enrolment. All children aged six months to five years living in seven adjacent Mandinka villages were examined by a physician and had a sample of blood taken for serological testing. Only those found to be uninfected were then randomized into the intervention (insecticide spraying of the child's dwelling) or control groups (Mayans et al., 1994).*

7.6 Informed consent

The eligible subjects must then be invited to participate in the trial. At this stage, they should be fully informed in simple language of the aims of the study, its procedures, what exactly will be required from them, and of possible risks and benefits. They should also be informed that they will be allocated to either the intervention group or the comparison group and that they may not know which group have they been allocated to until the end of the trial. Subjects should also be assured that their privacy will be respected, that their identity will not be revealed to anyone outside the research team, and that the investigators will not use any information obtained during the study to their detriment (for instance, to compile tax lists). Individuals should be given enough time to consider whether they are willing to participate and they should be allowed to refuse or to withdraw their participation at any time without any negative consequences to them.

If the subjects, provided with this information, still decide to participate in the study, they are said to have given their *informed consent*. In many countries, ethical committees and grant-giving bodies require that the participants sign a consent form (sometimes in the presence of a witness). This may be difficult to accomplish and of relatively little meaning in populations with low levels of literacy.

All efforts should be made to try to explain the nature of the study in a way that the individuals can understand and that it is appropriate to their cultural values and norms. What is appropriate in the 'western' world is not necessarily appropriate in other cultural settings. For example, in some societies, decisions about participation in a study may be taken at a communal rather than an individual level. Thus, permission to conduct a research project may be obtained through respected community leaders, instead of from individual community members. But even if communal consent is obtained for the study, the investigator still has the responsibility to explain the study procedures and the potential risks and benefits to every single individual who may participate and to ensure that each is aware that he/she is free to refuse to participate or to withdraw from the investigation at any time.

There is a parallel to this situation in western societies. Communal rather than individual consent is generally obtained in community trials, since it is generally impossible to obtain consent from every single member of the communities involved. Consent should be obtained from the local authorities and community leaders. Once these persons have agreed to the communities' participation, it is important for the investigator to inform the community members themselves that they will be participating in a study.

7.7 Study population

Those who are eventually found to be both eligible and willing to enrol in the trial compose the actual *study population* and are often a relatively small and selected subgroup of the experimental population (Figure 7.1). Participants in an intervention study are very likely to differ from non-participants in many ways that may affect the risk of development of the outcomes under investigation. Whether or not the subgroup of participants is representative of the entire experimental population will not affect the validity of the results of a trial conducted among that group. It may, however, affect the ability to generalize those results to either the experimental or the target population.

Example 7.6. The Physicians' Health Study was a randomized, placebo-controlled, double-blind clinical trial conducted in the United States to assess the effects of aspirin on total cardiovascular mortality, and of beta-carotene on cancer incidence. The trial began in 1982, when letters were mailed to 261 248 US male physicians aged 40–84 years asking them to participate. Roughly half of them responded, of whom half again indicated they were willing to participate. Men with a history of cancer (except non-melanoma skin cancer), myocardial infarction, stroke or transient cerebral ischaemia were considered as ineligible. Thus only 33 211 physicians who were both willing and eligible were enrolled in the run-in phase of the trial, lasting from 1 to 6 months, in which they were assigned to active aspirin and beta-carotene placebo treatment. The purpose of this run-in phase was to enhance compliance, since only those physicians who tolerated aspirin and complied with the medication regime were randomized. At the end of this run-in phase, 22 071 were considered eligible for the trial and were randomized (Hennekens et al., 1985, 1996; Stampfer et al., 1985).

In Example 7.6, less than 10% of the original experimental population ultimately entered the trial. Only those physicians who had proven to be good compliers and experienced no adverse effects were randomized, to increase the ability (power) of the study to test the two study hypotheses (see Chapter 15). Although the exclusion of poor compliers limited the generalizability of the results of the trial, it did not affect their validity. In this example, it was far more important to obtain clear answers to the questions being addressed than to try to ensure that it would be possible to extrapolate the results to a wider population.

An effort should be made, however, to obtain baseline data and/or to ascertain outcomes for subjects who are eligible but unwilling to participate. Such information is extremely valuable to assess the presence and extent of differences between participants and non-participants in a particular trial. This will help in judging whether the results among trial participants are generalizable to the target population.

7.8 Choice of the comparison intervention

A key characteristic of an intervention trial is the inclusion of at least one comparison group, against which the effect of the intervention under study is compared. Consideration must be given to what type of intervention the control group should receive. For instance, in a clinical trial, should the control group receive a placebo (a procedure that resembles the new treatment in all respects except that it does not contain the active ingredient(s)), the current best treatment, or nothing at all?

If there is already an established treatment of proven value, it would be unethical to use a placebo. Moreover, in these circumstances, the real pragmatic question is not so much to show whether the new treatment really works but whether it is any better than the existing one. If there is no standard treatment, a placebo is justifiable on the grounds that it makes it possible for the study to be double-blind (see Section 7.11). However, for many interventions it is not possible to devise a suitable placebo. For instance, it is not possible to find a suitable placebo for surgical interventions or for most health education programmes.

7.9 Allocation to the various study groups

Since participants and non-participants may differ in important ways related to the outcome under study, allocation to the various study groups should take place *only after subjects have been determined to be eligible and have expressed willingness to participate*. That is, the non-participants should be eliminated from the pool of potential subjects before allocation to the intervention and control groups is carried out.

7.9.1 Reasons for random allocation

Random allocation is the best method of allocating the study subjects to the different study groups. This method allows chance, and only chance, to determine the assignment of subjects to the various groups. It is, therefore, the only way of ensuring that any differences in the outcome measures of the trial are due to the effects of the intervention rather than to underlying differences between the groups. Randomization has two major advantages in relation to other methods of allocation:

(1) *Randomization eliminates selection bias on the part of the participants and investigators.*

Randomization eliminates the possibility of any subjective influence in the assignment of individuals to the different study groups. Methods based upon date of birth or date of entry have also been used in some trials, with one intervention being assigned to those who were born (or who report) on even dates and another to those who were born (or who report) on odd dates. The problem with these methods is that it is possible for the investigator to know in advance the group to which a participant will be allocated and this could introduce conscious or unconscious bias into the allocation procedure. An investigator who knows that a particular subject is going to be allocated to a particular intervention may be more or less likely to consider the subject eligible for entry into the study. Randomization can ensure that this does not happen, provided it is done only after subjects have been determined to be eligible and have expressed willingness to participate in the trial.

(2) *Randomization tends to create groups that are comparable in terms of the distribution of known and, more importantly, unknown factors that may influence the outcome.*

Randomization ensures that the distribution of known and, more importantly, of *unknown* confounding variables will be similar in the groups to be compared, provided that the sample size is relatively large. This is unique to experimental studies. Although it is possible in observational studies to take into account the effect of confounders in the analysis, this can only be done for variables which were known or suspected to be confounders at the beginning of the study and for which data were therefore collected (see Chapters 13 and 14). Trials may extend over many years and it is possible that new confounders will become known in the meantime. This would not affect the validity of the results from a randomized trial, however, in which the distribution of any unknown confounding variables would be similar in the study groups *provided that the number of subjects randomized was large.*

In this discussion of randomization, it is worth mentioning that confusion often exists in the use of the expressions 'random allocation' (or 'random assignment') and 'random sampling' (or 'random selection'). In this section we are dealing with 'random allocation', namely the process by which subjects are allocated to the study groups in a trial. This constitutes a fundamental principle on which intervention studies are based. Random selection refers to the process whereby a sample of subjects is selected at random from a larger population. Clinical trials rarely entail random selection; the investigator takes the patients available to him/her, provided they meet the criteria for entry into the study. In field trials, random selection may be used if the experimental population is larger than is required to ensure that the study will have the ability to answer the problem being addressed (that is, that the trial will have adequate power or precision—see Chapter 15). Methods for selecting random samples from a population are discussed in Chapter 10.

7.9.2 Methods of randomization

Various methods can be used to randomize the study subjects to the different study groups. Regardless of the method chosen, it is important to ensure from the earliest stages of the trial that the randomization procedure and the randomization list will be concealed from the persons who are responsible for recruiting the subjects, monitoring the effects of the intervention and assessing the outcomes of the trial.

Simple randomization

Simple randomization is the most elementary method of randomization. It is the equivalent of tossing a coin. However, randomization by tossing a coin should not be used because it cannot be checked or reproduced. The alternative is to use a table of random numbers (or a computer-generated randomization list) (Figure 7.2).

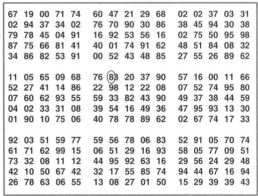

Figure 7.2.
Extract from a table of random numbers.

The first step in determining random group assignments is to set up a correspondence between the numbers in the table and the study groups. Let us assume that odd numbers correspond to the control group and even numbers to the new intervention. The second step is to define a convenient way of reading the table of random numbers, for instance, to read down the columns or across the rows.

The third step is to select a starting point, for instance, by closing your eyes and selecting a number with a pin. Once the starting point is established, numbers are then read from the table following the sequence defined in step two. Figure 7.2 is an extract of a table of random numbers (a full table is reproduced in Appendix 7.1). Suppose that the chosen starting point was the one circled in the table and that we have decided that numbers should be read column by column down the page. The first 10 numbers would have been 8, 9, 3, 5, 7, 5, 5, 9, 1, 0. The fourth step is to make the treatment assignments according to the system defined above (Table 7.1).

Random number tables are generated in such a way that each of the digits zero through nine is equally likely to occur. If equal numbers of participants are required in each intervention group, the same number of one-digit numbers should be assigned for each group, even if this means that some digits do not correspond to any group. Thus, in the case of three groups,

Patient no.	Sex	Random no.	Allocation
1	F	8	Intervention group
2	M	9	Control group
3	M	3	Control group
4	M	5	Control group
5	M	7	Control group
6	F	5	Control group
7	F	5	Control group
8	F	9	Control group
9	F	1	Control group
10	F	0	Intervention group

Table 7.1.
Example illustrating the use of a table of random numbers to allocate ten subjects to two study groups (see text).

three of the ten one-digit numbers are assigned to each group (e.g., numbers 1, 2, 3 to group A; 4, 5, 6 to group B; and 7, 8, 9 to group C). The remaining number (i.e., zero in our example) in the random tables is ignored and selection moves to the next number.

One of the disadvantages of simple randomization is that it may result in markedly unequal number of subjects being allocated to each group just by chance. For instance, in the above example, only two persons out of ten were assigned to the intervention group. Moreover, simple randomization may also result in the compositions of the different intervention groups being different with respect to factors that may affect the outcome measures in the trial. In the above example, not only was the number of persons allocated to the intervention small but the sex distribution was also quite different in the two groups. This is particularly likely to happen when the total number of subjects in a study is small. For trials involving several hundred participants or more, any such imbalance is likely to be small and can be taken into account in the analysis of the study. In a small trial, imbalance may make the trial more difficult to interpret and, hence, it is advisable to ensure balance by using the randomization methods described below.

Restricted randomization (or blocked randomization)

This method guarantees that the numbers of participants allocated to each study group are equal after every block of so many patients has entered the trial. Suppose that patients are going to be allocated to treatments A and B in such a way that after every fourth subject there are an equal number of participants on each treatment. There are only six possible combinations (permutations) of A and B in blocks of four:

No.	Combination
1	AABB
2	ABAB
3	ABBA
4	BBAA
5	BABA
6	BAAB

The combination for a particular block of four patients is chosen at random (by using a table of random numbers as described above) from the six possible (note that in the above example the digits 7, 8, 9 and 0 from the table of random numbers should be ignored). For instance, if the random numbers from the table were 2, 3, 6, 5 (and the blocks were assigned as listed), it would mean that patients 1–4, 5–8, 9–12, 13–16 would receive treatments ABAB, ABBA, BAAB and BABA, respectively. This procedure thus allocates eight patients to group A and eight to group B.

Stratified randomization

When the results of the trial are likely to vary between, say, the sexes or different age-groups, stratified randomization should be used. In this situation, strata or groups are formed and randomization occurs separately for the subjects in each stratum. As subjects become eligible for inclusion in the trial, their appropriate stratum is determined and they receive the next random-number assignment within that stratum. For example, patients may be classified according to sex and age (under 50, and 50 and over), yielding a total of four strata. Within each stratum, each patient will be randomly assigned to either the intervention or the control group. This could be done by using either simple or restricted randomization.

Stratified randomization has the advantage of assuring balance between the groups, at least on the characteristics that determine the strata. The use of this method of randomization in the example described above would ensure that the intervention and the control group would be balanced with respect to sex and age. If stratification had not been employed, the researcher would have run the risk that chance might produce imbalance with regard to these important factors, especially if the number of subjects in the trial was small. The disadvantage with stratified randomization is that it is administratively difficult and cumbersome to execute.

Matched-pair design

A matched-pair design is a special case of stratified randomization in which the strata are each of size 2. Individuals (or communities) are matched into pairs, chosen to be as similar as possible for potential confounding variables such that in the absence of any intervention they would be expected to be at similar risk of the disease under study. The intervention is assigned at random to one member of each pair, with the other member acting as a control.

Matching is unnecessary in large trials, as it is likely that any imbalance between the intervention groups, with respect to risk factors for the occurrence of the outcomes of interest, will tend to even out. Furthermore, it is possible to adjust for any residual imbalance during the data analysis without substantial loss of statistical power.

For small trials, more serious imbalance can arise for which it may be difficult to adjust fully in the analysis. This can be a special problem in trials in which communities are randomized, as it is unusual to be able to include large numbers of communities (more than 20) in such studies (Example 7.7). Pair-wise matching of similar communities (i.e., communities in which the rates of the disease are likely to be similar in the absence of the interventions to be applied) before the allocation of interventions is likely to be a useful strategy in such situations.

Example 7.7. In the Community Intervention Trial for Smoking Cessation (COMMIT) mentioned in Example 7.3, within each pair, communities were matched on factors such as population demographic characteristics (e.g., population size, age, sex and ethnic composition), degree of urbanization, socioeconomic factors, prevalence of smoking and access to media and health care services. The two paired communities were geographically close enough to permit monitoring by the investigators, but not so close that educational activities in the intervention community would affect the control community. One member of each of the 11 matched pairs was then randomly assigned to receive the health education programme and the other to the control surveillance (COMMIT Research Group, 1991).

7.9.3   Some special experimental designs
Factorial design

One technique to improve efficiency in intervention trials is to test two or more hypotheses simultaneously in a factorial design. A trial of two hypothesis can utilize a two-by-two factorial design, in which subjects are first randomized to intervention A or B to address one hypothesis, and then within each intervention group there is further randomization to interventions C and D to evaluate a second question (Example 7.8).

Example 7.8. The Physicians' Health Study described in Example 7.6 used a 2 × 2 factorial design. The physicians were assigned to one of four groups, as shown in Figure 7.3.

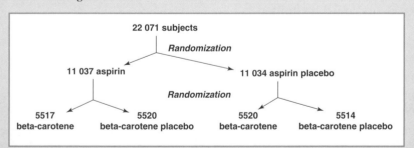

Figure 7.3.
Outline of the factorial design of the Physicians' Health Study.

This design allowed the study of two different questions related to two different diseases: (1) does aspirin reduce the risk of cardiovascular diseases? (2) does beta-carotene reduces the risk of cancer? In addition, it was possible to examine the combined effect of the two drugs on the occurrence of these two diseases (Hennekens et al., 1985; Stampfer et al., 1985).

The principal advantage of the factorial design is its ability to answer two or more questions in a single trial for only a marginal increase in cost. Moreover, the use of a factorial design also allows the assessment of interactions between interventions, which cannot be done in a single-factor study.

Crossover trials

Most trials have a *parallel* design, that is, a group of subjects receives the intervention and another parallel group receives the standard treatment or placebo. In contrast, in *crossover trials* each subject acts as his/her own control by receiving at least two different interventions (e.g., a new drug (treatment A) versus the standard drug (treatment B)) at different times during the trial (Figure 7.4). The order in which each individual receives them (A then B or B then A) should be determined by random allocation (Example 7.9). There should be a 'wash-out' period between each of the interventions to avoid 'carry-over effects' (also called 'spill-over effects'), that is, to ensure that there is no overlap of effects between the first and the second interventions. Consequently, this design is suitable only when neither of the interventions has long-term effects.

The main advantage of crossover trials is that each subject is compared with himself/herself and, therefore, confounding is eliminated from the comparison of the effects of the two treatments (provided that there is no carry-over effect). This design also increases statistical precision in the comparison, because it eliminates inter-subject variability in the outcome response. Hence, fewer subjects are needed than in a corresponding parallel trial.

Crossover trials are used mostly in the early phases of evaluation of new drugs in which their pharmacokinetic properties are investigated in healthy volunteers. They are not appropriate to assess the long-term effects of a treatment, as the nature of the design implies that the treatment period must be limited.

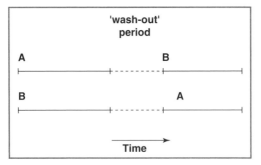

Figure 7.4.
Outline of a crossover trial

Example 7.9. *Thirty-one patients with a diagnosis of metastatic germ-cell tumour and receiving a four-day course of a chemotherapy regimen containing cisplatin were entered in a randomized, double-blind, crossover trial. The objective of this trial was to assess whether oral ondansetron (a serotonin antagonist) plus dexamethasone was more effective than oral ondansetron plus placebo in controlling the emesis associated with chemotherapy. During the first course of chemotherapy, patients were randomly allocated to one of the arms of the trial. Participants were given one of the treatments for eight days. A second course of chemotherapy was given 14 days after the start of the first during which patients crossed over to the alternative anti-emetic regimen (Smith et al., 1991).*

7.9.4. Conclusions

It should be emphasized that allocation of subjects to the study groups should be done only after having ascertained that individuals are both eligible and willing to participate. Otherwise subjects who refuse to participate or who withdraw from the study (because the treatment is inappropriate, etc.) will have to be excluded after the randomization, so that the groups may no longer be comparable. This is illustrated in Example 7.10.

Example 7.10. The effect of breast cancer screening on mortality from breast cancer was examined in a randomized trial. Women aged 40–64 years who were members of the Health Insurance Plan of New York were randomly allocated to two groups: an intervention group, whose members were offered four screening examinations (clinical examinations and mammography) at annual intervals; and a control group, who continued to receive their usual medical care. There were about 31 000 women in each group. The groups were very similar with respect to a wide range of demographic and other characteristics. Thirty-five per cent of those offered screening refused (Shapiro, 1977). Table 7.2 shows levels of mortality from causes other than breast cancer for each of the two study groups.

Study group	No. of deaths	Death rate (per 10 000 person-years)
Intervention group	850	57
Screened	421	42
Refused	429	86
Control group	877	58
[a] Data from Shapiro (1977).		

Table 7.2.
Mortality from causes other than breast cancer by the end of the first five years of follow-up.[a]

Table 7.2 shows that there was a large difference in mortality from causes other than breast cancer between women who actually received the intervention (i.e., who were screened) and those in the control group (42 versus 58 per 10 000 pyrs). Since the intervention under study (i.e., breast screening) should not have affected mortality from causes other than breast cancer, the observed difference seem to indicate that the two groups were different in relation to important baseline characteristics. However, if those who refused after randomization were included in the intervention group, as they should be, there is no longer a mortality difference between the two groups (57 versus 58 per 10 000 pyrs).

Random allocation does not necessarily guarantee that the groups will be similar. Discrepancies between the groups may arise just by chance, especially if the number of units being allocated (e.g., individuals, families, communities) is relatively small. Hence, it is essential to collect baseline data on the subjects. These baseline data should include all the variables which are known or thought to affect the outcome(s) of interest and can be used to check the degree of similarity of the groups. If the study groups differ, statistical techniques can be used that yield results 'adjusted' for any baseline differences (see Chapters 13 and 14).

7.10 Monitoring compliance and side-effects

The problem of achieving and maintaining high compliance is an important issue in the design and conduct of any trial. This is because non-compliance makes the intervention and the comparison groups more alike and, consequently, reduces the ability of the trial to detect any true difference between their outcome measures. A certain degree of non-compliance is acceptable in pragmatic trials, which are aimed at estimating the effectiveness of the intervention in real-life conditions. The aim of scientific trials, however, is to estimate the maximum potential benefit to be derived from the intervention in ideal circumstances, including compliance of 100%. One way of increasing compliance is to use a 'run-in phase' before randomization, as was illustrated in Example 7.6.

Compliance levels must be measured and monitored throughout the study. This can be done by using self-reports. This approach has the disadvantage that it relies exclusively on subjects' judgement and memory. Return of unused medication (e.g., tablets) to the investigators at regular intervals has been used in trials that involve administration of drugs or active substances. However, this method assumes that the subject has taken all the medication that was not returned. Self-reports are sometimes validated against laboratory measurements. Apart from being expensive, these methods also have limited value since they usually measure current and not long-term compliance.

In Example 7.11, the alpha-tocopherol and beta-carotene measurements made three years after entry into the trial were much higher than at baseline in those subjects who were allocated to receive these active ingredients, but changed little in those who were not allocated to receive them (Table 7.3). These findings indicate high levels of compliance.

In most trials, a proportion of participants inevitably become non-compliant for one reason or another (forgetting to take the drugs, developing secondary effects, etc). In such instances, maintaining any level of compliance is preferable to complete non-compliance. Moreover, as will be discussed in Section 7.12, every randomized subject should be included in the primary analysis of any intervention study, so that it is essential to obtain as complete follow-up information as possible on those who have discontinued the intervention programme. Investigators should follow up such individuals for the duration of the trial and obtain information on the relevant outcomes in the same way as for subjects who continue to comply.

Sometimes those who were randomized to one group may choose to obtain the alternative intervention on their own initiative. For instance, those allocated to the control group may adopt the active treatment under study. It is important to minimize this 'contamination' as much as possible. One way is to design the trial in such a way that opportunities of contamination are reduced. For instance, in Example 7.4, flights rather than

Example 7.11. The Alpha-Tocopherol, Beta-Carotene (ATBC) Cancer Prevention Study was a randomized, double-blind, placebo-controlled trial to determine whether daily supplementation with alpha-tocopherol, beta carotene or both would reduce the incidence of lung and other cancers. A total of 29 133 male smokers aged 50 to 69 years were randomly assigned to one of four regimens: alpha-tocopherol (50 mg per day) alone; beta-carotene (20 mg per day) alone; both alpha-tocopherol and beta-carotene; or placebo. Follow-up lasted for five to eight years. Compliance was assessed by counts of the remaining capsules at each visit, by measurement of serum levels of alpha-tocopherol and beta-carotene after three years of supplementation (Table 7.3), and by measurements in random serum samples throughout the study (Alpha-Tocopherol, Beta Carotene Cancer Prevention Study Group, 1994).

Treatment received	No. of subjects	Median	20th percentile	80th percentile
Serum alpha-tocopherol levels at baseline				
Alpha-tocopherol	14 472	11.5	9.3	14.2
No alpha-tocopherol	14 469	11.4	9.3	14.1
Serum alpha-tocopherol levels at three years				
Alpha-tocopherol	11 332	17.3	14.3	21.1
No alpha-tocopherol	11 258	12.4	10.2	15.1
Serum beta-carotene levels at baseline				
Beta-carotene	14 460	0.17	0.10	0.29
No beta-carotene	14 460	0.17	0.10	0.29
Serum beta-carotene levels at three years				
Beta-carotene	11 276	3.0	1.6	4.5
No beta-carotene	11 314	0.18	0.10	0.30
[a] Data from Alpha-Tocopherol, Beta Carotene Cancer Prevention Study Group (1994).				

Table 7.3.
Serum concentrations (milligrams per litre) of alpha-tocopherol and beta-carotene at baseline and after three years of supplementation by study group.[a]

individuals were chosen as the unit of randomization to minimize contamination. Similarly, in a community trial to evaluate the impact of a smoking cessation programme, it is important that the intervention and the control communities are geographically distinct units with stable populations and no migration between them (as in Example 7.7). Nevertheless, sometimes a certain degree of contamination is inevitable for reasons that are outside the control of the researchers.

In Example 7.12, no difference in the prevalence of oesophageal lesions was found by the end of the trial between the placebo and the treated groups. Laboratory measurements carried out at the time of entry into the study and two months later confirmed that there was a rise in vitamin levels in the active treatment group, but also revealed that the levels of retinol had improved in the placebo group. The change in the placebo group was probably due to better access to fresh fruits and vegetables (Muñoz *et al.*, 1985).

> *Example 7.12.* A randomized double-blind intervention trial was carried out in Huixian, People's Republic of China, to determine whether combined treatment with retinol, riboflavin and zinc for one year would reduce the prevalence of precancerous lesions of the oesophagus. A total of 610 subjects aged 35–64 years were randomized to the active treatment or placebo. Compliance was very good. At the end of the trial, the prevalence of oesophageal lesions was similar in the two groups: 45.3% in the placebo group and 48.9% in the intervention group (Muñoz et al., 1985).

A similar contamination problem occurred in the anti-smoking advice trial described in Example 7.2. During the 20-year period that the trial lasted, there was a progressive decline in the prevalence of smoking in the control group (Rose & Colwell, 1992) reflecting a general increase in the awareness of the negative health consequences of smoking. This contamination made the two study groups more alike and reduced the ability of the study to measure the health effects of stopping smoking.

It is also important to monitor any side-effects that might develop. A surveillance mechanism should be set up to allow the breaking of the randomization code if any subject develops serious side-effects. Monitoring side-effects not only is necessary to ensure the safety of the study participants, but also will help to assess the real benefits and hazards of the intervention under study.

7.11 Ascertainment of outcomes

The outcomes of interest should be clearly defined before the start of the trial. The choice of the outcome of interest has important implications for the duration of the trial. Most field trials in cancer epidemiology are aimed at reducing the risk of this disease. Since field trials are conducted among disease-free people, the probability of developing cancer is relatively small and may not be observable for several decades. The problem is less critical in cancer clinical trials, since most of the outcomes of interest (e.g., recurrence or death) tend to occur with a high probability.

One way of shortening the duration of a trial is to select a population that has an increased risk of developing the outcome of interest. For instance, in a field trial to assess the impact of a smoking cessation programme on lung cancer mortality rates, it makes sense to exclude all persons aged under 45 years, since lung cancer is rare at these ages.

Another possibility is to use intermediate endpoints as cancer surrogates, i.e., to use as outcome a biological event that is believed to lie on the causal pathway between exposure and cancer. Studies that use intermediate endpoints are quicker, smaller, and less expensive than studies that use malignancy as the outcome. However, the relevance of the results of the trial with respect to cancer depends on the strength of the association between the intermediate endpoint and the clinical cancer.

> **Example 7.13.** *A randomized, multicentre trial has been set up to test a dietary approach to decreasing the risk of recurrence of polyps of the large bowel. Patients with one or more histologically proven adenomatous polyps, who have had complete removal of polyps at colonoscopy, will be randomly assigned either to usual diet or to nutrition education and counselling aimed at a lifestyle change to a low-fat, high-fibre diet enriched with fruits and vegetables. The trial includes 2000 patients with planned follow-up of four years; colonoscopy will be repeated at years 1 and 4. The major outcome is recurrence of adenomas. The trial is based on the postulate that most large bowel cancers arise from adenomatous polyps. The results of the trial should provide useful evidence about the ability of dietary change to affect recurrence of adenomatous polyps and, hence, to affect indirectly the incidence of large bowel cancer (Chlebowski & Grosvenor, 1994).*

In Example 7.13, only 2000 individuals and a four-year follow-up were required, a substantially smaller number than would have been necessary for a trial having large bowel cancer as the outcome. The underlying assumption in these studies is that the observed relationship between exposure (e.g., diet) and intermediate endpoint (e.g., polyps) reflects a similar one between exposure and cancer *per se*. Clearly, this assumption needs to be validated before any intermediate endpoint can be used as a cancer surrogate (Lippman *et al.*, 1990).

The outcomes should be ascertained in such a way that measurement bias is minimized as far as possible. Blind or masking techniques provide the means for achieving this. When there is no standard intervention to be used in a blind study for comparison with the new intervention, placebos should be employed to maintain blindness. The placebo should be as similar as possible to the intervention itself (with respect to appearance, taste, etc.). Whenever possible, both the patient and the investigators should be unaware of who is assigned to each group until the end of the trial. Such a '*double-blind*' design (both the investigator and the participants are 'blind') eliminates the possibility that knowledge of which intervention an individual is allocated to will affect the way that individual is treated or monitored during the trial, the way the individual responds to the intervention or the way the individual is assessed at the end of the trial. A double-blind trial may not be feasible for the evaluation of programmes involving substantial changes in lifestyle, such as exercise, cigarette smoking or diet, surgical procedures, or drugs with characteristic side-effects. In these circumstances, a '*single-blind*' (the investigator knows to which group a participant belongs but the participant does not or vice-versa) or an unblinded design may be the only possibility.

The more subjective the outcome under study, the greater is the rationale for a double-blind trial. For example, if one deals with extremely subjective responses such as the relief of pain, or the improvement of psychological status, the use of double-blinding is crucial to the validity of the outcome measurements. When the outcome of a trial is more objective (for example, life or death, or perhaps the level of some substances in the blood or urine), the need for a double-blind trial is, obviously, less important.

The main strength of a double-blind design is to eliminate the potential for measurement bias. Of course, a concomitant limitation is that such trials are usually more complex and difficult to conduct. Procedures must be established for immediate 'unblinding' of a participant's physician in the event of serious side-effects or other clinical emergencies in which this information seems essential.

7.12 Analysis

7.12.1 Types of analysis

There are two main approaches to the analysis of a trial according to who should or should not be included. The 'intention to treat' analysis is based on outcomes that occur during the whole follow-up period, in the subjects originally allocated to each group, whether they persisted with their allocated intervention or not. The alternative is the 'on randomized treatment' analysis, which is confined to the outcomes observed while the subjects were on their allocated treatment. Exclusion of randomized subjects of a trial from the analysis may lead to serious bias that can arise from different levels of participation in the intervention and control groups and from the fact that individuals who withdraw or who were lost to follow-up are usually different from those who participate until the end. 'Intention to treat' analysis is the correct way of analysing the data, involving comparison of the outcomes in all the subjects originally allocated to each group (including those who did not have or who stopped having the specified intervention). This stringent approach may sometimes, however, dilute the true effect of the intervention.

7.12.2 On-going analysis

Analysis of results from a trial as data accumulate is an important way of monitoring its progress. Administrative analyses of the numbers of participants recruited each day or week and of the data collected by different field workers are important for quality control.

An independent data-monitoring committee is often set up in large trials to hold the randomization code of the study and to monitor the results of the trial as they come in, or at fixed intervals during the trial. This committee should have the power to stop further recruitment if there is evidence of a substantial risk of adverse reactions associated with any of the interventions under study. Similarly, if evidence accumulates that one intervention is substantially better than the others (or one is substantially worse), the committee can recommend that the intervention phase of the trial be stopped and all participants be given the better (or less harmful) treatment or intervention. It would be very difficult for the investigators to remain objective and impartial if they had to take these decisions themselves.

Example 7.14. The Beta Carotene and Retinol Efficacy Trial (CARET) is a multicentre, randomized, double-blind, placebo-controlled trial set up in 1983 to assess whether a combination of beta-carotene and retinol (vitamin A) could reduce the incidence of lung cancer in populations at high risk. A total of 14 254 heavy smokers and 4060 workers exposed to asbestos were randomized to the active intervention (beta-carotene and vitamin A) or placebo. The design of the trial stipulated that the administration of the intervention should last until late 1997. In January 1996, however, the data-monitoring committee decided to terminate the intervention because it became apparent that there was a 28% increase (95% confidence interval, 0.4% to 57%; P = 0.02) in the risk of lung cancer in the intervention group compared to the placebo group. Follow-up for additional cases is expected to continue for another five years (Omenn et al., 1996).

In Example 7.14, the intervention phase of the trial was terminated early. Post-intervention follow-up of the study subjects will continue for five years to identify additional lung cancer cases and to assess the long-term effects of the intervention.

7.12.3 Final analysis

The first step in the analysis of a trial is to examine the characteristics of the two (or more) groups at baseline to assess their comparability, determining whether randomization resulted in the formation of comparable and evenly balanced groups (Example 7.15). This comparison should constitute the first table of the results section of a paper.

Statistical tests are frequently carried out to assess whether baseline differences between the study groups are important. A statistical test yields the probability of finding by chance a difference at least as large as the one observed. We know, however, that all the observed differences, regardless of their magnitude, have arisen just by chance since the subjects were randomized. Thus, *statistical tests are superfluous and inappropriate to assess whether the study groups have similar baseline characteristics.*

Examination of the baseline characteristics of the groups can also help to reveal any unknown problems that may have occurred during the randomization procedure. For instance, if the baseline characteristics of the groups turn out to be very dissimilar, the entire randomization procedure should be checked for possible deception by some of those in charge of recruiting the subjects into the trial.

After ascertaining the comparability of the study groups, the investigator must determine whether the intervention was of any value. The two groups are compared and the size of the differences assessed. In general, the main results from a trial can be presented in a table similar to one of those shown in Table 7.5.

Table 7.4.

Distribution of baseline characteristics among heavy smokers and asbestos workers who participated in the CARET trial according to type of intervention received.[a]

Example 7.15. *The baseline characteristics of the participants in the CARET trial described in Example 7.14 are shown in Table 7.4. The intervention group and the placebo group were similar in relation to a large number of factors that might have influenced the main outcome of the study, i.e., the incidence of lung cancer.*

Characteristic	Workers exposed to asbestos		Heavy smokers	
	Intervention	Placebo	Intervention	Placebo
No. randomized	2044	2016	7376	6878
Age (yrs)[b]	57±7	57±7	58±5	58±5
Female[c]	0	0	3208 (43)	3081 (45)
Race or ethnic group[c]				
White	1805 (88)	1775 (88)	7000 (95)	6487 (94)
Black	152 (7)	153 (8)	103 (1)	122 (2)
Hispanic	36 (2)	43 (2)	101 (1)	95 (1)
Other/unknown	51 (2)	45 (2)	172 (2)	174 (3)
Smoking status[c]				
Never smoked	68 (3)	64 (3)	0	0
Former smoker	1195 (58)	1175 (58)	2473 (34)	2331 (34)
Current smoker	781 (38)	777 (39)	4903 (66)	4547 (66)
Cigarettes smoked/day[b]				
Former smoker	25±12	25±12	28±11	28±11
Current smoker	24±10	25±10	24±9	24±8
Pack-years of smoking (only former and current smokers)[b]	43±24	42±24	50±21	49±20
Years since quitting smoking (only former smokers)[b]	10±8	10±8	3±2	3±2

[a] Data from Omenn *et al.* (1996)
[b] Mean ± standard deviation.
[c] Number (%).

(a)

	Exposure	
	Intervention	Control
Outcome Yes	a	b
No	c	d

Risk in intervention group (p_1) = $a/(a+c)$
Risk in control group (p_0) = $b/(b+d)$
Risk ratio = p_1/p_0
Risk difference[a] = $p_0 - p_1$

(b)

	Exposure	
	Intervention	Control
Cases	a	b
Person-time at risk	y_1	y_0

Rate in intervention group (r_1) = a/y_1
Rate in control group (r_0) = b/y_0
Rate ratio = r_1/r_0
Rate difference[a] = $r_0 - r_1$

[a] In most trials the intervention is protective and thus it is appropriate to calculate the risk and rate difference as indicated (see Section 5.2.2). If the intervention is associated with an increase in incidence, the risk and rate difference should be calculated as $p_1 - p_0$ or $r_1 - r_0$, respectively.

Table 7.5.

Analysis of an intervention study: (a) by risk; (b) by rates.

If all or virtually all participants enter and leave the trial at the same time, the risk can be calculated (Table 7.5(a)). For example, if the follow-up period is uniformly three years, the three-year risk can be computed for each study group. The two study groups can be compared by calculating risk ratios and risk differences as measures of relative and absolute effect, respectively.

In Example 7.16, practically all participants entered the trial at the same point in time and were followed up until its end. If one assumes that, on average, the deaths in each treatment group occurred at similar points in time, the calculation of risk as a measure of disease occurrence is appropriate. The results from this trial were consistent with the null hypothesis of no treatment-associated difference in the risk of lung cancer, that is, a risk ratio equal to 1 (or a risk difference equal to zero).

Example 7.16. *In the Physicians' Health Study described in Examples 7.6 and 7.8, 22 071 US male physicians aged 40 to 84 years were randomized in 1982 to receive one of four treatments: (1) aspirin plus beta-carotene placebo; (2) beta-carotene plus aspirin placebo; (3) both active agents; (4) both placebos. The randomized aspirin complement of the trial was terminated early, in 1988, by the external data-monitoring board because it became apparent that there was a 44% reduction (P < 0.001) in the risk of a first myocardial infarction in those taking aspirin. The randomized beta-carotene component continued uninterrupted until its scheduled termination in 31 December 1995. A total of 11 036 physicians received beta-carotene and 11 035 received beta-carotene placebo and fewer than 1% were lost to follow-up. One of the main aims of this component of the study was to assess whether beta-carotene reduces the incidence of lung cancer (Hennekens et al., 1996). Table 7.6 shows the results.*

		Study group	
		Beta-carotene	Placebo
Lung cancer	**Yes**	82	88
	No	10 954	10 947
	Total	11 036	11 035

[a] Data from Hennekens *et al.*, 1996

$p_1 = 82/11\ 036 = 0.00743 = 7.43$ per 1000
$p_0 = 88/11\ 035 = 0.00797 = 7.97$ per 1000
$\chi^2 = 0.21$, 1 d.f.; $P > 0.50$
Risk ratio $(p_1/p_0) = 0.93$
95% confidence interval for the risk ratio = 0.69 to 1.26
Risk difference $(p_0 - p_1) = 7.97$ per 1000 $- 7.43$ per 1000 = 0.54 per 1000
95% confidence interval for the risk difference = -1.77 per 1000 to 2.85 per 1000

(Test statistics and confidence intervals were calculated using the formulae given in Appendix 6.1).

Table 7.6.
Distribution of lung cancer incident cases in the Physicians' Health Study, according to treatment group.[a]

Many intervention trials, however, involve varying periods of follow-up. Recruitment into the trial may take several years and if the follow-up is terminated at a specific point in calendar time, participants will have been observed for different lengths of time. Also, subjects are lost to follow-up or die at different points in time during the study, and consequently they will have been part of the trial for different periods.

Calculation of person-time of observation as the denominator for computation of rates is the method generally used in intervention trials when varying periods of observation (which result from persons entering and leaving the study at different ages and times) have to be taken into account. Results of the trial can be presented as in Table 7.5(*b*), and rate ratios and rate differences calculated as measures of relative and absolute effect, respectively.

Example 7.17. *The objective of the ATBC trial (described in Example 7.11) was to assess whether daily supplementation with alpha-tocopherol, beta-carotene or both would reduce the incidence of lung cancer and other cancers. A total of 29 133 male smokers aged 50 to 69 years from south-western Finland were recruited between 1985 and 1988. Follow-up continued for 5–8 years (median = 6.1), until death or 30 April 1993, when the trial ended (Alpha-Tocopherol, Beta Carotene Cancer Prevention Study Group, 1994). The results by type of treatment received are shown in Figure 7.5.*

Figure 7.5.
Number of cancer cases and incidence rates by site and type of treatment received (reproduced with permission from Alpha-Tocopherol, Beta Carotene Cancer Prevention Study Group, 1994).

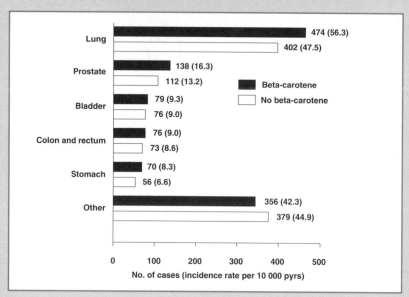

The results for lung cancer incidence in relation to beta-carotene supplementation can be presented as shown in Table 7.7.

Table 7.7.
Distribution of lung cancer cases and person-years at risk according to treatment received.[a]

	Study group	
	Beta-carotene	No beta-carotene
Lung cancer cases	474	402
Person-years at risk	84 192	84 632

[a] Data from Alpha-Tocopherol, Beta Carotene Cancer Prevention Study Group, 1994

r_1 = 474/84 192 = 56.3 per 10 000 pyrs

r_0 = 402/84 632 = 47.5 per 10 000 pyrs

χ^2 = 6.30; 1 d.f.; $P \approx 0.01$

Rate ratio (r_1/r_0) = 1.19

95% confidence intervals for the rate ratio = 1.04 to 1.36

Rate difference (r_1-r_0) = 8.8 per 10 000 pyrs

95% confidence interval for the rate difference = 1.9 to 15.7 per 10 000 pyrs

(Test statistics and confidence intervals were calculated using the formulae given in Appendix 6.1).

In Example 7.17, the duration of follow-up varied from subject to subject. Thus it is more appropriate to calculate person-time at risk and rates as the measure of occurrence of disease. The results of this trial did not support the study hypothesis that beta-carotene reduces the incidence of lung cancer. In fact, they provide evidence that administration of beta-carotene may increase the risk of lung cancer.

Statistical tests and, more importantly, confidence intervals for measures of relative and absolute effect should always be calculated and reported. In Examples 7.16 and 7.17, we used the formulae presented in Appendix 6.1.

The *prevented fraction* (see Section 5.2.2) is another important measure in intervention trials. It measures the proportion of cases of disease that were prevented by the intervention under study among those who received it.

Prevented fraction (%) = 100 × [rate (or risk) difference/rate (or risk) in the unexposed]

If the aim of the trial is to assess the value of a vaccine, this measure is called *vaccine efficacy*. For instance, if the risk of developing a particular disease among those who were vaccinated was 40 per 100 000 and 70 per 100 000 among those not vaccinated, the vaccine efficacy would be

Vaccine efficacy (%) = 100 × [(70 per 100 000 – 40 per 100 000)/70 per 100 000]
= 43%

Thus, 43% of cases could have been prevented among the unvaccinated if they had been vaccinated.

If baseline differences between the study groups need to be taken into account in the analysis, one of the statistical techniques discussed in Chapter 14 should be used.

If we are particularly interested in the distribution of *time until occurrence of the event of interest* (e.g., time from treatment to death or time from treatment to recurrence), as is the case in many clinical trials, the most appropriate approach is *survival analysis*. The techniques used in survival analysis derive from the life-table methods which are discussed in Chapter 12.

Subgroup analysis

It is usual for investigators to perform subgroup analyses to assess whether the intervention has an effect on subgroups of individuals with certain characteristics (e.g., males, elderly people, patients with particular clinical features, etc.). These subgroup analyses raise important problems, however. If the *subgroups are defined according to the baseline characteristics* of the patients, the main concern involves loss of ability of the trial to detect an effect (that is, loss of statistical power or precision (see Chapter

15)), since the results will be based on only a small proportion of the total numbers of randomized subjects. On the other hand, if multiple analyses are performed, some will inevitably achieve 'statistical significance' just by chance. Their interpretation will depend very much on the existence of *a priori* hypotheses based on biological plausibility, existence of supporting evidence from laboratory experiments and from other epidemiological observations.

Analyses performed on *subgroups defined on the basis of individual characteristics which develop after randomization* are of much greater concern, because potential confounding variables will no longer be distributed at random among the subgroups. For instance, analyses restricted to persons who reached a certain serum concentration of the active treatment or who developed a well known secondary effect (e.g., skin yellowing after ingesting beta-carotene) should be treated with extreme caution. Their findings should never be reported as main results of the trial but just as interesting observations that might be worth investigating in specifically designed trials.

7.13 Interpretation

The interpretation of results from a well conducted intervention study should be relatively straightforward, since the two major problems of concern in observational studies, bias and confounding, are greatly reduced by using an experimental design.

This is not to say that trials are exempt from problems. The lung cancer beta-carotene story provides a good illustration of this. Data from three large-scale chemoprevention trials conducted in western countries to assess this question have now been published. The ATBC Cancer Prevention Study (Example 7.11) was set up in Finland to test the hypothesis that a high intake of beta-carotene and alpha-tocopherol reduces the risk of lung cancer. This was a reasonable hypothesis given the substantial evidence available from observational epidemiological studies suggesting that beta-carotene was associated with a lower risk of lung cancer. The results of this trial failed to show any benefit of beta-carotene (or alpha-tocopherol) in the prevention of this malignancy; instead, men who took beta-carotene had an unexpected 'statistically significant' increase in the risk of lung cancer (as we saw in Example 7.17). The authors did consider alternative explanations for this unexpected finding. Confounding could be discarded given the large sample size and the random allocation of subjects to the various study groups. Moreover, the treatment groups were well balanced in relation to relevant baseline characteristics. Since this result was not supported by biological or previous epidemiological evidence, the authors were reluctant to reject the null hypothesis of no effect. They stated at the end of their paper:

"In summary, we found no overall reduction in the incidence of lung cancer or in mortality due to this disease among male smokers who received dietary supplementation with alpha-tocopherol, beta-carotene, or both in this large trial in Finland. The results of this study raise the possibility that these substances may have harmful effects as well as beneficial effects. Longer observation of the participants in this trial and data from other studies of people at normal or high risk for cancer will be required to determine the full spectrum of effects of these agents. Public health recommendations about supplementation with these micronutrients would be premature at this time" (Alpha-Tocopherol, Beta Carotene Cancer Prevention Study Group, 1994).

Results from two other trials were subsequently published. The active-intervention phase of the CARET trial (Example 7.14) was terminated early because its results confirmed the unexpected increase of lung cancer risk among those who took beta-carotene reported by the ATBC trial. There was again no obvious explanation for this unexpected finding. The Physicians' Health Study (Example 7.8) had a much longer follow-up (12 years) than the other two trials (average of 6 and 4 years for the ATBC and CARET trials, respectively). Its results were consistent with the null hypothesis of no effect of beta-carotene on the risk of lung cancer; in other words, they did not provide evidence of either a beneficial or a harmful effect of beta-carotene. Thus, the lung cancer beta-carotene story shows that results from a single trial should not be considered in isolation.

The results of a trial cannot be translated directly into public health decisions. Other factors that need to be taken into account include issues such as generalizability of the results to different populations, acceptability of the intervention, feasibility, costs, available resources and competing public health priorities. Furthermore, the overall impact of an intervention in a particular population depends not only on the magnitude of the effect of the intervention on the risk of developing a particular condition, but also on the frequency (and severity) of the condition in the population. This issue is further discussed in Chapter 16.

Further reading

* The book by Smith & Morrow (1996) provides a comprehensive coverage of the design, implementation and monitoring of field trials, with particular emphasis on practical aspects. Although the focus is on developing countries, most of the issues discussed in this book are also relevant to developed countries.

* The book by Pocock (1983) provides a good and accessible reference for those interested in the design, analysis and interpretation of clinical trials.

* A short review of methodological issues in design, analysis and interpretation of cancer clinical trials can be found in two papers by Peto *et al.* (1976, 1977).

Box 7.1. Key issues

• Intervention trials are characterized by the fact that investigators are responsible for allocating subjects to the different study groups.

• The main advantages of this type of study are:

  1. *Random allocation* of subjects ensures that allocation of subjects to the different study groups is unaffected by selection bias.

  2. *Random allocation* ensures that the groups are well balanced in relation to known and, more importantly, unknown factors that may affect the outcome(s) of the study (provided the study is sufficiently large).

  3. If the allocation is *double-blind*, measurement bias is also minimized.

  4. *Multiple outcomes* can be studied for any one intervention.

  5. Incidence of disease can be measured in the various study groups.

• The main disadvantages of this type of study are:

  1. Intervention trials, particularly field trials, are large enterprises. They are very expensive and time-consuming.

  2. They may raise important ethical problems.

  3. It may be difficult to ensure compliance and avoid contamination throughout the trial, particularly in trials of long duration.

Appendix 7.1
Table of random numbers

16 22 77 94 39	49 54 43 54 82	17 37 93 23 78	87 35 20 96 43	84 26 34 91 64
84 42 17 53 31	57 24 55 06 88	77 04 74 47 67	21 76 33 50 25	83 92 12 06 76
63 01 63 78 59	16 95 55 67 19	98 10 50 71 75	12 86 73 58 07	44 39 52 38 79
33 21 12 34 29	78 64 56 07 82	52 42 07 44 38	15 51 00 13 42	99 66 02 79 54
57 60 86 32 44	09 47 27 96 54	49 17 46 09 62	90 52 84 77 27	08 02 73 43 28
18 18 07 92 46	44 17 16 58 09	79 83 86 19 62	06 76 50 03 10	55 23 64 05 05
26 62 38 97 75	84 16 07 44 99	83 11 46 32 24	20 14 85 88 45	10 93 72 88 71
23 42 40 64 74	82 97 77 77 81	07 45 32 14 08	32 98 94 07 72	93 85 79 10 75
52 36 28 19 95	50 92 26 11 97	00 56 76 31 38	80 22 02 53 53	86 60 42 04 53
37 85 94 35 12	83 39 50 08 30	42 34 07 96 88	54 42 06 87 98	35 85 29 48 39
70 29 17 12 13	40 33 20 38 26	13 89 51 03 74	17 76 37 13 04	07 74 21 19 30
56 62 18 37 35	96 83 50 87 75	97 12 25 93 47	70 33 24 03 54	97 77 46 44 80
99 49 57 22 77	88 42 95 45 72	16 64 36 16 00	04 43 18 66 79	94 77 24 21 90
16 08 15 04 72	33 27 14 34 09	45 59 34 68 49	12 72 07 34 45	99 27 72 95 14
31 16 93 32 43	50 27 89 87 19	20 15 37 00 49	52 85 66 60 44	38 68 88 11 80
68 34 30 13 70	55 74 30 77 40	44 22 78 84 26	04 33 46 09 52	68 07 97 06 57
74 57 25 65 76	59 29 97 68 60	71 91 38 67 54	13 58 18 24 76	15 54 55 95 52
27 42 37 86 53	48 55 90 65 72	96 57 69 36 10	96 46 92 42 45	97 60 49 04 91
00 39 68 29 61	66 37 32 20 30	77 84 57 03 29	10 45 65 04 26	11 04 96 67 24
29 94 98 94 24	68 49 69 10 82	53 75 91 93 30	34 25 20 57 27	40 48 73 51 92
16 90 82 66 59	83 62 64 11 12	67 19 00 71 74	60 47 21 29 68	02 02 37 03 31
11 27 94 75 06	06 09 19 74 66	02 94 37 34 02	76 70 90 30 86	38 45 94 30 38
35 24 10 16 20	33 32 51 26 38	79 78 45 04 91	16 92 53 56 16	02 75 50 95 98
38 23 16 86 38	42 38 97 01 50	87 75 66 81 41	40 01 74 91 62	48 51 84 08 32
31 96 25 91 47	96 44 33 49 13	34 86 82 53 91	00 52 43 48 85	27 55 26 89 62
56 67 40 67 14	64 05 71 95 86	11 05 65 09 68	76 83 20 37 90	57 16 00 11 66
14 90 84 45 11	75 73 88 05 90	52 27 41 14 86	22 98 12 22 08	07 52 74 95 80
68 05 51 18 00	33 96 02 75 19	07 60 62 93 55	59 33 82 43 90	49 37 38 44 59
20 46 78 73 90	97 51 40 14 02	04 02 33 31 08	39 54 16 49 36	47 95 93 13 30
64 19 58 97 79	15 06 15 93 20	01 90 10 75 06	40 78 78 89 62	02 67 74 17 33
05 26 93 70 60	22 35 85 15 13	92 03 51 59 77	59 56 78 06 83	52 91 05 70 74
07 97 10 88 23	09 98 42 99 64	61 71 62 99 15	06 51 29 16 93	58 05 77 09 51
68 71 86 85 85	54 87 66 47 54	73 32 08 11 12	44 95 92 63 16	29 56 24 29 48
26 99 61 65 53	58 37 78 80 70	42 10 50 67 42	32 17 55 85 74	94 44 67 16 94
14 65 52 68 75	87 59 36 22 41	26 78 63 06 55	13 08 27 01 50	15 29 39 39 43

Table A7.1.
Table of random numbers (from Table XXXIII of Fisher and Yates (1963)).

Chapter 8
Cohort studies

A cohort study is an observational study in which a study population (a cohort) is selected and information is obtained to determine which subjects either have a particular characteristic (e.g., blood group A) that is suspected of being related to the development of the disease under investigation, or have been exposed to a possible etiological agent (e.g., cigarette smoking). The entire study population is then followed up in time, and the incidence of the disease in the exposed individuals is compared with the incidence in those not exposed.

Thus cohort studies resemble intervention studies in that people are selected on the basis of their exposure status and then followed up in time, but differ from them in that the allocation to the study groups is not under the direct control of the investigators.

> *Example 8.1.* *A cohort study of 22 707 Chinese men in Taiwan was set up to investigate the association between the hepatitis B surface antigen (HBsAg) and the development of primary hepatocellular carcinoma. The study was conducted among male government employees who were enrolled through routine health care services. All participants completed a health questionnaire and provided a blood sample at the time of their entry into the study. Participants were then followed up for an average of 3.3 years (Beasley et al., 1981).*

In Example 8.1, a group of 22 707 Chinese male government employees (the 'cohort') was assembled and their HBsAg status (the 'exposure') determined at the start of the study. They were then followed up for several years to measure (and compare) the incidence of hepatocellular carcinoma (the 'outcome') in subjects who were HBsAg-positive or HBsAg-negative at the time of entry into the study.

8.1   Definition of the objectives
As in any other study design, it is essential that a clear hypothesis is formulated before the start of a cohort study. This should include a clear definition of the exposure(s) and outcome(s) of interest. Since cohort studies in cancer epidemiology often involve follow-up of a large number of people for a long period of time, they tend to be very expensive and time-consuming. Consequently, such studies are generally carried out after a hypothesis has been explored in other (cheaper and quicker) types of

study (e.g., cross-sectional or case–control studies). For instance, the cohort study in Taiwan (Example 8.1) was set up only after a series of case–control studies of hepatocellular carcinoma had been carried out in the early and mid-1970s (IARC, 1994b).

8.2 Choice of the study population
8.2.1 Source of the study population

The choice of a particular group to serve as the study population for any given cohort study depends on the specific hypothesis under investigation and on practical constraints. The cohort chosen may be a general population group, such as the residents of a community, or a more narrowly defined population that can be readily identified and followed up, such as members of professional or social organizations (e.g., members of health insurance schemes, registered doctors and nurses). Alternatively, the cohort may be selected because of high exposure to a suspected etiological factor, such as a source of ionizing radiation, a particular type of treatment (e.g., chemotherapy, radiotherapy) or an occupational hazard.

A *general population cohort* may be drawn from a geographically well defined area (as in Example 8.2), which is initially surveyed to establish baseline exposure status with respect to a number of factors and then examined periodically to ascertain disease outcomes.

> **Example 8.2.** *A cohort of 10 287 individuals resident in the Ernakulam district of Kerala (India) were followed up for a 10-year period to assess the effect of tobacco chewing and smoking habits on overall mortality. Participants were initially identified through a baseline survey in which a number of villages in the district were randomly selected. All residents in the selected villages aged 15 years and over were interviewed about their tobacco habits in a house-to-house survey and entered into the cohort. Refusals were negligible (Gupta et al., 1984).*

One of the great advantages of this type of cohort study is that it allows a large number of common exposures to be considered in relation to a large number of outcomes. The Framingham Study is a classical example of this. Approximately 5000 residents of the town of Framingham, in Massachusetts (USA), have been followed up since 1948 (Dawber *et al.*, 1951). There were several reasons for selecting this location for the study, mainly determined by logistic and other practical considerations to ensure that it would be feasible to identify and follow participants for many years. At the time the study was set up, Framingham was a relatively stable community including both industrial and rural areas, with a number of occupations and industries represented. The town was small enough to allow residents to come to one central examining facility and there was only one major hospital. Follow-up of this cohort has permitted assessment of the effects of a wide variety of factors (e.g., blood pressure, serum cholesterol, alcohol intake, physical exercise, smoking) on the risk of numerous diseases, ranging from cardiovascular diseases and cancer to gout, gallbladder disease and eye conditions.

Alternatively, it can be preferable for logistic reasons to draw a general population cohort from a well defined socio-professional group of individuals. For instance, the Taiwan study described in Example 8.1 was conducted among civil servants not because they were thought to have a higher exposure to hepatitis B virus than the rest of the population, but because this group of people was easier to identify and to follow than any other potential study population.

> *Example 8.3.* *A postal questionnaire was sent in 1951 to all men and women whose names were at that time on the British Medical Register and who were believed to be resident in the United Kingdom. In addition to name, address and age, they were asked a few simple questions about their smoking habits. A total of 34 439 male and 6194 female doctors provided sufficiently complete replies. These doctors have been followed up since then (Doll & Hill, 1954; Doll & Peto, 1976; Doll et al., 1980, 1994a,b).*

Similarly, when Richard Doll and Bradford Hill set up a cohort study in England and Wales to assess the health effects of smoking, the choice of the British physicians as the study population (Example 8.3) was determined mainly by logistic considerations. Physicians were registered with the British Medical Association and were therefore easy to identify and follow up. Besides, they were more likely to cooperate and the cause of death to be properly investigated.

If the *exposure is rare*, a study of the general population will have little ability to detect an effect (i.e., the study would have insufficient statistical power (see Chapter 15)), since very few people would have been exposed to the factor of interest. This problem can be overcome by deliberately selecting a *highly exposed group* of people as the study population. For example, exposure to dyestuffs is rare in the general population. However, by choosing a group of workers with high exposure, the full range of effects of the exposure on their health can be studied, including outcomes that are rare in the general population but not in those heavily exposed. The general public health impact of the exposure may be small, but such studies can give insight into common biological mechanisms in disease.

> *Example 8.4.* *The Life Span Study is an on-going cohort study which was set up to investigate the long-term health effects of exposure to high levels of ionizing radiation among survivors of the atomic bomb explosions in Japan. It comprises a sample of 120 128 subjects who were resident in Hiroshima and Nagasaki in 1950, when the follow-up began (Shimizu et al., 1990).*

The follow-up of the survivors of the atomic bomb explosions in Japan (Example 8.4) has not only clarified many of the long-term health effects of acute exposure to high levels of ionizing radiation, but has also contributed to our understanding of the effects of chronic exposure to low-level radiation.

8.2.2 Choice of the comparison group

Once the source of exposed subjects has been determined, the next step is to select an appropriate comparison group of unexposed individuals. This selection is the most critical aspect in the design of a cohort study. The unexposed group should be as similar as possible to the exposed group with respect to the distribution of all factors that may be related to the outcome(s) of interest except the exposure under investigation. In other words, if there were really no association between the exposure and the disease, the disease incidence in the two groups being compared would be essentially the same. Two main types of comparison group may be used in a cohort study: *internal* and *external*.

General population cohorts tend to be heterogeneous with respect to many exposures and, hence, their members can be classified into different exposure categories. In such circumstances, an *internal comparison group* can be utilized. That is, the experience of those members of the cohort who are either unexposed or exposed to low levels can be used as the comparison group. For example, in the cohort study of British physicians (Example 8.3), it was possible to categorize individuals in terms of their smoking habits and then compare the mortality from lung cancer (and other conditions) in smokers with mortality in non-smokers.

> *Example 8.5. The Nurses' Health Study was established in 1976, when a cohort of 121 700 US female registered nurses aged 30–55 years completed a questionnaire on medical conditions and lifestyle practices. A total of 1799 newly diagnosed breast cancer cases occurred during the first 10 years of follow-up from mid-1976 to mid-1986. Analyses were then conducted to investigate the relationship between oral contraceptive use and risk of breast cancer. Women who reported in the initial questionnaire in 1976 and in subsequent ones to have never taken oral contraceptives were considered as the 'unexposed' group in this analysis (Romieu et al., 1989).*

In Example 8.5, a portion of the cohort of US registered female nurses was taken as the 'unexposed group' to examine the relationship between oral contraceptive use and risk of developing breast cancer.

In general population cohorts, it is possible to examine the effect of more than one exposure. Thus, the choice of the group of people in the cohort who will be regarded as 'unexposed' depends on the particular exposure under investigation. For instance, the Nurses' Health Study has also allowed examination of the relationship between dietary total fat intake and the risk of breast cancer. For this purpose, nurses were asked to complete a dietary questionnaire and the distribution of fat intake in the whole cohort was examined and divided into five groups of equal size ('quintiles'); women in the lowest quintile of fat intake were taken as the 'unexposed group' (Willett *et al.*, 1987).

In occupational cohorts, an internal comparison group might consist of workers within the same facility with other types of job not involving exposure to the factor under investigation.

> *Example 8.6.* A cohort of all 14 282 workers employed at the Sellafield plant of British Nuclear Fuels at any time between the opening of the site in 1947 and 31 December 1975 was identified retrospectively from employment records. Employees who worked in areas of the plant where they were likely to be exposed to external radiation wore film badge dosimeters and these personal dose records were kept by the industry. These workers were considered in the present study as 'radiation workers', while those who never wore film badges were taken as 'non-radiation' workers. It was initially planned to follow up the workers from the time they joined the workforce up to the end of 1975, but the follow-up period was later extended to the end of 1988. The mortality experienced by the 'radiation workers' was then compared with that experienced by the 'non-radiation workers' (Smith & Douglas, 1986; Douglas et al., 1994).

In Example 8.6, it was possible to identify a group of workers who could be regarded as unexposed to external radiation on the basis of personal dose records.

When the cohort is essentially homogeneous in terms of exposure to the suspected factor, a similar but unexposed cohort, or some other standard of comparison, is required to evaluate the experience of the exposed group. For example, in some occupational cohorts it is not possible to identify a subgroup of the cohort that can be considered as 'unexposed' for comparison. In this instance, an *external comparison group* must be used. A potential comparison group is a cohort of similar workers in another occupation which does not involve exposure to the factor of interest. For instance, many occupational exposures only occur among certain workforces and therefore it can often be assumed that the level of exposure of other workforces is virtually zero. We can therefore choose people in employment from the same geographical area, who are not exposed to the risk factor of interest, as a comparison group. It is important to ensure that the risk of disease in these workforces is not affected by their own occupational exposures.

Alternatively, the general population of the geographical area in which the exposed individuals reside may be taken as the external comparison group. In this case, the disease experience observed in the cohort is compared with the disease experience of the general population at the time the cohort is being followed. Comparison with rates in the general population avoids the need to follow up a large number of unexposed individuals, but it has several disadvantages. First, it can be done only for outcomes for which such information exists for the general population. Second, it assumes that only a very small proportion of the general population is exposed to the risk factor of interest, otherwise the presence of the exposure in the comparison group will lead to a gross underestimation of its true effect. Third, even if the general population is chosen to be as similar as possible to the exposed cohort in relation to basic demographic and geographic characteristics, it may well differ with respect to other risk factors for the disease, such as diet, smoking, etc. Since this information is not available on individuals in a general population, any observed differences may in fact be due to the effects of confounding that cannot be controlled.

The advantage of using another special group of people as the external unexposed comparison group rather than making comparison with disease rates of the general population is that the group can be selected to be more similar to the exposed cohort than the general population would be. Moreover, information on potential confounding factors can be obtained from all exposed and unexposed individuals in the study and differences controlled for in the analysis.

In many cohort studies, it may be useful to have *multiple comparison groups*, especially when we cannot be sure that any single group will be sufficiently similar to the exposed group in terms of the distribution of potential confounding variables. In such circumstances, the study results may be more convincing if a similar association were observed for a number of different comparison groups. For instance, with some occupational cohorts both an internal comparison group (people employed in the same factory but having a different job) and the experience of the general population (national and local rates) may be used.

In Example 8.7, the all-cause mortality of the cohort of rubber workers was compared with the mortality of another industrial cohort and with local (state) and national rates. Note that both the rubber and the steel workers experienced lower age-specific death rates than either the state or the national populations. This is because people who work tend to be healthier than the general population, which includes those who are too ill or disabled to work (although for steel workers the difference may be due partly to changes in mortality over time). This well known selection bias is called the 'healthy worker effect'.

The healthy worker effect may conceal true increases in the risk of a disease in relation to a particular exposure. It is known to vary with type of disease, being smaller for cancer than for other major diseases, and it tends to disappear with time since recruitment into the workforce (see Section 13.1.1). If rates in the occupational cohort remain lower than those from the general population throughout the follow-up period, this is more likely to be due to sociodemographic and lifestyle differences between the workforce and the general population than to the selection of healthy individuals at the time of recruitment.

Example 8.7. A cohort of workers in a major tyre-manufacturing plant in Akron, Ohio (USA) was set up to examine their overall and cause-specific mortality. A total of 6678 male rubber workers aged 40 to 84 at 1 January 1964 were identified retrospectively from pension, payroll, death claims and other company files. These workers were followed from 1964 to 1972. The age-specific mortality experienced by this cohort was then compared with that experienced by three comparison groups—an industrial cohort of steel workers, the population of the state where the plant is located (Ohio) and the US national population (Table 8.1) (McMichael et al., 1974).

Age-group (years)[b]	Age-specific mortality rate (per 100 000 pyrs)			
	Rubber worker cohort (1964–72)	Steel worker cohort (1953–61)	Ohio state (1972)	USA (1968)
45–54	852	907	940	980
55–64	2317	2166	2365	2370

[a] Data from McMichael *et al.* (1974).

[b] Only data for these two age-groups were available for all the four populations.

Table 8.1.
Male age-specific mortality rates from all causes in the rubber worker cohort and in three other comparison groups: steel workers, Ohio state population and USA national population.[a]

This health selection effect is not restricted to occupational cohorts. A similar phenomenon has been observed in many other types of cohort study. In the British doctors study described in Example 8.3, those who replied to the initial questionnaire had a much lower mortality in the first years of follow-up than those who did not reply (Doll & Hill, 1954). Less health-conscious people, or those already suffering from health problems, might have felt less motivated to participate.

8.3 Measurement of exposure

Measurement of the exposure(s) of interest is a crucial aspect in the design of a cohort study. Information should be obtained on age at first exposure, dates at which exposure started and stopped, dose and pattern of exposure (intermittent versus constant), and changes over time (see Section 2.3).

Information on the exposure(s) of interest may be obtained from a number of sources, including records collected independently of the study (e.g., medical, employment or union records); information supplied by the study subjects themselves, through personal interviews or questionnaires; data obtained by medical examination or other testing of the participants; biological specimens; or direct measurements of the environment in which cohort members have lived or worked. The advantages and limitations of each of these sources were discussed in Chapter 2.

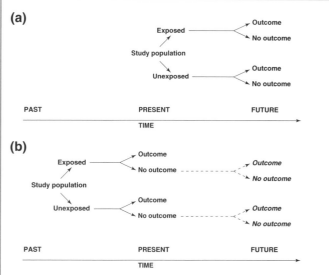

Figure 8.1.
Outline of (a) a prospective cohort study and (b) a historical cohort study.

There are two main types of cohort study, defined according to the point in time when information on exposure was collected: present or past. In *prospective cohort studies*, data on exposure is collected now, once the study population has been defined. In this instance, it is possible to use the most up-to-date methods of exposure measurement so that bias in exposure classification can be minimized. The main disadvantage of this type of cohort study, however, is that the time from exposure to onset of disease (i.e., the induction period) may be too long (many decades for most cancers). Examples 8.1 to 8.5 are examples of prospective cohort studies which involved the follow-up of large numbers of people for very long periods of time.

The alternative, particularly useful for conditions with long induction periods, is to rely on exposure measurements made many years before the study was set up, which may be available from medical, employment or other personal records. By use of data from existing records, the time we have to wait for the exposure to have any effect on the risk of disease may be considerably reduced or even eliminated. This type of cohort study is called a *historical cohort study*.

> **Example 8.8.** *In the early 1950s, Case and his co-workers set up a cohort study to assess whether men engaged in the manufacture of certain dyestuff intermediates had an excess risk of bladder cancer. They began by constructing a list of all men who had ever been employed in the chemical industry in the United Kingdom for at least six months since 1920. The age and the dates between which exposure to dyestuffs occurred were recorded. A search was made retrospectively for all bladder cancer cases occurring among men who had been employed in the chemical industry, in or after 1921 until 1 February 1952. The number of observed bladder cancer cases among these workers was then compared with the number that would have been expected if these workers had the same mortality experience as the general population of the United Kingdom (Case et al., 1954; Case & Pearson, 1954).*

The study described in Example 8.8 is a classic example of the use of this historical approach. Examples 8.6 and 8.7 are also illustrations of historical cohort studies, since both relied on preexisting employment records to identify the cohort members and to classify them according to their exposure status. Historical cohort studies are particularly useful in occupational epidemiology because, if there is concern that a particular exposure may be a hazard, it is not reasonable to wait decades for clarification in a prospective cohort study. However, if at the time the historical cohort is identified, a large proportion of members are still alive, the follow-up period can be extended into the future (as in Example 8.6) to ensure that all possible long-term health effects are properly assessed.

One of the main limitations of historical cohort studies is that the exposure data available in past records are generally less accurate and detailed than if they were collected prospectively. Thus, in historical occupational cohorts, for example, past exposure measurements made in the working environment are rarely available and therefore variables such as work assignment or membership in a union or professional society are generally used to classify individual exposure. These proxy variables are, at best, only crude markers of the true exposure levels and the available detail may be insufficient to address adequately specific research questions. It is, however, unlikely that the accuracy or completeness of these records would be different for those who developed the outcome of interest and those who did not, since the data were recorded before the individuals developed the outcome under study, and, in most cases, for reasons totally unrelated to the investigation. As long as exposure misclassification is independent of the outcome status (i.e., is non-differential), it will tend to dilute any true association between the exposure and the outcome (see Sections 2.7 and 13.1.2).

The historical approach can be particularly successful when biological specimens were stored in the past, so that up-to-date laboratory techniques can be used to measure past exposure. Access to serum banks, for example, permits measurement of exposure to infectious agents (as in Example 8.9) or chemical substances. This method minimizes inaccuracies in past exposure measurement, but the number of such biological specimen banks is limited and the stability of the biological marker during long periods of storage is often unknown.

Example 8.9. Many studies have reported elevated titres of IgG antibody against capsid antigen of Epstein–Barr virus (EBV) and high prevalence of antibodies against early antigen in patients with Hodgkin's disease. However, the blood samples analysed had been collected after diagnosis and treatment for Hodgkin's disease. To evaluate whether enhanced activation of EBV preceded the development of Hodgkin's disease, a study was undertaken in collaboration with five serum banks located in the USA, Norway and Sweden, holding samples from over 240 000 persons. Patients who had subsequently been diagnosed with cancer were identified by linkage to hospital records and cancer registry records. Forty-three cases of Hodgkin's disease were identified and their stored serum samples were then tested for EBV (Mueller et al., 1989).

In many cohort studies, a single classification of exposure is made for each individual at the time of his/her entry into the study. This is appropriate for attributes that do not change with time. Frequently, however, changes in exposure levels for the factors of interest occur during the course of long-term follow-up. Individuals may change jobs, decide to stop smoking (as in Example 8.10), or adopt a low-fat diet. It may be possible to repeat the exposure measurements at intervals during the follow-up period, or information on changes may be available from historical records, allowing the risk of developing the disease to be studied in relation both to the initial exposure status and to subsequent changes.

There may be other reasons for re-assessing the exposure status of the study subjects, particularly in long-term prospective studies. More refined methods of measuring the exposures of interest may become available in the course of the study or new scientific information about the disease may indicate the importance (or desirability) of measuring additional variables that were not measured initially.

Example 8.10. In the British doctors study described in Example 8.3, the first questionnaire was sent to all registered British doctors in 1951. Further inquiries about changes in smoking habits were made in 1957, 1966, 1972, 1978 and 1990–91. The two last questionnaires also included additional questions on alcohol consumption and some other personal characteristics. To assess the extent of changes in smoking habits during the 40-year follow-up period, the smoking habits of the men who replied to the 1990–91 questionnaire were compared with the habits they reported in the initial questionnaire in 1951 (Table 8.2) (Doll et al., 1994a).

Table 8.2.
Smoking habits of male participants in the British doctors study who replied to the 1951 and 1990–91 questionnaires.[a]

Smoking habits, 1951	Smoking habits, 1990-91					
	Non-smoker	Former smoker	Current smoker			No. (%) in 1951
			Cigarette only	Cigarette and other	Pipe or cigar	
Non-smoker	2361	198	17	4	86	2666 (25)
Former smoker	0	1374	10	3	66	1453 (13)
Current smoker						
Cigarettes only	0	3355	535	47	446	4383 (41)
Cigarettes and other	0	897	74	31	308	1310 (12)
Pipe or cigar	0	695	16	2	287	1000 (9)
No. (%) in 1990–91	2361 (22)	6519 (60)	652 (6)	87 (1)	1193 (11)	10 812 (100)

[a] Data from Doll et al. (1994a).

In Example 8.10, there were marked changes in the smoking habits of the male British doctors during the 40-year follow-up period (Table 8.2). Sixty-two per cent of the male doctors reported to be current smokers in 1951. The corresponding figure in 1990–91 was only 18%. Such changes in exposure status can be taken into account in the analysis of cohort studies (see Section 8.7).

8.4 Measurement of potential confounding variables

Cohort studies are observational studies and therefore participants are not randomly allocated to the various exposure categories. This may lead to differences between the groups in terms of exposures other than the one being studied. This is of importance only if these other exposures are also risk factors for the particular disease (or other outcome) under study, i.e., if these exposures are confounding variables. Thus, if we are studying an occupational exposure in relation to lung cancer, it is necessary to be sure that the 'exposed' and 'unexposed' groups have a similar smoking history. If they do not, *statistical adjustment* for differences in smoking must be made (see Chapters 13 and 14). In order to carry out this adjustment, data on smoking for each individual are required. These data must be as accurate as possible and of similar quality to the data on the exposure of primary interest.

In historical cohort studies, information on confounding factors is frequently missing. This is one of their main limitations. For instance, in many of the historical occupational cohorts set up to investigate the relationship between asbestos exposure and respiratory cancers, information on smoking habits was not available. In contrast, the collection of data on potential confounders can be built into the design of most prospective cohort studies, except when local or national rates are taken as the unexposed comparison group.

8.5   Measurement of outcome(s)

A major advantage of cohort studies is that it is possible to examine the effect of a particular exposure on *multiple outcomes*.

Many cohort studies make use of existing routine surveillance systems to ascertain the outcomes of interest. Such systems include cancer registries, death certification and other specialized surveillance systems. They allow tracing of study subjects and ascertainment of their outcomes at much lower cost than if it is necessary to personally contact the subjects. However, it is only possible to examine outcomes of the type which are recorded routinely by these systems and according to the way in which they are coded there. This is particularly important in studies that last for several decades, since major changes may be introduced during the study period in the way diseases are ascertained and coded by these surveillance systems (see Appendix A.2.2).

When no form of disease surveillance system exists, or when the outcome of interest is not routinely recorded by them, some form of surveillance of disease within the cohort has to be set up. For instance, the ascertainment of the outcomes of interest may be done through self-administered questionnaires sent regularly to all study subjects, through personal interviews, or by regular physical examination of all members of the cohort.

Regardless of the method chosen to ascertain the outcome(s) of interest, it is vital to ensure that it is used identically for subjects exposed and those not exposed. If possible, interviewers and any other persons involved in the ascertainment of the outcomes should be kept blind to the exposure status of the study subjects. Otherwise, there is potential to introduce measurement bias (see Section 13.1.2).

Cohort studies focus on disease development. In order for a disease to develop, it must, of course, be absent at the time of entry into the study. An initial examination of the potential study population may be required to identify and exclude existing cases of disease. Even so, it may still be impossible to be absolutely certain that all individuals were disease-free at entry to the study, particularly for conditions with a long latent period (i.e., with a long interval from disease initiation to onset of clinical symptoms and signs). It is therefore usual to exclude disease events occurring during some time period immediately following entry into the study. For cancer, this is often the first 2–3 years of follow-up.

8.6   Follow-up

The *criteria for entry* into the cohort must be defined before the start of the study in a clear and unambiguous way. Individuals should enter the cohort, and contribute person-time at risk, only after all the entry criteria have been satisfied. In most cohort studies, participants will join the cohort at different points in time and therefore the exact date of entry of each subject should be recorded.

Methods must be set up at the start of the study to ensure adequate follow-up of the study subjects. In general, these involve periodic contacts with the individuals such as home visits, telephone calls or mailed questionnaires. Cohort studies of conditions which have a long induction period require follow-up of a very large number of subjects over many years. This is obviously a huge and costly enterprise. To minimize these difficulties, many cohorts are defined in terms of membership of a particular group (professional body, occupational pension plan, union, health insurance plan, college alumni), in which the study population can be more easily followed. Any routine surveillance system that exists may be used to trace and follow up the study subjects at much lower cost than if the investigators had to contact them personally.

The *criteria for exit* from the cohort should also be clearly defined. A date should be specified as the end of the follow-up period (at least for the current analysis). For instance, if death is the outcome of interest, the vital status on that date must be ascertained for all cohort members. All subjects whose vital status is known at that date should contribute person-time at risk until that date (or until their date of death if it occurred earlier). Those whose vital status is not known at that date should be considered as 'lost to follow-up' and the last date for which their vital status was known should be taken as the end of their contribution to person-time at risk.

It is essential that as high a proportion of people in the cohort as possible is followed up. Some people will migrate, some die and some change employment, but every effort should be made to ascertain their outcome(s). All of these factors may be influenced by the exposure and so incomplete follow-up may introduce selection bias (see Section 13.1.1).

8.7   Analysis

The first step in the analysis of a cohort study is to measure the incidence of disease (or of any other outcome of interest) in those exposed and in those unexposed and compare them.

(a)

Outcome		Exposure	
		Yes	No
Outcome	Yes	a	b
	No	c	d

Risk in exposed group (p_1) = $a/(a+c)$
Risk in unexposed group (p_0) = $b/(b+d)$
Risk ratio = p_1/p_0
Risk difference[a] = $p_1 - p_0$

(b)

		Exposure	
		Yes	No
Cases	Yes	a	b
Person-time at risk	No	y_1	y_0

Rate in exposed group (r_1) = a/y_1
Rate in unexposed group (r_0) = b/y_0
Rate ratio = r_1/r_0
Rate difference[a] = $r_1 - r_0$

[a] If the exposure is protective, the risk and rate differences should be calculated as $p_0 - p_1$ or $r_0 - r_1$, respectively (see Section 5.2.2)

Table 8.3.
Analysis of a cohort study (*a*) by risks; (*b*) by rates.

If all, or virtually all, cohort members were followed up for the same period of time, we can calculate risk as the measure of disease occurrence in each group (Table 8.3(*a*)). For example, if the period is uniformly five years, the five-year risk can be computed separately for the exposed and unexposed groups. Risk ratio and risk difference can then be calculated as measures of relative and absolute effect, respectively.

If study subjects have unequal follow-up periods, this must be taken into account in the analysis. Follow-up durations may differ markedly if subjects were recruited into the study population over a relatively long period of time, or if some were lost to follow-up during the course of the study (for example, by moving out of the area). One way of handling variable follow-up periods is to calculate rates which use person-years at risk (or person-months or person-days, etc.) as the denominator (Table 8.3(*b*)). With this approach, each subject contributes to the population at risk only as many years of observation as he/she is actually observed; thus if the subject leaves after one year, he/she contributes 1 person-year; if after 10, 10 person-years (see Section 4.2.2).

People may contribute person-years of observation to more than one subgroup. Suppose, for example, that in a five-year study, disease incidence is determined for each 10-year age subgroup. A person entering the cohort when he or she reaches the age of 48 years will contribute 2 person-years of observation to the 40–49 year-old subgroup and 3 person-years of observation to the 50–59 year-old subgroup (see Section 4.3.2). This may also happen with exposure categories if the study subjects change their exposure status over time. For instance, a person may be a smoker for a few years and then give up.

Example 8.11. The Nurses' Health Study described in Example 8.5 is a cohort study of 121 700 US female registered nurses aged 30–55 years when the cohort was established in mid-1976. A total of 1799 newly diagnosed breast cancer cases were identified during the first 10 years of follow-up from mid-1976 to mid-1986. Analyses were then conducted to investigate the relationship between oral contraceptive use and risk of breast cancer. On the baseline questionnaire in mid-1976, the following question was asked: "If you are now using or have used oral contraceptives, please indicate intervals of oral contraceptive use starting from first use and continuing until the present time. If applicable, please indicate reasons for stopping". The same question was asked on subsequent biennial follow-up questionnaires.

In response to the 1976 questionnaire, 7133 women reported that they were using oral contraceptives. Responses to the 1978, 1980, and 1982 questionnaires showed that 2399, 1168, and 302 women, respectively, were still using oral contraceptives. In 1984, none of the women were current users.

The information given in the 1976 questionnaire was used to classify nurses according to categories of oral contraceptive use ('non-users', 'past users' and 'current users') and each nurse started contributing person-time at risk to that category. Similarly, for each subsequent two-year interval, women contributed additional person-time of follow-up to each updated report of oral contraceptive use. The follow-up of women who developed breast cancer was truncated at the time their breast cancer was diagnosed (Romieu et al., 1989).

In Example 8.11, women who changed their oral contraceptive status during the follow-up period would have contributed person-time at risk to different exposure categories. For instance, a woman who began using oral contraceptives at the start of 1978 and stopped by the end of 1984 would have contributed approximately 1.5 person-years to the non-user category (from the start of the study in mid-1976 to the end of 1977), 7 person-years to the current user category (from the start of 1978 to the end of 1984), and 1.5 person-years to the past user category (from the start of 1985 until the end of the follow-up in mid-1986). If that woman had developed breast cancer at the end of 1982, her person-time contribution would have been 1.5 person-years to the non-user category but only 5 person-years to the current user category (her person-time contribution would have been stopped at the time she developed breast cancer).

The outcomes of interest also need to be allocated to the different exposure categories. In our previous example, the breast cancer case should have been allocated to the current user category since it occurred during the time the woman was contributing person-years to this category. Once the person-time at risk and the outcomes are allocated to the relevant exposure categories, it is possible to estimate breast cancer incidence rates for each oral contraceptive use category by dividing the number of breast cancer cases in each category by the corresponding total number of person-years (Example 8.12).

The results in Example 8.12 show that there was no statistically significant difference in the incidence of breast cancer between ever-users (past and current users were pooled in this analysis) and never-users of oral contraceptives.

Example 8.12. *In Example 8.11, the incidence of breast cancer among nurses aged 45–49 years at the time of their entry into the cohort was examined in relation to use of oral contraceptives.*

	Oral contraceptive use		Total
	Ever (current or past use)	Never	
Cases	204	240	444
Person-years at risk	94 029	128 528	222 557
Rate per 100 000 pyrs	217	187	199

[a] Data from Romieu *et al.* (1989)

Rate ratio = 217 per 100 000 pyrs/187 per 100 000 pyrs = 1.16

95% confidence for the rate ratio = 0.96 to 1.40

Rate difference = 217 per 100 000 pyrs − 187 per 100 000 pyrs = 30 per 100 000 pyrs

95% confidence interval for the rate difference = − 8 to 68 per 100 000 pyrs

$\chi^2 = 2.48$; 1 d.f.; $P=0.12$.

(Test statistics and confidence intervals were calculated using the formulae given in Appendix 6.1).

Table 8.4.
Distribution of breast cancer cases and person-years at risk among US female nurses aged 45–49 years at the time of their entry into the cohort according to oral contraceptive use.[a]

Most often the exposures we are interested in can be further classified into various levels of intensity. Smokers may be classified by number of cigarettes smoked per day, oral contraceptive users by total duration of use, and occupational exposures by intensity of exposure (often estimated indirectly from data on type of job or place of work in the factory) or duration of employment. If various levels of exposure are used in the cohort, we can examine *trends* of disease incidence by level of exposure. The conclusions from a study are strengthened if there is a trend of increasing risk (or decreasing, if the exposure is protective) with increasing level of exposure (i.e., if there is an *exposure–response* relationship).

In Example 8.13, non-users of oral contraceptives were taken as the unexposed baseline category. Rate ratios for each timing and duration category were calculated by dividing their respective rates by the rate of the baseline category. Thus, the rate ratio for current users who had used oral contraceptives for 48 or less months was calculated as 1220 per 100 000 pyrs/187 per 100 000 pyrs = 6.52 (95% confidence interval 2.43–17.53) (Table 8.5). This result suggests that risk might be raised among current

Example 8.13. In Example 8.11, the risk of developing breast cancer was also examined according to timing and duration of oral contraceptive use (Table 8.5).

Table 8.5.
Incidence of breast cancer among nurses aged 45–49 years at the time their entry into the cohort by timing and duration of oral contraceptive use.[a]

Timing Duration of use	Cases	Person- years	Rate (per 100 000 pyrs)	Rate ratio (95% confidence interval)
Non-users[b]	240	128 528	187	1.00
Current users				
≤ 48 months	4	328	1220	6.52 (2.43–17.53)
> 48 months	4	2263	177	0.95 (0.35–2.55)
				χ^2 test for trend = 0.46; $P = 0.50$
Past users[c]				
≤ 48 months	106	54 080	196	1.05 (0.84–1.32)
> 48 months	86	36 039	239	1.28 (1.00–1.64)
				χ^2 test for trend = 3.33; $P = 0.07$

[a] Data from Romieu *et al.* (1989).
[b] Taken as the baseline category.
[c] Information on duration is missing for four past users.
(The 95% confidence intervals and the χ^2 test for a linear trend in rates were calculated using the formulae given in Appendix 6.1.)

short-term users, but this estimate was based on only four breast cancer cases (hence, the wide confidence interval).

To assess whether there was a linear (positive or negative) trend in rates with increasing duration of use, a special statistical test (χ^2 test for a linear trend) was performed separately for current and past users (using the formula given in Section A6.1.3). There was moderate evidence of a positive trend among past users, but no evidence of a linear trend among current users (Table 8.5).

It should be noted that the shape of an exposure–response relationship does not have to be linear. This is clearly illustrated in Example 8.14. For instance, the relationship between alcohol consumption and all-cause mortality (Figure 8.2(a)) is U-shaped, with men who reported drinking 8–14 units of alcohol a week having the lowest mortality. By contrast, the relationship between alcohol consumption and mortality from alcohol-related disorders (Figure 8.2(b)) is basically linear, with a progressive increase in mortality with increasing alcohol consumption among regular drinkers. Thus, lack of a linear trend (as assessed by the χ^2 test for trend) does not imply absence of a relationship. The form of an exposure–outcome relationship should primarily be identified by plotting the data as in Figure 8.2. If the shape is suggestive of a non-linear trend, special statistical procedures, which are outside the scope of this book, should be used to assess its statistical significance.

Since the allocation of the study subjects to the different exposure categories is not random in cohort studies, the exposure groups are likely to differ in many respects other than the exposure of interest. These differences must be taken into account in the analysis. For instance, age is an

Example 8.14. In the British doctors study described in Examples 8.3 and 8.10, additional questions on alcohol consumption were included in the 1978 questionnaire. Doctors were asked about frequency of drinking and, if they were regular drinkers (i.e., they drank in most weeks), about how much they drank in an average week. By 1991, almost a third of the 12 321 men who replied had died. The risk of death in men was then examined in relation to self-reported alcohol consumption (Doll et al., 1994b). Some of the results are shown in Figure 8.2.

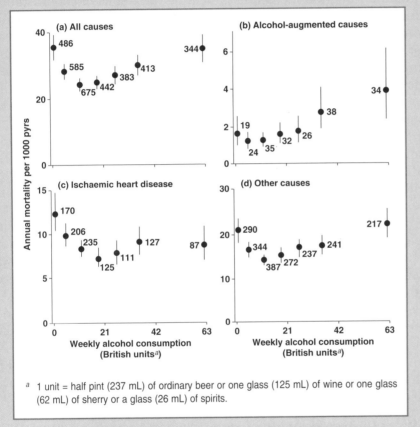

Figure 8.2.
Male mortality from various causes by weekly alcohol consumption: (*a*) all causes; (*b*) conditions known to be alcohol-related (e.g., cancers of the liver, mouth, pharynx, oesophagus and larynx, cirrhosis, alcoholism, and external causes); (*c*) ischaemic heart disease; (*d*) other known causes (cerebrovascular diseases, respiratory diseases, all other cancers not included in (*b*), and others). Points and bars are rates and 95% confidence intervals adjusted for age, smoking habits and history of previous disease; the values are numbers of deaths (reproduced, by permission of BMJ Publishing Group, from Doll *et al.*, 1994b).

^a 1 unit = half pint (237 mL) of ordinary beer or one glass (125 mL) of wine or one glass (62 mL) of sherry or a glass (26 mL) of spirits.

important confounding factor of the relationship between oral contraceptive use and breast cancer, since it is strongly associated with oral contraceptive use, and it is in itself an independent risk factor for breast cancer. Thus differences in the age distribution between women in different oral contraceptive categories may distort the relationship between oral contraceptive use and breast cancer incidence. To minimize this potential confounding effect, we deliberately restricted the analysis in Examples 8.12 and 8.13 to a narrow age-stratum (women aged 45–49 years at the time of their entry into the cohort). It is, however, possible (and desirable) to obtain summary measures (for all ages combined) that are 'adjusted' for age and any other potential confounding variable by using more complex statistical methods. Standardization is one of these methods, as we shall see below. The interpretation of these 'adjusted summary measures' is similar, regardless of the method used. In Example 8.14 (and Figure 8.2), rates were adjusted for age and smoking habits. This means that differences in mortality between the different alcohol consumption categories cannot be explained by differences in their age or smoking distributions, provided the measurements of these confounding variables were valid. These issues are discussed further in Chapters 13 and 14.

Another common method of presenting the results of cohort studies, particularly those based on the disease experience of the general population as the comparison group, is to calculate *standardized mortality (or incidence) ratios* (see Section 4.3.3). Imagine that a total of 24 deaths from lung cancer were observed among a cohort of 17 800 male asbestos insulators. This observed number (O) is then compared with the number that would have been expected (E) if the cohort had the same age-specific mortality rates from lung cancer as the whole male population resident in the same area. Calculations similar to those shown in Section 4.3.3 indicate that only seven deaths would have been expected. Thus, the SMR is equal to $O/E = 24/7 = 3.4$ (or 340 if the SMR is expressed as a percentage). This measure is, in fact, an *age-adjusted rate ratio*. In this example, asbestos insulators were 3.4 times more likely to die from lung cancer than the entire male population resident in the same area, and this difference in mortality is not due to differences in the age-structure between the cohort and the general population. A similar approach was used in Example 8.15. Although this method is often used to adjust for age, it can also be used to adjust for any other confounding variable (e.g., calendar time, smoking habits). Statistical tests and 95% confidence intervals for an SMR can be calculated as shown in Sections A6.1.2 and A6.1.3.

Another way of analysing cohort data, which also takes into account different lengths of follow-up, is to use *survival analysis* methods. These are discussed in Chapter 12.

8.8 Cohort studies with nested case–control studies

In a traditional cohort study, all study individuals are subjected to the same procedures—interviews, health examinations, laboratory measurements, etc.—at the time of their entry into the study and throughout the follow-up period. Alternatively, a cohort may be identified and followed up until a sufficient number of cases develop. More detailed information is then collected and analysed, but only for the 'cases' and for a sample of the disease-free individuals ('controls'), not for all members of the cohort. This type of case–control study conducted within a fixed cohort is called a *nested case–control study* (see Chapter 9). This approach is particularly useful if complex and expensive procedures are being applied. For instance, blood samples for all members of the cohort can be collected at the time of entry and frozen. However, only the blood samples of

Example 8.15. In the occupational cohort described in Example 8.7, the mortality experience of 6678 male rubber workers was compared with that of the 1968 US male population (McMichael et al., 1974). Mortality from selected causes of death is shown in Table 8.6.

Cause of death (ICD-8 code)	Observed deaths (O)	Expected deaths (E)[b]	SMR (%) ($100 \times O/E$)[c]	95% confidence interval
All causes	489	524.9	93	85–102
All neoplasms (140–239)	110	108.9	101	83–122
All malignant neoplasms (140–209)	108	107.3	100	82–120

[a] Data from McMichael *et al.*, 1974.

[b] Expected deaths calculated on the basis of the US male age-specific death rates, 1968.

[c] $P > 0.10$ for all the SMRs shown in the table.

(Test statistics and confidence intervals were calculated using the formulae given in Appendix 6.1.)

Table 8.6.
Mortality from selected causes of death among a cohort of male rubber workers.[a]

the cases (i.e., those individuals in the cohort who contract the disease under study) and of a subgroup of individuals who remained disease-free (the controls), are analysed at the end of the follow-up.

Example 8.16. In 1972, a cohort of 42 000 children was established in the West Nile District of Uganda in order to investigate the etiological role of the Epstein–Barr virus (EBV) in Burkitt's lymphoma. A blood sample was obtained from each child at the time of entry into the study. By the end of the follow-up in 1979, 16 new Burkitt's lymphoma cases had been detected among the cohort members. The level of EBV antibodies in the serum sample taken at entry from each of these cases was then compared with the levels in the sera of four or five children of the same age and sex who were bled in the neighbourhood at the same time as the Burkitt's lymphoma case but who did not develop the disease ('controls') (Geser et al., 1982).

In Example 8.16, blood samples were obtained and stored from all 42 000 children who participated in the study but the rather complex and expensive virus tests were carried out only on the serum samples from the 16 children who developed the lymphoma and from a sample of about 80 selected disease-free members who acted as controls.

Similarly, in nutritional cohort studies, food diaries may be used to measure the subjects' usual dietary intake. As the coding and analysis of food diaries is very labour-intensive, a nested case–control study may be conducted in which only the diaries of the cases and of a sample of disease-free members of the cohort ('controls') are examined.

This type of study design and the analysis of its data are discussed further in Sections 9.3 and 9.5.

8.9   Interpretation

The main advantage of cohort studies is that the *time sequence* between exposure to a factor and occurrence of the disease is clearly observed.

Cohort studies may, however, suffer from important bias. Knowledge of the presence or absence of exposure to a particular factor may affect the subsequent assessment of disease and introduce *measurement bias*. This can occur if the decision as to the presence or absence of disease is made by persons who are aware of the subject's status with regard to the study factor. Cohort studies are also potentially prone to *selection bias* due to loss of study subjects. Such losses may occur initially if a portion of the target study population does not participate, or later on as members of the study population are lost to follow-up. These losses do not necessarily invalidate the study. However, the investigators should consider whether the reasons for loss might have affected the study results. Sometimes it is possible to gather information concerning lost subjects, particularly about whether they left because of illness or death possibly related to the exposures and outcomes under investigation.

As with any other observational study, *confounding* is a critical issue in the interpretation of cohort studies. Special statistical techniques can be used to take into account the effect of potential confounding variables, but only if these variables were known at the time of the data collection and if they were properly measured. If these data were not collected, we have to judge how much the observed findings are likely to have been affected by confounding in the light of all available biological and epidemiological evidence.

In Example 8.17, uranium miners had significantly elevated mortality for cancers at three sites relative to the general population (Table 8.7). Before concluding that these raised risks are due to exposures in the mines, we need to consider alternative explanations for the observed findings. A possible explanation for the high risk of lung cancer among miners is that they were heavier smokers than the general population. No information on smoking habits was available for the miners, but a survey of 697 men in other Czech uranium mines in 1974 showed that 76% were smokers, slightly more than the average (66%) for Czechoslovakian males at that time (see Tomášek *et al.* (1994)). The results from this survey indicate that differences in smoking habits are unlikely to have fully accounted for the estimated five-fold higher lung cancer risk in the miners than in the general population. Moreover, Table 8.8 (Example 8.18) shows that there was a significant positive trend of mortality from lung cancer with increasing cumulative exposure to radon. This trend provides considerable support for a true association between exposure to radon and lung cancer. Similar findings have been found in other radon-exposed miners.

Example 8.17. *A cohort of uranium miners in western Bohemia was identified by a retrospective search in 1970 of employment records. Workers were eligible for entry into the study if: (a) they started to work underground during 1948–59; (b) they worked there for at least four years; and (c) personnel and employment records were available. A total of 4320 miners were eligible. They were exposed to high radon levels, dust and, in one of the two major mines, also high levels of arsenic. The mortality experience of these miners up to the end of 1990 (an average of 25 years of follow-up) was then compared with that of the general population of the former Czechoslovakia. Information on the smoking and alcohol drinking habits of the miners was not available (Tomášek et al., 1993, 1994). Mortality in this cohort from selected cancer sites is shown in*

Cause of death	Observed deaths (O)	Expected deaths (E)[b]	SMR (O/E)[b] (95% confidence interval)
Lung cancer	704	138.6	5.08 (4.71–5.47)
Liver cancer	22	13.2	1.67 (1.04–2.52)
Cancer of gallbladder and extrahepatic bile ducts	12	5.3	2.26 (1.16–3.94)

[a] Data from Tomášek *et al.* (1993).

[b] Expected number of deaths (E) calculated using national male age-specific mortality rates for the former Czechoslovakia

Table 8.7.

Number of observed deaths (O) from selected cancer sites in the West Bohemian uranium miners cohort compared with the number expected (E) if the miners had the same mortality as the general male population of the former Czechoslovakia.[a]

Example 8.18. *In the cohort of uranium miners described in Example 8.17, the cumulative exposure to radon gas (and its progeny) was estimated for each miner. The exposure, measured in terms of 'working level months' (WLM), was calculated by considering the time spent in each mineshaft in conjunction with about 39 000 shaft-specific measurements of radon gas made in 1949–63 (Tomášek et al., 1993). Mortality according to exposure levels is shown in Table 8.8.*

Site		Cumulative radon exposure (WLM)					P-value for trend
		<110	110–149	150–209	210–329	≥330	
Lung cancer	O	86	100	139	161	181	<0.001
	O/E [b]	3.07	3.66	4.98	6.23	8.10	
Liver cancer	O	7	3	4	5	3	0.57
	O/E [b]	2.70	1.18	1.53	2.04	1.40	
Cancer of gallbladder and extrahepatic bile ducts	O	0	2	1	3	6	0.003
	O/E [b]	0.00	1.92	0.93	3.03	6.73	

[a] Data from Tomášek *et al.* (1993)

[b] Expected number of deaths (E) calculated using national male age-specific mortality rates for the former Czechoslovakia.

Table 8.8.

Number of observed deaths (O) and standardized mortality ratio (O/E) from selected cancers by cumulative radon exposure.[a]

There was also a positive trend in mortality from gallbladder and extra-hepatic bile duct cancer with increasing levels of cumulative exposure to radon (Table 8.8), but there is little supporting evidence in favour of this finding from other epidemiological studies, and further investigation is needed. By contrast, mortality from liver cancer did not increase with cumulative radon exposure, making it unlikely that the excess in the miners was caused by radon. No information was available on the alcohol consumption of the miners, but they were well paid compared with other Czech workers and, therefore, it is likely that their alcohol consumption was higher than in the general population. They also had a significant excess of deaths from liver cirrhosis, probably caused by alcohol consumption and, for six of the liver cancer deaths, cirrhosis was also mentioned on the death certificate (Tomášek *et al.*, 1993).

The issues that need to be addressed in interpreting results from cohort studies are further discussed in Chapter 13.

Box 8.1. Key issues

- Cohort studies are studies in which subjects are selected on the basis of their exposure status and then followed up in time. In contrast with intervention studies, however, the allocation of exposure is not determined by the investigators.

- The main advantages of this type of study are:

    1. Exposure is measured before disease onset and is therefore likely to be unbiased in terms of disease development.

    2. Rare exposures can be examined by appropriate selection of study cohorts.

    3. Multiple outcomes (diseases) can be studied for any one exposure.

    4. Incidence of disease can be measured in the exposed and unexposed groups.

- The main disadvantages of this type of study are:

    1. They can be very expensive and time-consuming, particularly if conducted prospectively.

    2. Changes in exposure status and in diagnostic criteria over time can affect the classification of individuals according to exposure and disease status.

    3. Ascertainment of outcome may be influenced by knowledge of the subject's exposure status (*information bias*).

    4. Losses to follow-up may introduce *selection bias*.

- Cohort studies in cancer epidemiology generally involve the follow-up of a large number of individuals for long periods of time. They therefore tend to be very expensive and time-consuming. Various approaches may be used to reduce the costs:

    1. Use preexisting records (or biological specimens) to identify retrospectively a suitable study population and obtain information on the exposure status of their members *(historical cohort study)*.

    2. Use available surveillance systems (e.g., death certification, cancer registration) to follow up subjects and obtain information on the outcomes of interest.

    3. Use national (or local) rates as the comparison unexposed group.

    4. Conduct a *nested case–control study*.

Further reading

* The book by Breslow & Day (1987) provides a very comprehensive coverage of the role, design, analysis and interpretation of cohort studies in cancer epidemiology. Some of the material is presented at a relatively advanced level.

* Discussion of the healthy worker effect can be found in papers by Carpenter (1987) and McMichael (1976).

Chapter 9
Case–control studies

A case–control study involves the identification of individuals with ('cases') and without ('controls') a particular disease or condition. The prevalence (or level) of exposure to a factor is then measured in each group. If the prevalence of exposure among cases and controls is different, it is possible to infer that the exposure may be associated with an increased or decreased occurrence of the outcome of interest (see Section 9.5).

> **Example 9.1.** *The relationship between use of conjugated estrogens and the risk of endometrial cancer was examined among 188 white women aged 40–80 years with newly diagnosed endometrial cancer and 428 controls of similar age hospitalized for non-malignant conditions requiring surgery at the Boston Hospital for Women Parkway Division, Massachusetts, between January 1970 and June 1975. The data on drug use and reproductive variables were extracted from hospital charts and from the medical records of each woman's private physician. Thirty-nine per cent of the cases and 20% of the controls had used conjugated estrogens in the past (Buring et al., 1986).*

In Example 9.1, women with endometrial cancer ('cases') or without ('controls') were identified and information on their past use of conjugated estrogens ('exposure') was extracted from hospital and other medical records. The prevalence of use of conjugated estrogens was much higher among the cases (39%) than among the controls (20%), suggesting that the use of this drug was associated with an increase in the incidence of endometrial cancer.

The major difference between cohort and case–control methods is in the selection of the study subjects. In a cohort study, we start by selecting subjects who are initially free of disease and classify them according to their exposure to putative risk factors (see Chapter 8), whereas in a case–control study, we identify subjects on the basis of presence or absence of the disease (or any other outcome) under study and determine past exposure to putative risk factors.

Case–control studies are particularly suitable for the study of relatively rare diseases with long induction period, such as cancer. This is because a case–control study starts with subjects who have already developed the condition of interest, so that there is no need to wait for time to elapse between exposure and the occurrence of disease, as in prospective cohort studies. Historical cohort studies allow similar savings in time, but can be conducted only in the rare situations when past records with data on relevant exposures have been kept or when banks of biological specimens have been properly stored and appropriate laboratory assays are available for measurement of the exposures of interest.

9.1 Study hypothesis

As with any other type of study, the specific hypothesis under investigation must be clearly stated before a case–control study is designed in detail. Failure to do this can lead to poor design and problems in interpretation of results. Case–control studies allow the evaluation of a wide range of exposures that might relate to a specific disease (as well as possible interactions between them). Example 9.2 clearly illustrates this feature.

Example 9.2. A population-based case–control study was carried out in Spain and Colombia to assess the relationship between cervical cancer and exposure to human papillomavirus (HPV), selected aspects of sexual and reproductive behaviour, use of oral contraceptives, screening practices, smoking, and possible interactions between them. The study included 436 incident cases of histologically confirmed invasive squamous-cell carcinoma of the cervix and 387 controls of similar age randomly selected from the general population that generated the cases (Muñoz et al., 1992a).

Case–control studies often constitute one of the first approaches to study the etiology of a disease or condition, as in Example 9.3. This is partly because of their ability to look at a wide range of exposures and partly because they can be conducted relatively cheaply and quickly.

Example 9.3. Because of their rarity, very little is known about the etiology of malignant germ-cell tumours in children. To explore risk factors for these malignancies and generate etiological hypotheses, a population-based case–control study of 105 children with malignant germ-cell tumours and 639 controls was conducted (Shu et al., 1995).

The results from these *exploratory* case–control studies may suggest specific hypotheses which can then be tested in specifically designed studies.

9.2 Definition and selection of cases

9.2.1 Case definition

Precise criteria for the definition of a case are essential. It is usually advisable to require objective evidence that the cases really suffer from the disease or condition of interest, even if, as a result, some true cases have to be eliminated. For instance, a histologically confirmed diagnosis should be required for most cancers. By accepting less well documented cases, the investigator runs the risk of diluting the case group with some non-cases and lessening the chances of finding real exposure differences between cases and controls.

It is sometimes impossible to eliminate all cases whose diagnosis is not properly documented, particularly if the pool of available cases is relatively small. In these circumstances, it may be possible to classify the cases according to diagnostic certainty. Such classification allows assessment of the extent to which the results are likely to be affected by disease misclassification (see Chapter 13). Suppose, for instance, that cases in a particular case–control study are classified as 'definite', 'probable' or 'possible'. If there is disease misclassification, a gradual decline in relative risk from the 'definite' to the 'possible' category should become apparent in the analysis, since the probability that non-cases may have been misdiagnosed as cases increases from the 'definite' to the 'possible' category.

The case definition should be established in such a way that there is no ambiguity about types of cases and stages of disease to be included in, or excluded from, the study. The choice of cases should be guided more by concern for validity than for generalizability. For example, in a study of breast cancer, we may learn more by limiting the cases (and the controls) to either pre- or post-menopausal women than by including women of all ages (unless the number of cases in each group is large enough to allow separate analyses), since the risk factors for pre- and post-menopausal breast cancers may be different. By ensuring that the cases are a relatively homogeneous group, we maximize the chances of detecting important etiological relationships. The ability to generalize results to an entire population is usually less important than establishing an etiological relationship, even if only for a small subgroup of the population.

Cases should also be restricted to those who have some reasonable possibility of having had their disease induced by the exposure under investigation.

Example 9.4. A multinational, hospital-based case–control study was conducted to evaluate the relationship of combined oral contraceptive use to the risk of developing five different site-specific cancers. The study was conducted in 10 participating centres in eight countries (Chile, China, Colombia, Israel, Kenya, Nigeria, Philippines and Thailand) from October 1979 to September 1986. Women with newly diagnosed cancers of the breast, corpus uteri, cervix uteri, ovary and liver were eligible if born after 1924 or 1929 (depending on when oral contraceptives became locally available) and had been living in the area served by the participating hospital for at least one year (WHO Collaborative Study of Neoplasia and Steroid Contraceptives, 1989).

In Example 9.4, cases were restricted to women born since the 1920s because only women born since then could have been exposed to the factor of interest (oral contraceptives).

Although most case–control studies include only one case group, it is possible to study simultaneously two or more cancers whose risk factors are thought to share the same, or related, risk factors. Example 9.4 illustrates this point. Such multiple-disease case–control studies may be regarded as a series of case–control studies. This approach provides two main advantages. First, it provides the possibility of studying more than one cancer for relatively little extra cost. Second, the control groups may be combined to give each case–control comparison increased statistical power, that is, the ability of the study to detect a true effect, if one really exists, is enhanced because of the larger number of controls per case (see Chapter 15).

If the disease or condition of interest is very rare, the study may have to be carried out in various participating centres, possibly located in various countries. The study cited in Example 9.4 was conducted in 10 centres in eight countries. Despite this, only 122 newly diagnosed liver cancers were accrued during the seven-year study period. Some studies deliberately include participating centres from low- and high-incidence areas to assess whether the risk factors are similar. For instance, the cervical cancer study mentioned in Example 9.2 was conducted in Colombia and Spain, countries with an eight-fold difference in cervical cancer incidence (Muñoz *et al.*, 1992a).

The eligibility criteria should include not only a clear case definition but also any other inclusion criteria (Example 9.5). Persons who are too ill to cooperate or for whom the study procedures may cause considerable physical or psychological distress should be excluded. It is also usual to exclude elderly people in cancer case–control studies because their diagnosis is likely to be less valid and because of their difficulty in recalling past exposures.

> *Example 9.5. In the cervical cancer case–control study mentioned in Example 9.2, eligible cases were incident, histologically confirmed, invasive squamous-cell carcinomas of the cervix identified among patients resident in the study areas for at least six months. Patients were excluded if their physical and/or mental condition was such that interview and/or collection of specimens was inadvisable or if they were older than 70 years (Muñoz et al., 1992a).*

Usually, the inclusion of all patients who meet the eligibility criteria is not possible for a variety of reasons. Subjects may move out of the area, die or simply refuse to cooperate. The investigator should report how many cases met the initial criteria for inclusion, the reasons for any exclusion, and the number omitted for each reason (as in Example 9.6). This information allows us to assess the extent to which the results from the study may have been affected by selection bias (see Chapter 13).

Example 9.6. A large multi-centre case–control study was conducted in high- and low-risk areas of Italy to evaluate the role of dietary factors in the etiology of gastric cancer and their contribution to the marked geographic variation in mortality from this cancer within the country. All patients with new histologically confirmed gastric cancer diagnosed between June 1985 and December 1987, resident in the study areas, and aged 75 years or less were eligible as cases. A total of 1129 eligible cases were identified in surgery and gastroenterology departments and outpatient gastroscopic services of private and public hospitals. Approximately 83% of these cases were successfully interviewed using a structured questionnaire (Buiatti et al., 1989a,b). Table 9.1 shows the numbers of eligible patients in each recruitment centre, how many were recruited and the reasons for exclusion.

Recruitment centre	Eligible cases	Recruited No. (%)	Excluded due to		
			Refusal No. (%)	Poor health No. (%)	Deceased[b] No. (%)
Cagliari	104 (100)	82 (78.9)	3 (2.9)	4 (3.8)	15 (14.4)
Cremona	71 (100)	66 (93.0)	0 (0.0)	4 (5.6)	1 (1.4)
Florence	435 (100)	382 (87.8)	9 (2.1)	28 (6.4)	16 (3.7)
Forli	255 (100)	232 (91.0)	8 (3.1)	14 (5.5)	1 (0.4)
Genoa	155 (100)	122 (78.7)	3 (1.9)	24 (15.5)	6 (3.9)
Imola	76 (100)	47 (61.8)	9 (11.8)	8 (10.5)	12 (15.9)
Siena	133 (100)	85 (63.9)	18 (13.5)	29 (21.8)	1 (0.8)
Total	**229 (100)**	**1016 (82.7)**	**50 (4.1)**	**111 (9.0)**	**52 (4.2)**

[a] Data from Buiatti *et al.* (1989a).
[b] Deceased after being identified as potential cases.

Table 9.1.
Recruitment levels among gastric cancer cases and reasons for non-participation by recruitment centre[a].

Information on the entire eligible case series should be sought, whenever possible, regarding characteristics such as age, gender, education, socioeconomic status, so that selection factors for the non-participating subjects may be evaluated. This information may be available from routine data sources such as hospital records and cancer registries (as in Example 9.7).

9.2.2 Incident versus prevalent cases

An important issue to consider at the design stage of a case–control study is whether to include *prevalent* or only *incident* cases. Incident cases are all *new* cases occurring in a population within a fixed period of time. Prevalent cases are all *existing* (new and old) cases who are present in a population at a particular point in time (or within a very short period) (see Section 4.2). The main disadvantage of using a prevalent case series is that patients with a long course of disease tend to be over-represented since, by

Example 9.7. In the stomach cancer case–control study discussed in Example 9.6, the number and characteristics of the cases recruited in each participating centre were compared with the information collected by local cancer registries or pathology departments. Table 9.2 shows that the cases recruited to the study in Florence were slightly younger and more often females than the cases notified to the local cancer registry. This was because cases without histological confirmation were excluded from the study, and these were generally men in older age-groups (Buiatti et al., 1989a, b).

Table 9.2.
Age and sex distribution (%) of gastric cancer cases recruited by the Florence centre during 1985–87 and of gastric cancer cases notified to the local cancer registry in 1985.[a]

Age (years)	Males (M)				Females (F)				M:F ratio
	<45	45–54	55–64	65–74	<45	45–54	55–64	65–74	
Cases recruited, 1985-87	4.4	13.3	33.2	49.1	3.8	12.1	18.2	65.9	1.7
Cases notified to the registry, 1985	2.6	10.7	33.2	53.6	3.1	13.5	20.8	62.5	2.0

[a] Data from Buiatti *et al.* (1989a,b). (The numbers of cases on which these percentages are based were not given in these papers).

definition, all those with a short duration leave the pool of prevalent cases because of either recovery or death. Unless we can justify the assumption that the exposure being studied is not associated with recovery or survival, every effort should be made to limit recruitment to incident cases. By using only newly diagnosed (incident) cases and selecting controls to be representative of subjects from the population from which the cases arise, the case–control study aims to identify factors responsible for disease development, much like a cohort study. Moreover, prevalent cases may not be representative of all cases if some affected patients are institutionalized elsewhere or move to another city where there are special facilities for treatment.

There are other advantages to the use of incident cases. Recall of past events in personal histories tends to be more accurate in newly diagnosed cases than in prevalent cases. Besides, incident cases are less likely to have changed their habits (or 'exposures') as a result of the disease.

If constraints on time or resources make the use of prevalent cases inevitable, we should choose those that were diagnosed as close as possible to the time of initiation of the study. A check on the characteristics of the prevalent cases may be possible by comparing the frequency (or level) of exposure among subjects with different times of diagnosis. If, among the cases, the frequency of exposure to a factor suspected of being associated with the disease changes with time since diagnosis, we should suspect *survival bias*. For instance, if those cases who were exposed to the factor under study have poorer survival than those unexposed, they will become underrepresented in a prevalent case series as time since diagnosis increases. As a result, the prevalence of exposure among the surviving cases will decrease.

Prevalent cases may have to be used for conditions for which it is difficult to establish a specific date of onset. For instance, case–control studies to examine risk factors for *Helicobacter pylori* infection have to be based on prevalent cases, because it is difficult to establish the date of onset of this condition.

9.2.3   Source of cases

Which cases are to be recruited into a study needs to be carefully considered. The study may be *'hospital-based'* and the cases taken from all patients fulfilling the eligibility criteria and attending a certain hospital or a group of hospitals. In Example 9.1, the cases were white women, aged 40–80 years, who were admitted to a certain hospital in Boston from January 1970 to June 1975 with a first diagnosis of endometrial cancer.

Alternatively, the study may be *'population-based'* and cases taken from a defined population over a fixed period of time. This is illustrated in Example 9.8.

> **Example 9.8.** *In the cervical cancer case–control study mentioned in Example 9.2, an active case-finding network was organized with periodic visits to all hospitals, clinics and pathology departments in the public and private sector in each study area to identify and interview the cases before any treatment was applied. All cervical intraepithelial neoplasia (CIN) III cases diagnosed during the study period were also identified and the histological slides were reviewed by a panel of pathologists to ensure completeness of recruitment of the invasive cancer cases (Muñoz et al., 1992a).*

In population-based case–control studies, it is essential to ensure completeness of case-finding. Issues that need to be considered are completeness of patient referral to health centres (which is likely to be a minor problem in cancer studies in countries where medical care is generally available but a much greater one elsewhere), difficulty in tracing the subjects, and refusal to participate.

Population-based cancer registries may be used to recruit all incident cases from their catchment population, but their value as a source of cases may be limited if there is a substantial time lag between diagnosis and registration. Moreover, cases with poor survival may have died in the meantime and others may have moved out of the catchment area as a result of their disease. Thus, by the time cases are registered, it may not be possible to regard them as incident.

9.3   Definition and selection of controls

9.3.1   Definition of controls

Controls must fulfil all the eligibility criteria defined for the cases apart from those relating to diagnosis of the disease. For example, if the cases are women with breast cancer aged 45 years and over, the controls must be selected from women in the same age group without the disease.

If the disease being studied is uncommon in the group serving as a source of controls, little, if any, diagnostic effort or documentation is needed to rule out the disease in the selected controls. A simple interview question will often suffice. However, if the disease is common, a greater effort to minimize misclassification, such as a review of the individuals' medical records, is desirable (as in Example 9.9).

> *Example 9.9. In the cervical cancer case–control study mentioned in Example 9.2, controls were eligible if they were 70 years of age or younger, had not received previous treatment for cervical cancer or had not been hysterectomized, and if the cytological smear taken at the time of recruitment was normal or had only inflammatory changes (Pap classes I and II) (Muñoz et al., 1992a).*

9.3.2 Source of controls

In case–control studies, controls should represent the population from which the cases are drawn, i.e., they should provide an estimate of the exposure prevalence in the population from which the cases arise. If not, the results of the study are likely to be distorted because of *selection bias*.

In a *nested case–control study*, it is relatively straightforward to ensure that the cases and controls are drawn from the same study population, since both will arise from a clearly defined population—the cohort (see Section 8.8). In general, all the cases arising as the cohort is followed prospectively become the 'cases' in the case–control study, while a sample of unaffected members of the cohort become the 'controls'.

In Example 9.10, both the cases and the controls were drawn from the same population—the cohort of 5908 Japanese American men living in Hawaii.

Conceptually, we can assume that all case–control studies are 'nested' within a particular population. In a *population-based case–control*

> *Example 9.10. The relationship between* Helicobacter pylori *infection and gastric carcinoma was examined in a cohort of Japanese American men living in Hawaii. A total of 5908 men were enrolled from 1967 to 1970. At that time each man provided a blood sample. By 1989, a total of 109 new cases of pathologically confirmed gastric carcinoma had been identified among the cohort members. The stored serum samples from all the patients with gastric carcinoma ('cases') and from a selection of subjects who did not develop gastric cancer ('controls') were then tested for the presence of serum IgG antibody to* Helicobacter pylori *(Nomura et al., 1991).*

study, a study population can be defined from which all incident cases are obtained; controls should be randomly selected from the disease-free members of the same population. Consider, for example, all the newly diagnosed cases of childhood cancer in the catchment area of a regional cancer registry. Controls for these cases would appropriately be drawn from the population of the same area in the same sex- and age-groups. Even when the cases are identified exclusively from hospitals, it still may be reasonable to assume that they represent all the cases in the catchment area if the disease is serious enough that all cases end up in hospital (which is likely to be true for most cancer cases in countries with good health care).

It is generally expensive and time-consuming to draw controls from a random sample of the catchment population. A list of all eligible subjects or households must be available for sampling, or has to be created (as in Example 9.11). (Methods to select a random sample from the study population are discussed in Chapter 10.) Besides, healthy people may be disinclined to participate, which may introduce selection bias due to non-response.

> **Example 9.11.** *In the cervical case–control study mentioned above, controls were randomly selected from the general population that generated the cases. In Colombia, up-to-date aerial pictures of the city were used as the sampling frame. From these pictures, houses were selected at random and door-to-door searching following pre-determined routines was employed to identify suitable controls. In Spain, the provincial census of 1981, the latest available, was used as the sampling frame (Muñoz et al., 1992a).*

Controls may also be selected from close associates of the case, such as *friends and relatives* who are from the same catchment population as the cases. Although a relatively small effort is required to identify these controls and obtain their cooperation, there is a danger that they will be too similar (overmatched) to cases in terms of exposures and other characteristics (see Section 9.3.4). *Neighbourhood controls* can also be used, but people living in the same neighbourhood are likely to be similar in many respects, so such controls may also be overmatched. Moreover, if the interviewer has to visit each neighbourhood to contact these controls, the cost of the study may become extremely high.

When using hospital-based cases, it may not be possible to define the population from which the cases arose, either because the exact catchment area of the hospital cannot be defined or because not all the cases in the area are referred to the hospital, and those referred may be selected according to particular criteria (e.g., the more serious). In these circumstances, *hospital-based controls* may be used because the study population can then be defined as potential 'hospital users'.

Hospitalized controls have several advantages. There are many selective factors that bring people to hospitals (e.g., financial standing, area of residence, ethnicity, religious affiliation) and by selecting controls from the same pool of patients that gave rise to the cases, we reduce the effect of these factors. These controls are generally easily identified and they tend to be cooperative. In addition, since they have also experienced illness and hospitalization, they may resemble the cases with respect to their tendency to give complete and accurate information, thus reducing potential differences between cases and controls in the quality of their recall of past exposures.

Choosing suitable hospital controls is often difficult and great care must be taken to avoid selection bias. A major disadvantage of a control group selected from diseased individuals is that some of their illnesses may share risk factors with the disease under study, that is, they may have a higher, or lower, exposure prevalence compared with the population from which the cases arise. For instance, in a study investigating the role of alcohol and breast cancer, the use of controls from the accident and emergency department of the same hospital would introduce bias because this group is known to have a higher alcohol consumption than the general population from which the cases arise. One way of minimizing this bias is to select controls with different conditions so that biases introduced by specific diseases will tend to cancel each other out.

Choice of a suitable control group is the most difficult part of designing a case–control study. Some studies use more than one type of control group. The conclusions from a study are strengthened if similar results are obtained with each of the control groups.

After the source and number of control groups for a study have been determined, it is necessary to decide how many controls per case should be selected. This issue is considered in detail in Chapter 15, but when the number of available cases and controls is large and the cost of obtaining information from both groups is comparable, the optimal control-to-case ratio is 1:1. When the number of cases available for the study is small, or when the cost of obtaining information is greater for cases than controls, the control-to-case ratio can be altered to ensure that the study will be able to detect an effect, if one really exists (i.e., that the study has the necessary statistical power). The greater the number of controls per case, the greater the power of the study (for a given number of cases). However, there is generally little justification to increase this ratio beyond 4:1, because the gain in statistical power with each additional control beyond this point is of limited magnitude. Sample size issues (and the concept of 'statistical power' of a study) are discussed in Chapter 15.

As for cases, it is important to collect information on reasons for non-participation of controls and, whenever possible, to obtain additional information on their sociodemographic characteristics (e.g., sex, age, socioeconomic status) (as in Example 9.12).

Example 9.12. *In the Italian gastric cancer case–control study mentioned in Examples 9.6 and 9.7, controls were randomly selected from population lists within five-year age and sex strata. A total of 1423 population-based controls were sampled, of whom 1159 (81%) were successfully interviewed using the same structured questionnaire as for the cases (Buiatti* et al., *1989a,b). Table 9.3 shows the numbers of controls that were sampled, how many were recruited and the reasons for non-participation by recruitment centre.*

Recruitment centre	Sampled No. (%)	Recruited No. (%)	Excluded due to	
			Refusal No. (%)	Poor health No. (%)
Cagliari	118 (100)	108 (91.5)	8 (6.8)	2 (1.7)
Cremona	61 (100)	51 (83.6)	5 (8.2)	5 (8.2)
Florence	547 (100)	440 (80.4)	74 (13.6)	33 (6.0)
Forli	291 (100)	259 (89.0)	20 (6.9)	12 (4.1)
Genoa	205 (100)	137 (66.8)	17 (8.3)	51 (24.9)
Imola	74 (100)	61 (82.4)	10 (13.5)	3 (4.1)
Siena	127 (100)	103 (81.1)	6 (4.7)	18 (14.2)
Total	**1423 (100)**	**1159 (81.4)**	**140 (9.9)**	**124 (8.7)**

[a] Data from Buiatti *et al.* (1989a).

Table 9.3.
Recruitment levels among controls and reasons for non-participation by recruitment centre.[a]

9.3.3. Sampling schemes for controls

If the source of incident cases is a closed cohort with a fixed follow-up period (as is the case in nested case–control studies), controls may be selected in three different ways, as illustrated in Example 9.13.

In this example, the first option for the investigators is to sample controls from the population still at risk by the end of the study, that is from those subjects who were still disease-free by the end of the follow-up period (A in Figure 9.1). In this design, each woman can be either a case or a control, but not both.

The second option is to sample controls from those who are still at risk at the time each case is diagnosed, that is, controls are *time-matched* to the cases (see Section 9.3.4) (B in Figure 9.1). In this sampling design, a subject originally selected as a control can become a case at a later stage. The opposite cannot happen, since once a woman has acquired endometrial cancer she is no longer at risk, and therefore not eligible for selection as a control. Subjects selected as controls who then become cases should be retained as, respectively, controls and cases in the appropriate sets.

Thirdly, controls can be a sample from those who were at risk at the start of the study (C in Figure 9.1). Studies of this type are called 'case–cohort studies'. Since the control group reflects the total population and not just those who did not get the disease, a woman ascertained as a case may also be selected as a control, and vice versa. Such women should

Example 9.13. Suppose that a cohort of 200 000 healthy women was followed up for ten years to assess the relationship between lifestyle variables and the risk of developing various types of cancer and that a total of 60 women were diagnosed with endometrial cancer during the follow-up period. Suppose also that the investigators decided to conduct a case–control study nested within this cohort to assess whether oral contraceptive use protected against endometrial cancer. The investigators could sample the controls in three different ways, as indicated in Figure 9.1: (1) from those who were still disease-free by the end of the follow-up period (situation A); (2) from those who were still at risk at the time each case was diagnosed (situation B); or (3) from those who were at risk at the start of the study (situation C).

Figure 9.1.
Sampling schemes for controls when the source of incident cases is a closed cohort with a fixed follow-up (x=incident case).

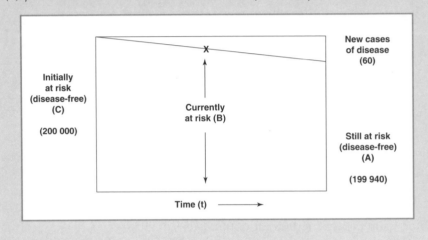

be included in the study as both cases and controls.

If the source of incident cases is a dynamic population, as in most hospital and population-based case–control studies, it may be difficult to establish the exact population at risk at the start and end of the follow-up period, so the preferred method is to choose for each incident case one or more controls from those subjects who are members of the same population and still at risk of developing the disease at the time of the diagnosis of the case.

As we shall see later in this chapter (Section 9.5), the specific relative measure of effect (rate ratio, risk ratio or odds (of disease) ratio) that can be estimated from a case–control study depends on the type of sampling design used in the selection of the controls.

9.3.4. Matching

Individual matching refers to the procedure whereby one or more controls are selected for each case on the basis of similarity with respect to certain characteristics other than the exposure under investigation. Since cases and controls are similar on the matching variables, their difference with respect to disease status may be attributable to differences in some other factors. It is, however, important that *matching is restricted to con-*

founding factors and is not performed for the exposure under investigation. The characteristics generally chosen for matching are those that are known to be strong *confounders*. Common matching variables are age, sex, and ethnicity but others might be place of residence, or socioeconomic status.

Let us suppose that we are interested in examining the relationship between current use of oral contraceptives and ovarian cancer. In this example, it is appropriate to match on age, since age is associated with the exposure of interest (current oral contraceptive use) and is an independent risk factor for ovarian cancer. In other words, age is a confounding factor. Failure to match, or otherwise control, for age would result in a biased assessment of the effect of oral contraceptive use.

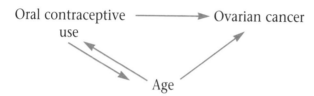

When controls are chosen so as to be similar to the cases for a characteristic and when this similarity tends to mask the disease's association with the exposure of interest, cases and controls are said to be *overmatched*. This can happen when controls are matched to cases for a characteristic that is part of the pathway through which the possible cause of interest leads to disease. Imagine a case–control study conducted in West Africa to investigate the role of hepatitis B virus in the etiology of liver cancer in which controls were matched to cases on the basis of previous history of liver disease.

Hepatitis B virus ⟶ Chronic liver disease ⟶ Liver cancer

If chronic liver disease is on the pathway between hepatitis B infection and liver cancer, matching on that condition would result in an underestimation of the effect of the virus on the occurrence of liver cancer, since controls would have been made similar to the cases in relation to this variable.

Another form of overmatching relates to matching for a variable which is correlated to the exposure of interest but is not an independent risk factor for the disease under study (and so cannot be a confounding factor) and is not on its causal pathway. For instance, suppose we wish to examine the relationship between smoking and lung cancer in a population where smoking levels are positively correlated with alcohol intake, that is, the more someone drinks the more he/she is likely to smoke. In this example, matching on alcohol intake would result in overmatching because controls would be made similar to the cases not only in relation to their alcohol intake but also in relation to their smoking habits, which is the exposure of interest in this study.

Hence, caution should be exercised in determining the number of variables selected for matching, even when there are no practical restrictions. If the role of a variable is in doubt, the preferable strategy is not to match but to adjust for it in the statistical analysis (see Chapters 13–14).

In most case–control studies, there are a small number of cases and a large number of potential controls to select (or sample) from. In practice, each case is classified by characteristics that are not of direct interest, and a search is made for one or more controls with the same set of characteristics.

Example 9.14. Adenocarcinoma of the vagina in young women was recorded rarely until the report of several cases treated at the Vincent Memorial Hospital (in Boston, MA, USA) between 1966 and 1969. The unusual diagnosis of this tumour in eight young patients led to the conduct of a case–control study to search for possible etiological factors. For each of the eight cases with vaginal carcinoma, four matched female controls born within five days and on the same type of hospital service (ward or private) as the case were selected from the birth records of the hospital in which the case was born. All the mothers were interviewed personally by a trained interviewer using a standard questionnaire (Herbst et al., 1971).

In Example 9.14, cases and controls were individually matched on date of birth (and, hence, age), hospital of birth and type of hospital service (ward versus private). If the factors are not too numerous and there is a large reservoir of persons from which the controls can be chosen, case–control individual matching may be readily carried out. However, if several characteristics or levels are considered and there are not many more potential controls than cases, matching can be difficult and it is likely that for some cases, no control will be found. Moreover, when cases and controls are matched on any selected characteristic, *the influence of that characteristic on the disease can no longer be studied.* The number of characteristics for which matching is desirable and practical is actually rather small. It is usually sensible to match cases and controls only for characteristics such as age, sex and ethnicity whose association with the disease under study is well known.

As an alternative to individual matching, we may *frequency match* (or *group match*). This involves selecting controls so that a similar proportion to the cases fall into the various categories defined by the matching variable. For instance, if 25% of the cases are males aged 65–75 years, 25% of the controls would be taken to have similar characteristics. Frequency matching within rather broad categories is sufficient in most studies.

9.4   Measuring exposures

Data on the relevant exposures can be obtained by personal, postal or telephone interview, by examining medical, occupational or other records, or by taking biological samples. Whatever method is chosen, it is fundamental to ensure that the information gathered is unbiased, i.e., it is not influenced by the fact that an individual is a case or a control. Ideally, the investigator or interviewer should be 'blind' to the hypothesis under study and to the case/control status of the study subjects. In practice, this may be difficult to accomplish, but all possible efforts should be made to ensure unbiased collection of data to minimize *observer bias*. Particular effort is required in multicentric studies to ensure standardization of data collection techniques across the different participating centres.

Bias can also occur when the validity of the exposure information supplied by the subjects differs for cases and controls (*responder bias*). Subjects with a serious disease are likely to have been thinking hard about possible causes of their condition and so cases may be inclined to give answers that fit with what they believe (or think is acceptable to say) is the cause of their illness. This type of responder bias is called *recall bias*. Responder bias can be minimized by keeping the study members unaware of the hypotheses under study and, where possible, ensuring that both cases and controls have similar incentives to remember past events. These issues are further discussed in Chapter 13.

9.5   Analysis

The analysis of data from case–control studies depends on their design. Individual-matched studies require a different type of analysis from ummatched (or frequency-matched) studies.

9.5.1 Unmatched (and frequency-matched) studies

The first step in the analysis of an unmatched case–control study is to construct a table showing the frequency of the variables of interest separately for cases and controls. The frequency of some of these variables in the controls may help to judge whether they are likely to represent the population from which the cases arise. For instance, in Example 9.15, the distribution of schooling, parity, smoking, etc. in the control group of this population-based study may be compared with governmental statistics or results from surveys conducted in the same areas.

In Example 9.15, the distributions of some of the variables known to be risk factors for cervical cancer are consistent with those found in other studies in that cases were more likely to have a lower educational level, higher parity and a greater number of sexual partners than controls. They were also more likely to have ever used oral contraceptives or smoked.

Table 9.4.
Distribution of selected socio-demo-graphic and reproductive variables among cervical cancer cases and controls in each of the participating centres[a].

Example 9.15. In the cervical cancer case–control study described in Example 9.2, the distribution of variables known to be risk factors for cervical cancer was examined among cases and controls. Table 9.4 shows the results for some of these variables.

	Spain		Colombia	
	Cases No. (%)	Controls No. (%)	Cases No. (%)	Controls No. (%)
Age (years)				
<30	7 (2.8)	7 (2.9)	15 (8.1)	10 (6.7)
30–39	41 (16.4)	39 (16.4)	48 (25.8)	30 (20.1)
40–44	30 (12.0)	27 (11.3)	27 (14.5)	24 (16.1)
45–54	61 (24.4)	58 (24.4)	50 (26.9)	40 (26.9)
55+	111 (44.4)	107 (45.0)	46 (24.7)	45 (30.2)
Schooling				
Ever	162 (64.8)	179 (75.2)	155 (83.3)	140 (94.0)
Never	88 (35.2)	59 (24.8)	31 (16.7)	9 (6.0)
Parity				
0–2	102 (40.8)	136 (57.1)	41 (22.0)	45 (30.2)
3–5	119 (47.6)	86 (36.1)	62 (33.3)	53 (35.6)
6+	29 (11.6)	16 (6.7)	83 (44.6)	51 (34.2)
Number of sexual partners				
0–1	189 (75.6)	218 (91.6)	76 (40.9)	87 (58.4)
2–5	48 (19.2)	16 (6.7)	77 (41.4)	58 (38.9)
6+	13 (5.2)	4 (1.7)	33 (17.7)	4 (2.7)
Oral contraceptives				
Never	182 (72.8)	175 (73.5)	109 (58.6)	95 (63.8)
Ever	64 (25.6)	53 (22.3)	77 (41.4)	53 (35.6)
Unknown	4 (1.6)	10 (4.2)	0 (0.0)	1 (0.6)
Smoking				
Never	184 (73.6)	198 (83.2)	92 (49.5)	90 (60.4)
Ever	66 (26.4)	40 (16.8)	94 (50.5)	59 (39.6)

[a] Data from Bosch *et al.* (1992)

In an unmatched study, the numbers of cases and controls found to have been exposed and not exposed to the factor under investigation can be arranged in a 2 × 2 table as shown in Table 9.5:

Table 9.5.
Layout of a 2 × 2 table showing data from an unmatched case–control study

	Exposed	Unexposed	Total
Cases	a	b	n_1
Controls	c	d	n_0
Total	m_1	m_0	N

In Section 4.2.2, we presented the three measures of incidence (risk, odds of disease and rate) that can be estimated from a cohort study. These three measures use the same numerator—the number of new cases that occurred during the follow-up period—but different denominators. Risk takes as the denominator people who were at risk at the start of the follow-up; odds of disease takes those who were still disease-free by the end of the follow-up; and the rate uses the total person-time at risk, which takes into account the exact time when the cases occurred. Comparison of these measures of incidence in those exposed relative to those unexposed yields three different measures of relative effect: the risk ratio, the odds (of disease) ratio and the rate ratio, respectively (see Section 5.2.1).

In case–control studies, it is not possible to directly estimate disease incidence in those exposed and those unexposed, since people are selected on the basis of having or not having the condition of interest, not on the basis of their exposure status[a]. It is, however, possible to calculate the odds of exposure in the cases and in the controls:

Odds of exposure in the cases = a/b

Odds of exposure in the controls = c/d

The *odds (of exposure) ratio* can then be calculated as

$$\text{Odds (of exposure) ratio} = \frac{\text{Odds of exposure in the cases}}{\text{Odds of exposure in the controls}} = \frac{a/b}{c/d}$$

Example 9.16. In the case–control study illustrated in the previous example, the risk of cervical cancer was examined in relation to education (schooling). Data from Spain and Colombia were pooled in this analysis (Table 9.6) (Bosch et al., 1992).

| | Schooling | | Total |
	Never ('exposed')	Ever ('unexposed')	
Cervical cancer cases	119 (a)	317 (b)	436 (n_1)
Controls	68 (c)	319 (d)	387 (n_0)
Total	187 (m_1)	636 (m_0)	823 (N)

[a] Data from Bosch *et al.* (1992)

Odds ratio = (119 / 317) / (68 / 319) = 1.76

95% confidence interval = 1.24–2.46

$\chi^2 = 11.04$, 1 d.f.; $P = 0.0009$

(Confidence intervals and test statistics for the odds ratio were calculated as shown in Appendix 6.1.)

Table 9.6.
Schooling among cervical cancer cases and controls.[a]

It can be shown algebraically that the odds (of exposure) ratio obtained from a case–control study provides an unbiased estimate of one of the three relative measures of effect that can be obtained from

[a] Indirect calculations are possible in population-based case–control studies (see Appendix A16.1)

a cohort study, depending on the sampling scheme used to select the controls (see Section 9.3.3). If controls are selected from all those who are initially at risk, the case–control study will directly estimate the *risk ratio*. If controls are sampled from those who are still disease-free by the end of the follow-up, the study will estimate the *odds (of disease) ratio*. If controls are selected from those still at risk at the time each case is ascertained, the study will provided an unbiased estimate of the *rate ratio*. In this last instance, the analysis should respect the fact that cases and controls are *matched* with respect to time. (An unmatched analysis will also yield an unbiased estimate of the rate ratio if the rates of acquiring disease remain constant over time among both the exposed and unexposed populations and the total numbers at risk remain relatively constant in both populations.)

As we saw in Section 5.2.1, when the disease is rare, as with cancer, cases constitute a negligible fraction of the population. The number of people at risk in a cohort study remains practically constant over time and therefore the three measures of effect yield similar results. Consequently, the three sampling schemes used to select controls in a case–control study will also provide similar results. If the disease is common, however, different control sampling schemes will yield different results and the choice of the most appropriate one will depend on the specific problem being addressed (Smith *et al.*, 1984; Rodrigues & Kirkwood, 1990).

In strict terms, the odds ratio obtained from a case–control study tells us how many more (or less, if the exposure is associated with a reduced risk) times likely the cases are to have been exposed to the factor under study compared with the controls.

In Example 9.16, cervical cancer cases were 76% more likely to have never attended school than controls. Since the odds ratio obtained from a case–control study provides an estimate of one of the three relative measures of effect that can be calculated from a cohort study, we can also interpret it as an indication of the likelihood of developing the disease in the exposed individuals relative to those unexposed. In our example, the odds ratio indicates that women who never attended school were 76% more likely to develop cervical cancer than those who attended.

As in other types of study, inferences about the association between a disease and a factor are considerably strengthened if there is evidence of a gradient between the level (or intensity) of exposure and risk of the disease in question. Odds ratios can be computed separately for each level of the exposure. The general approach is to treat the data as a series of 2 × 2 tables, comparing controls and cases at different levels of exposure, and then calculating the odds ratio at each level.

In Example 9.17, there is a trend of increasing risk of cervical cancer with increasing number of sexual partners.

Table 9.7.
Number of lifetime sexual partners among cases and controls.[a]

Example 9.17. *In the cervical cancer case–control study conducted in Colombia and Spain and described in Examples 9.2 and 9.15, the risk of developing cervical cancer was examined in relation to the lifetime number of sexual partners (Bosch et al., 1992). Data from Spain and Colombia were pooled together in this analysis (Table 9.7).*

Number of sexual partners	Cervical cancer cases	Controls	Odds ratio (95% confidence interval)
0–1[b]	265	305	1.0[c]
2–5	125	74	1.94 (1.39–2.70)
6+	46	8	6.62 (3.07–14.27)

[a] Data from Bosch *et al.* (1992)
[b] Taken as the baseline (reference) category.
[c] χ^2 test for trend = 39.48; 1 d.f.; $P<0.00001$
(Confidence intervals and χ^2 test for trend in odds ratio calculated as shown in Appendix 6.1.)

The odds ratios for each category of exposure were calculated in the following way:

	Number of sexual partners	
	2–5 ('exposed')	0–1 ('unexposed')
Cervical cancer cases	125	265
Controls	74	305

Odds ratio = (125 / 265) / (74 × 305) = 1.94

	Number of sexual partners	
	6+ ('exposed')	0–1 ('unexposed')
Cervical cancer cases	46	265
Controls	8	305

Odds ratio = (46 / 265) / (8 / 305) = 6.62

Special statistical techniques can be used to adjust for potential confounding factors in the analysis. These are discussed in Chapters 13 and 14. One of these techniques was used to examine the association between schooling and the risk of developing cervical cancer found in Example 9.16. The *crude odds ratio* was 1.8 (Table 9.6). After taking into account differences in age, participating centre, human papillomavirus status, number of sexual partners, education, age at first birth, and history of previous screening between cases and controls, the resulting *adjusted odds ratio* was 2.5 (95% confidence interval = 1.6–3.9). Thus, the association between never having attended school and cervical cancer observed in the crude analysis could not be explained by differences in the distribution between cases and controls of any of these factors (in fact, the adjusted odds ratio was higher than the crude odds ratio) (see Section 13.2 and Chapter 14 for further discussion of these issues).

9.5.2 Individual-matched studies

Individual-matched studies require a special type of analysis, in which the 2×2 table takes a different form. Let us consider the simplest situation where there is only one control per case. The status of the cases with regard to the presence or absence of the exposure of interest is cross-tabulated against the exposure status of their respective controls (Table 9.8).

Table 9.8.
Layout of a 2×2 table with data from an individual-matched case–control study (control-to-case ratio = 1:1).

		Controls		Total
		Exposed	Unexposed	
Cases	Exposed	r	s	a
	Unexposed	t	u	b
	Total	c	d	$N/2$

In this table, r, s, t, u represent the number of pairs in which

r = case exposed and control exposed (+ +)
s = case exposed but control not exposed (+ –)
t = case not exposed and control exposed (– +)
u = case not exposed and control not exposed (– –)

The marginal totals (a, b, c, d) of this table correspond to the entries in the cells of the table for the unmatched studies. The total for the entire table is $N/2$ pairs, where N represents the total number of paired individuals.

The *matched odds ratio* can be calculated as

$$\text{Odds ratio} = s/t \text{ (provided } t \text{ is not equal to 0)}$$

This odds ratio calculation considers only the discordant pairs. It can be explained intuitively: pairs where both case and control were exposed or where both were unexposed give no information about the relationship of the exposure to disease (Example 9.18).

The analysis is more complex than shown here if there is more than one control per case (see Breslow & Day (1980), chapter 5).

9.6   Interpretation of results

Case–control studies are well suited to study diseases of long induction, because no lengthy follow-up is involved. They are also suitable for studying rare diseases, since a prospective cohort study would require the recruitment of a very large number of individuals and a long follow-up period to ensure the accrual of a sufficient number of cases.

The interpretation of case–control studies is, however, less straightforward than that of cohort studies and the investigator must always consider

Example 9.18. *A case–control study was carried out in Canada to assess whether artificial sweeteners, particularly saccharin, increased the risk of bladder cancer. Newly diagnosed cases of bladder cancer that occurred among residents in the provinces of British Columbia, Nova Scotia and Newfoundland between April 1974 and June 1976 were identified through provincial cancer registries and cooperative pathologists and urologists. A total of 821 eligible cases were ascertained, and 632 of these were personally interviewed in their homes using a structured questionnaire. Reasons for failure to interview included death (56), refusal (65), too ill to be interviewed (25), and refusal of permission by the attending physician (34). Most interviews were done within three months of diagnosis, and all within six months. For each case, an individual matched on sex, age (within 5 years), and neighbourhood residence was interviewed (Howe et al., 1977). The main results are shown in Table 9.9.*

		Controls		Total
		Exposed	**Unexposed**	
Cases	Exposed	468 (*r*)	87 (*s*)	555 (*a*)
	Unexposed	73 (*t*)	4 (*u*)	77 (*b*)
	Total	**541 (*c*)**	**91 (*d*)**	**632 (*N/2*)**

[a] Data from Howe *et al.* (1977)

Matched odds ratio = 87/73 = 1.19

95% confidence interval for the matched odds ratio = 0.86–1.65

McNemar's χ^2 = 1.23; *P* = 0.27.

(The calculation of confidence intervals and significance tests for matched case–control studies is explained in Breslow & Day (1980)).

Table 9.9.
Frequency of exposure to artificial sweeteners among 632 bladder cancer cases and their individual-matched controls.[a]

whether the result could have arisen as a result of selection bias in the choice of cases and controls, information bias in the gathering of exposure data, or failure to take proper account of confounding factors.

The most serious potential problem in case–control studies is that the procedures used to select cases and controls may produce groups that are not truly comparable.

In Example 9.19, selection bias could have affected the results of this study since only 62% (314/510) of all eligible patients were included in the final analysis. Low participation levels can introduce bias if cases who used oral contraceptives were more or less likely to participate in the study. If, for instance, users of oral contraceptives were more likely to have a less aggressive form of breast cancer than non-users and, hence, a better survival, this would lead to over-estimation of the effect of oral contraceptives since a high proportion of the deaths would have occurred among non-users.

Selection of an appropriate control group is one of the most difficult problems in case–control studies. Controls must come from the same defined population as the cases. The use of hospital-based controls works only if patients with different diseases came from the same general population (i.e.,

Example 9.19. The relation between use of oral contraceptives by young women and their risk of breast cancer was investigated in a population-based case–control study conducted in Los Angeles County. The cases were patients with histologically confirmed breast cancer, first diagnosed between July 1972 and May 1982, diagnosed before age 37 years, and without a prior history of malignancy. A total of 510 eligible cases were identified through the local population-based cancer registry, of whom 458 were still alive at the time of the first contact through their doctors. Physicians gave permission to contact 393 (86%) of these patients. Of these, 26 could not be located and 37 refused to be interviewed. Thus, completed questionnaires were obtained from 330 patients. Sixteen of these patients were later excluded because no suitable individually matched control was found (Pike et al., 1983).

if the referral patterns are the same for the disease under investigation and the control diseases) and if the control diseases are themselves unrelated to the exposure. In many situations, it is difficult to be sure that these conditions are satisfied. The use of population-based controls avoids these problems, but selection bias may still be introduced if the levels of non-response are high either because some eligible controls cannot be traced or because they refuse to participate (as in Example 9.20). In this instance, the control series may not be representative of the population from which the cases arise.

Example 9.20. The possible association between oral contraceptive use and the risk of breast cancer at young ages (under 45 years) was investigated in a population-based case–control study conducted in Sweden and Norway. In Norway, where notification of all cancer diagnoses is mandatory, cases were identified from population-based cancer registries. A total of 114 eligible women were identified of whom 105 (92%) participated. For each case who agreed to participate, two controls were chosen from an up-to-date national population register. Potential controls were mailed a request to participate. If an answer was not received within four weeks or if the control refused to participate, a new control was selected. Nine controls were never located; 34 never answered the letter; 38 refused to participate; 4 were either temporarily abroad and could not be reached or had mental disorders. Thus, to obtain two controls for each case, it was eventually necessary to select 295 controls from the population register. Only 72% of the women with whom contact was sought were interviewed (Meirik et al., 1986).

Another problem of case–control studies is that accurate measurements of past exposures are usually difficult to obtain, and the degree of accuracy and completeness of these measurements may be different for cases and controls. For instance, recall bias can arise in case–control studies because patients with the disease under study may be inclined to answer questions more carefully than control subjects. Comparison of the exposure histories obtained from cases and controls with an independent source of information (e.g., medical records) may help to determine whether there was a systematic difference in recall by cases and controls.

> **Example 9.21.** *In the study described in the Example 9.20, an introductory letter with a brief description of the aim and scope of the study was sent initially to cases and controls. If they agreed to participate, they were interviewed personally by specially trained professional female interviewers (Meirik et al., 1986).*

In Example 9.21, the aim of the investigation was explained to the women involved. This may have increased recall bias, particularly since the study was carried out during a time of great public concern about oral contraceptives and breast cancer. This problem could have been minimized to a certain extent by not disclosing the study hypothesis to the study subjects.

The other potential source of bias in a case–control study is *diagnostic bias*. For instance, if women using oral contraceptives are more likely than non-users to examine their breasts, or to have them examined by a physician or nurse, or to undergo mammography, diagnostic bias may be introduced. Thus, if a positive association between oral contraceptives and breast cancer is found in a study, it may just be due to the fact that oral contraceptive users are more investigated and therefore more likely to be diagnosed with breast cancer than non-users. One way of minimizing diagnostic bias is to obtain information on the frequency of breast examinations for each of the study subjects so that any effects of more frequent surveillance of oral contraceptive users can be controlled for in the analysis.

A well conducted case–control study that has taken into account all the methodological concerns can yield valid and informative results. As discussed earlier in this chapter (see Sections 9.3.3 and 9.5), if cases and controls are selected independently of exposure and controls are sampled randomly from a defined study population from which the cases arose, the results from a case–control study provide an unbiased estimate of the measure of effect that would be obtained from an equivalent cohort study. Nevertheless, it is important to remember that case–control studies always have the potential for bias and that each study should be evaluated individually to determine whether bias influenced the results. Usually, the difficulty lies in the fact that although it is easy to identify potential sources of bias in any particular case–control study, it is rarely possible to estimate the true impact that these biases may have had on the results.

An important limitation of case–control studies is that they cannot provide direct estimates of the incidence of disease in those exposed and in those unexposed (unless they are population-based; see Appendix 16.1). Thus, it is usually not possible to calculate the absolute impact of the exposure on the occurrence of the disease.

Case–control studies are not suitable for studying rare exposures because very few cases will have been exposed, unless a large proportion of the total

Further reading

* A brief history of the development and use of case–control studies in epidemiology is given in Lilienfeld & Lilienfeld (1979).

* Breslow & Day (1980) provides a comprehensive treatment of the analysis of case–control studies in cancer epidemiology.

* Detailed discussions of sampling schemes for selection of controls are given by Miettinen (1976), Greenland & Thomas (1982), Smith *et al.* (1984) and Rodrigues & Kirkwood (1990).

cases of disease are attributable to that particular exposure (i.e., the population excess fraction is high (see Section 16.2.1)). For instance, the prevalence of asbestos exposure is rare in the general population and accounts for a small proportion of lung cancers. Therefore a case–control study would not be appropriate to investigate the relationship between this exposure and lung cancer because very few cases would have been exposed to asbestos. However, this study design would be appropriate to investigate the relation between asbestos and pleural cancer because this exposure is responsible for a large proportion of these cases.

Finally, the temporal sequence between exposure and disease may be difficult to establish. The possibility that the exposure is the result (rather than the cause) of the disease should always be considered (*reverse causality*). For instance, even if an association between diet and stomach cancer is found in a case–control study, there is a possibility that dietary differences are a consequence rather than a cause of the cancer.

Box 9.1. Key issues

- Case–control studies are studies in which a group of people with the condition of interest ('cases') and a group without that condition ('controls') are identified and the prevalence (or level) of the relevant exposure is measured in the two groups and compared.

- The main advantages of these studies are:

  1. They are efficient in time and cost (at least compared with prospective cohort studies)

  2. They provide the possibility to investigate a wide range of possible risk factors.

  3. They are particularly suitable to investigate rare diseases or diseases with a long induction period.

- The main disadvantages of these studies are:

  1. It may be difficult to select an appropriate control group (*selection bias*).

  2. It is difficult to obtain accurate unbiased measures of past exposures (*information bias*).

  3. The temporal sequence between exposure and disease may be difficult to establish (*reverse causality*).

  4. They are not suitable for investigating rare exposures (unless the exposure is responsible for a large proportion of cases, i.e., the population excess fraction is high).

  5. It is not possible to obtain estimates of disease incidence among those exposed and those unexposed to a putative risk factor (except if the study is population-based).

Chapter 10
Cross-sectional surveys

Cross-sectional surveys are studies aimed at determining the frequency (or level) of a particular attribute, such as a specific exposure, disease or any other health-related event, in a defined population at a *particular point in time*. For instance, we can carry out a cross-sectional survey to estimate the prevalence of hepatitis B infection, the prevalence of smoking or the proportion of women of childbearing age who are breast-feeding in a given population at the time of the survey (Example 10.1).

Example 10.1. The World Fertility Surveys (WFS) were national surveys of human reproductive behaviour conducted in about 40 developing and 20 developed countries in the late 1970s. Among other aspects of reproductive behaviour, these surveys collected information on breast-feeding practices (United Nations, 1987). Table 10.1 shows the percentages of women aged 15–49 years who were breast-feeding around the time of these surveys in selected countries.

Region and country	Year of survey	Sample size	Percentage of women aged 15–49 years currently breast-feeding
Africa			
Egypt	1980	8788	34.3
Ghana	1979–80	6125	37.7
Kenya	1977–78	8100	43.2
Latin America and the Caribbean			
Colombia	1976	5378	17.1
Mexico	1976	7310	19.8
Venezuela	1977	4361	15.3
Asia and Oceania			
Bangladesh	1975–76	6513	51.1
Indonesia	1976	9155	15.9
Pakistan	1975	4996	40.5
[a] Data from United Nations (1987)			

Table 10.1.
Proportion of women aged 15–49 years in selected countries who were breast-feeding at the time the World Fertility Surveys were conducted, 1975–80.[a]

In this type of study, subjects are contacted at a fixed point in time and relevant information is obtained from them. On the basis of this information, they are then classified as having or not having the attribute of interest.

213

Example 10.2. In the World Fertility Surveys, breast-feeding practices were examined in relation to socioeconomic factors such as mother's education (Table 10.2).

Table 10.2.
Mean duration of breast-feeding (months) by mother's years of schooling in selected countries. World Fertility Surveys, 1975–80.[a]

Region and Country (sample size)	Year of survey	Years of schooling			
		Zero	1–3	4–6	7+
Africa					
Egypt (8788)	1980	21.2	19.5	16.3	10.2
Ghana (6125)	1979–80	21.3	n.a.	19.2	15.7
Kenya (8100)	1977–78	19.6	17.4	15.2	12.5
Latin America and the Caribbean					
Colombia (5378)	1976	11.9	11.4	8.3	5.3
Mexico (7310)	1976	12.9	10.9	8.3	3.8
Venezuela (4361)	1977	11.6	10.0	6.7	3.5
Asia and Oceania					
Bangladesh (6513)	1975–76	34.4	30.4	n.a.	n.a.
Indonesia (9155)	1976	28.4	27.0	24.7	13.7
Pakistan (4996)	1975	22.0	n.a.	19.8	n.a.

[a] Data from United Nations (1987)

n.a. = data not available because of small sample sizes.

In some instances, cross-sectional surveys attempt to go further than just providing information on the frequency (or level) of the attribute of interest in the study population by collecting information on both the attribute of interest and potential risk factors. For instance, in a cross-sectional survey conducted to estimate the prevalence of hepatitis B in a given population, it is also possible to collect data on potential risk factors for this condition such as socioeconomic status, intravenous drug use, sexual behaviour, etc.

Example 10.3. A national survey was conducted in the USA in 1966 to assess the prevalence of smoking, and attitudes and beliefs towards the use of tobacco and other related variables. The questionnaire included, among others, questions on the following topics: smoking behaviour (past and present); attempts to stop and/or cut down cigarette smoking; self-estimation of future smoking behaviour; beliefs about ability to change, and willingness to change; rationale for cigarette smoking behaviour; attitudes and beliefs about smoking as a health hazard in general, and to respondents in particular; gratification derived from smoking; and social pressures for continuation or cessation (US Department of Health, Education, and Welfare, 1969).

In Example 10.2, breast-feeding duration was examined by years of schooling of the mother. In all countries where the comparison could be made, breast-feeding duration decreased consistently with increasing educational level of the mother.

Cross-sectional surveys are also useful in assessing practices, attitudes, knowledge and beliefs of a population in relation to a particular health-related event (Example 10.3). The results from these surveys not only give an indication of the magnitude of the problem in a particular population at a particular point in time, but also provide a basis for designing appropriate public health measures (e.g., health education campaigns).

Surveys are also a valuable method of obtaining information on the patterns of morbidity of a population, as well as on the utilization of preventive and curative health services (Example 10.4). Their results help health planners to establish health priorities.

> *Example 10.4.* *The Danfa Comprehensive Rural Health and Family Planning Project was set up to assess health care and family-planning delivery systems in southern Ghana. As part of this project, a baseline household morbidity cross-sectional survey was undertaken in the study area to provide data on patterns of illness and disability, amount of work lost and use of health care services during the two-week period preceding the survey (Belcher* et al., *1976).*

10.1 Target population and study sample

As for the other types of epidemiological design, the aims of the study must be clearly established before its start. This process requires a precise definition of the attribute of interest (whether disease, exposure or any other health-related event) and of potential risk factors, and a clear consideration of the *target population*, i.e., the population to which the main results of the study will be extrapolated. For instance, if we were planning a study of the dietary habits of Seventh Day Adventists (a religious group who do not eat meat or drink alcohol), it would be necessary to decide whether to include children, recent converts to the church or those who had recently left.

Next, a suitable *source population* needs to be identified (Figure 10.1). For practical and logistic reasons, the source population is generally more limited than the target population. For instance, although our target population comprises all Seventh Day Adventists, it would be impossible to include all of them in the study. The choice of the source population should be determined by the definition of the target population and by logistic constraints. For logistic reasons, we might decide to conduct the study in California (USA), where a large number of Seventh Day Adventists live. If this source population is small enough to be studied using the human and financial resources available, the entire population can be included. If the source population is still too large, a *representative sample* has to be selected.

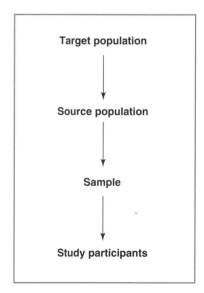

Figure 10.1.
Diagram illustrating the relationship between the target population and the study participants.

10.1.1 How to select a sample?

In order to select a sample from the source population, we need to decide on the *sample design*, i.e., on the method to be used for selecting the sampling units from the population. Samples are sometimes chosen by *judgement* (i.e., what the investigator judges to be a 'balanced' or 'representative' sample) or by *convenience* (i.e., the most easily obtained subjects such as volunteers or people who attend a clinic).

None of these methods provides any guarantee against the possibility that (conscious or unconscious) selection bias may be introduced. Some people may be more likely than others to get into the sample, and the sample will become unrepresentative. For example, clinic attenders may be different from non-attenders (as in Example 10.5).

> *Example 10.5. A survey was conducted in Seoul, Republic of Korea, to determine the prevalence of* Helicobacter pylori *infection in the population of the city. The sample consisted of asymptomatic healthy adults and children who visited a health screening centre at Guro Hospital for routine health examination. The majority of the individuals served by the centre were from the middle class, with fewer private patients and families from lower socioeconomic classes (Malaty* et al., *1996).*

The best approach is to use *random sampling*. In this method, chance alone determines who will be included in the sample, removing any possibility of selection bias.

In order to draw a random sample from the source population, we need to have a *sampling frame*, i.e., a complete enumeration of the sampling units in the study population. The sampling unit may be an individual person, a household, or a school. Electoral registers may be a suitable sampling frame for adults but not for children. If the sampling frame is based on official statistics, some groups may be under-represented, such as recent immigrants, the homeless, and slum dwellers. A sampling frame may not exist for other groups such as gypsies and other nomad groups. In certain countries it may be impossible to enumerate everyone in the study population. As we shall see later in this chapter (Section 10.1.4), special techniques can be used in these circumstances to ensure the attainment of a representative sample.

10.1.2 Simple random sampling

The most elementary kind of random sample is a simple random sample, in which each sampling unit has an equal chance of being selected directly out of the source population.

The first step is to define who are the sampling units, i.e., the people or items (e.g., households) who are to be sampled. These units need to be defined clearly in terms of their particular characteristics. The next step is to draw up a sampling frame, i.e., a list of all the sampling units in the source population. The sampling frame should be comprehensive, complete and up-to-date, to keep selection bias to a minimum. Common examples of sampling frames include census lists and electoral registers. Once a suitable sampling frame has been identified, its sampling units should be given a number. If the source population is formed by 2000 individuals, each one should be assigned a unique number between 1 and 2000. Random number tables can then be used to select a random sample out of the total sampling units who make up the source population. First, a random starting place in the table and a random direction should be selected. Then all the sequential digits found on the table should be recorded, stopping only when the required sample size is reached (see Section 7.9.2 for an illustration of how to use tables of random numbers). Alternatively, sequences of random numbers can be generated by a calculator or a computer package. The sample will be formed by the sampling units which correspond to these random numbers.

The main feature of simple random sampling is that it is relatively simple as compared with other methods (such as those described in Sections 10.1.4 and 10.1.5). Its main limitation is that it is only practicable when the population is relatively small and concentrated in a small geographical area and where the sampling frame is complete.

Example 10.6. A cross-sectional survey was performed on random samples of women in a high-risk area for cancer of the cervix uteri (Nuuk, Greenland) and in a low-risk area (Nykøbing Falster) of Denmark to assess the prevalence of infections by specific types of human papillomavirus (HPV) and herpes simplex virus (HSV) infection. The Danish Central Population Registry is a computerized record of everyone who was alive in 1968 or who was born in or immigrated into Denmark thereafter and includes information on vital status and emigration. A sample of 800 women aged 20–39 years, born in Greenland and residing in the municipality of Nuuk/Godthåb, was drawn at random from this population registry. Similarly, a random sample of 800 women aged 20–39 years, born in Denmark and resident in Nykøbing Falster municipality, was also drawn from the same registry (Kjaer et al., 1988).

In Example 10.6, a sample of women was selected by simple random sampling in each of the two municipalities. This method was adequate and convenient since there was a proper sampling frame (i.e., the computerized list) for each area and both populations were concentrated in relatively small geographical areas.

Although it is not usually feasible to use simple random sampling for selecting the whole sample in a survey covering a large geographical area, it is often used for the final selection of the study units (e.g., selecting households in communities, after communities have been selected) within more complex schemes as described in Section 10.1.4.

10.1.3 Systematic sampling

Sometimes it may be more convenient to draw a systematic sample rather than a simple random sample. To do this, the units must be arranged in some kind of sequence as in a directory or in a series of index cards, or houses along a street, or patients as they arrive at a clinic. Then we need to decide what fraction of the population is to be studied. Suppose, for example, we wish to select a sample of 40 from a population of size 200. This will be a 1 in 5 sample. We choose a number at random between 1 and 5—let us suppose it was 2. Then starting at the beginning of the list, we select the sampling unit number 2 and then every fifth subsequent unit. The sample will include units 2, 7, 12, 17,... and so on.

The main advantage of systematic sampling is convenience. It generally provides a good approximation to simple random sampling provided that the intervals do not correspond with any recurring pattern in the source population. If particular characteristics arise in the sampling frame at regular intervals, bias will be introduced. Consider what would happen if the population were made up of a series of married couples with the husband always listed first. Picking every fourth person would result in a sample constituted exclusively by men if one started with the first or third subject or exclusively by women if one started with the second or fourth. Similarly, every 20th house on a list of addresses or houses might be a corner house with different characteristics to the other houses.

10.1.4 Multi-stage sampling

In many situations, it is not feasible or practical to draw a simple random sample or a systematic sample from the whole source population. This is either because a sampling frame is unavailable and the effort involved in drawing one up would be too great, or because the population is dispersed over a very large geographical area. For example, it would be unrealistic to try to draw a simple random sample of 200 people from the population of an entire country. Even if a proper sampling frame did exist, most of the sample would live in different communities far away from each other, and the time and expense involved in contacting them would be prohibitive. One solution is to use *two-stage sampling* as follows:

1. The population is first divided into *clusters*, for example regions, villages or districts, and a list of these *first-stage units* (or primary sample units) drawn.

2. A random sample of first-stage units is then selected from this list.

3. In each of the selected first-stage units, a sampling frame of the *second-stage units* (e.g., households or individuals) is drawn up, and a random sample of these selected.

Example 10.7. A large cross-sectional survey was carried out in China in 1983 at the end of the harvest season to provide information on diet and lifestyle. A multi-stage sampling procedure was used to select the participants.

(1) Sixty-five rural counties (almost all with populations over 100 000 in 1973–75) were selected from a total of 2392 counties. The county selection was not random, but designed to produce geographical areas with a wide range of cancer rates for seven of the most common cancers and wide geographical scatter.

(2) Two communes in each of the 65 counties were selected, i.e., a total of 130 communes. Although the selection of the communes was random, a decision was made to keep all communes within four hours' travel time from the survey station (in the commune) to the county laboratory, resulting in replacement of six communes.

(3) One production brigade in each commune was randomly selected, i.e., a total of 130 production brigades.

(4) Two production teams in each of the 130 production brigades were randomly selected, i.e., a total of 260 production teams.

(5) Within each of the 260 production teams, 25 households were randomly selected from an official registry of residences (yielding a total of 100 households per county and 50 households per commune).

(6) For each household, either one male or one female aged 35–64 years of age was then invited to donate blood and to complete a questionnaire about their dietary, drinking, smoking, and reproductive histories. A total of 6500 subjects participated in the study (Chen et al., 1990).

This strategy can be extended to several stages *(multi-stage sampling)*, as in Example 10.7.

If no frame of households exists and it is not practical to create one, some selection method has to be used which ensures that the sample is as representative as possible. This usually involves two phases: a method of selecting one household to be the starting point and a procedure for selecting succeeding households after that. One possibility is to choose some central point in a town, such as the market or the central square; choose a random direction from that point (e.g., by throwing a pencil in the air and seeing which way it lands); count the number of households between the central point and the edge of town in that direction; select one of these houses at random to be the starting point of the survey. The remaining households in the sample should be selected to give a widespread coverage of the town. The precise method used is not too important, as long as it does not result in all the chosen households being very close to one another, and as long as the rule for selecting households after the first is simple and unambiguous, to remove the possibility of interviewers introducing bias by avoiding certain areas.

If the objective of the study is to obtain an overall estimate of the prevalence or level of an attribute across the whole target population, it is sensible to select the various geographical areas in such a way that the probability of selection is proportional to the size of their population. For instance, a town with a population of 200 000 should stand ten times the chance of being selected as a town with a population of 20 000. A similar number of individuals or households should then be taken from both small and large towns. This *probability proportional to size sampling* approach ensures that individuals (or households) in both large and small towns stand an equal probability of being selected at the start of the sampling procedure.

The advantages of multiple-stage sampling are obvious in terms of costs and time. Thus, should all samples be obtained by selection of convenient clusters? One drawback of this method is that in many situations the clusters are likely to be formed by sets of individuals that are more homogeneous than the population as a whole. For instance, people living in the same neighbourhood or village are likely to be similar in terms of their lifestyle characteristics. If this is the case, individuals in a sample of neighbourhoods provide less information than a sample of similar size obtained from the whole study population.

10.1.5 Stratified random sampling

A stratified random sample involves dividing the population into distinct subgroups according to some important characteristics, such as sex, age or socioeconomic status, and selecting a random sample out of each subgroup. Each subgroup is known as a *stratum* (plural: *strata*), and a separate random sample (simple or multi-stage) is selected in each one.

> **Example 10.8.** *The seroprevalences of immunoglobulin G (IgG), M (IgM), and A (IgA) antibodies to* Helicobacter pylori *were assessed by enzyme-linked immunosorbent assay techniques in a survey conducted in the western part of Copenhagen County (Denmark). In 1982, an age- and sex-stratified sample consisting of 4807 men and women born in the years 1922, 1932, 1942, and 1952 (i.e., aged 30, 40, 50 or 60 years) and residing in the western part of Copenhagen County was randomly drawn from the Danish Population Registry, in which all persons living in Denmark are registered (Andersen et al., 1996).*

In Example 10.8, eight sex and age strata were formed (1, males born 1922; 2, males born 1932; 3, males born 1942; 4, males born 1952; 5, females born 1922; 6, females born 1932; 7, females born 1942; 8, females born 1952), and a random sample selected within each stratum.

There are many situations where this type of sampling is the most appropriate. Sometimes we may wish to have independent results for different strata, and to ensure an adequate sample size in each one. Also, there may be indications that prevalence will vary between strata (as in Example 10.8). Since different sampling schemes can be used in different strata, stratified random sampling is particularly convenient when, for instance, sampling frames are available only for some subgroups of the population (as in Example 10.9).

Example 10.9. The World Fertility Surveys mentioned in Examples 10.1 and 10.2 used a general sampling design to select samples in the various participating countries. Firstly, a sampling frame of geographical area units whose boundaries were reasonably well defined was identified in each country. Secondly, a sample of these area units was randomly selected with probability proportional to the size of their population. Thirdly, a list of dwellings or households in the selected area units was drawn up. Fourthly, a similar number of dwellings or households was randomly chosen from each selected area unit and in these households all women meeting the criteria for entry into the survey were interviewed. Stratification was also used in some countries to ensure that both urban and rural areas were properly represented or because of the need to use different sampling designs in different geographical areas. For instance, population lists were available for some urban areas from which women could be randomly selected without the need to draw up a list of dwellings or households (Scott & Harpham, 1987).

10.1.6 Study participants

Not everyone in the selected random sample will end up participating in the study. Some subjects will refuse to participate despite all reasonable efforts; others will have died or moved out of the area. Thus, participants are usually a subset of the initial random sample (as in Example 10.10).

All possible efforts should be made to ensure a high level of response and participation to minimize selection bias. The number of people or households interviewed, not just the number in the original sample, should always be reported so that non-response levels can be computed. What response level should be considered as acceptable in a survey? For an uncommon condition, a response rate of 85% might be unacceptable, because a few cases in the unexamined 15% might greatly alter the findings; on the other hand, in a survey of a relatively common attribute, this response level might be considered good.

Participants in any survey are likely to differ in some of their characteristics from those who do not respond. The important issues are whether this will introduce bias into the study and if such bias exists, how much it is likely to affect the results. In order to assess the bias introduced by non-response, it is essential to try to obtain some information

Example 10.10. In the cross-sectional survey described in Example 10.6, a random sample of women was selected in each of two geographical areas to assess (and compare) their prevalence of infections by human papillomavirus (HPV) and herpes simplex virus (HSV). The researchers described the method of enrolment of the study participants in each area as follows:

"Eight hundred women aged 20–39 years, born in Greenland and residing in the municipality of Nuuk/Godthåb, were drawn at random from the computerized Central Population Register for the Danish Kingdom as a whole. Of these women, 104 had moved out of the municipality and one had died before they could be contacted, leaving 695 eligible for our study. [...] General information about the study was provided in local news media (newspaper, radio), after which each [randomly selected] woman was invited, by a personal letter, for a visit to the local health clinic. Reminders were sent 2–3 weeks later and non-responders were finally contacted by a personal messenger from the clinic. Of the 695 eligible women, 586 (84.3%) were included in the study; 93 (13.4%) could not be reached and 16 (2.3%) did not want to participate. The relatively high proportion of women that could not be traced may be attributable to errors in the municipal population register and weaknesses of the postal service.

[...] From the Central Population Register a random sample of 800 women, born in Denmark, was drawn from the female population aged 20–39 years in Nykøbing Falster municipality. Fourteen of these women had moved out of the municipality and one had died prior to enrolment, leaving 785 women eligible for investigation. General information about the study was provided through local and national news media. Each [randomly selected] woman was then invited by personal letter to participate in the study and scheduled for a visit to the local hospital. Reminders were sent 2–3 weeks later and non-responders were finally approached by telephone. A total of 661 women (84.2%) were enrolled; 58 (7.4%) could not be contacted and 66 (8.4%) did not want to participate." (Kjaer et al., 1988)

about the individuals who initially refused to participate or could not be contacted. Two approaches are possible. Firstly, a small random sample may be drawn from the non-respondents, and special efforts, including home visits, made to encourage their participation. The findings from this small random sample will indicate the extent of bias among non-respondents as a whole. Secondly, some information may be available for all persons listed in the study population; from this it will be possible to compare respondents and non-respondents with respect to basic characteristics such as age, sex, residence and socioeconomic status.

In Example 10.11, the age distribution of the participants was fairly similar to that of the total female population living in each of the two selected areas, with a slight under-representation of women in the youngest age-group.

Example 10.11. *Consider again the study described in Example 10.10. The age distributions of the total female population in the two selected geographical areas, of the two random samples selected from them, of the women who were eligible and of those who actually participated in the study are shown in Table 10.3.*

Age	Number (%) of women			
	Total female population	Random sample	Eligible women	Participants
Nykøbing Falster (Denmark)				
20–24	975 (27.9)	228 (28.5)	222 (28.3)	166 (25.1)
25–29	774 (22.2)	158 (19.8)	153 (19.5)	132 (20.0)
30–34	825 (23.6)	195 (24.4)	194 (24.7)	172 (26.0)
35–39	920 (26.3)	219 (27.3)	216 (27.5)	191 (28.9)
Total	**3494 (100)**	**800 (100)**	**785 (100)**	**661 (100)**
Nuuk (Greenland)				
20–24	582 (37.0)	281 (35.1)	227 (32.7)	193 (32.9)
25–29	439 (27.9)	226 (28.3)	192 (27.6)	171 (29.2)
30–34	328 (20.8)	167 (20.8)	156 (22.4)	127 (21.7)
35–39	225 (14.3)	126 (15.8)	120 (17.3)	95 (16.2)
Total	**1574 (100)**	**800 (100)**	**695 (100)**	**586 (100)**

[a] Data from Kjaer *et al.* (1988)

Table 10.3.
Age distribution of the female resident populations of Nykøbing Falster (Denmark) and Nuuk (Greenland), of the two random samples selected from them, and of the study participants.[a]

10.1.7 Final comments

Methods for selecting an appropriate sample constitute an important and well developed field of statistics that cannot be covered fully in this chapter. It is worth emphasizing, however, that the sampling design should be appropriate to the specific objectives of the study. To develop and implement a proper sampling scheme requires not only statistical expertise but also familiarity with the field conditions. For instance, if the survey uses 'households' as one of its sampling units, this term needs to be clearly defined in the context of the population where the survey is going to be carried out. A 'household' is usually defined as a group of people who live and eat together. However, in many societies, this definition will not be easily translated into practice. In such instances, it is crucial to obtain a good understanding and clear definition of the different living arrangements of the population to be surveyed before the study begins.

Other practical problems should be foreseen at the design stage of the study and unambiguous instructions written in the protocol and given to the interviewers. For instance, if there is no-one at home when the interviewer arrives, he/she should come back again rather than go to the house next door, because households with a person at home in the day-time tend to differ from those without.

Although a random method to select the study sample is generally the most appropriate, in a large number of epidemiological surveys it is not possible to select a sample in such a way for ethical or logistic reasons. For instance, studies that require the use of invasive diagnostic techniques that can only be performed in a hospital may have to rely on hospital attenders. The conclusions from such studies can be extrapolated to the population of 'hospital attenders', but the extent to which they can be generalized to the whole target population requires careful judgement.

The choice of an appropriate sampling design in cancer epidemiology will also depend on the aims of the survey. If the main objective is to obtain an overall estimate of the prevalence (or level) of an attribute in the target population, random sampling methods should be used at all stages of the sampling process to ensure that selection bias is not introduced. If, however, the main objective of the study is to examine potential exposure–outcome relationships, it may be more appropriate to select the main sampling units in a non-random way since, in these situations, informativeness is usually more important than representativeness. For instance, the selection of the 65 participating Chinese counties in Example 10.7 was not done randomly because the main objective of the survey was not to provide an overall estimate of the prevalence (or level) of the various lifestyle attributes for the whole of China. The intention was rather to compare the distribution of lifestyle attributes in counties known to have very different levels of mortality from certain cancer sites. It was, however, necessary to obtain unbiased lifestyle prevalence estimates for each of the selected counties and thus random methods were used to select the participants in each county.

Another issue that needs to be considered in the sampling design is the size of the sample. The sample should be sufficiently large to address the main objectives of the study with adequate precision, but not excessively larger than required, so that resources are not wasted. Sample size issues are discussed in Chapter 15.

10.2 Data collection

The methods used to collect the relevant data in cross-sectional studies are basically those discussed in Chapter 2. Questionnaires, sometimes supplemented by diagnostic tests and collection of biological samples, are most frequently used to obtain information from the study subjects in this type of study. Most questionnaires include questions about past exposures as well as current exposures. Information on past exposures considerably strengthens the ability of surveys to identify exposure–outcome relationships.

10.3 Analysis

Prevalence[a] is the measure of occurrence of a disease, condition or characteristic that can primarily be obtained from cross-sectional surveys (see Section 4.2.1). This is illustrated in Example 10.12

[a] When the characteristic of interest is a quantitative variable (such as duration of breast-feeding, weight, height, etc.), prevalence can be calculated only if the observations are classified into categories. Otherwise, means or median levels can be used.

Example 10.12. Suppose that a cross-sectional survey was carried out to assess the prevalence of breast cysts in a particular female population. A sample of 5891 women randomly selected from that population were examined and a total of 201 were found to have breast cysts. The prevalence of breast cysts in this population at the time of the survey was thus: 201 / 5891 = 3.4%.

To examine the association between a putative risk factor for the attribute of interest and the attribute itself, the population is first subdivided into those exposed and those not exposed to the factor under study and the prevalence of the attribute in each group is calculated and compared. A *prevalence ratio* can then be computed as the ratio of the prevalence of the attribute of interest in those exposed to the putative risk factor relative to the prevalence in those unexposed.

Example 10.13. Suppose that in the hypothetical survey described in the Example 10.12, the investigators wished to assess whether the prevalence of breast cysts was associated with having ever used oral contraceptives. The results are shown in Table 10.4.

| Breast cysts | Lifetime use of oral contraceptives | | Total |
	Ever used	Never used	
Yes	124	77	201
No	3123	2567	5690
Total	**3247**	**2644**	**5891**

Prevalence of breast cysts among ever-users = 124 / 3247 = 3.8%

Prevalence of breast cysts among never-users = 77 / 2644 = 2.9%

Prevalence ratio = 1.3

Table 10.4.
Breast cysts and lifetime use of oral contraceptives: data from a hypothetical cross-sectional survey.

In Example 10.13, the prevalence of breast cysts was 30% higher in ever-users of oral contraceptives compared to never-users. It should be noted that prevalence ratio is a good estimate of the incidence rate ratio only if the prevalence of the outcome of interest among those unexposed is low (less than 10%) and the duration of the disease is the same among those who were exposed and those who were unexposed to the factor of interest.

Most often the exposures we are interested in can be further classified into various levels of intensity as in Example 10.14. We can then examine trends in prevalence by level of exposure.

It is also usual to measure the strength of the association between a putative risk factor and the outcome of interest in a cross-sectional study by calculating the *odds ratio*. This is the ratio of the odds of exposure to a putative risk factor in subjects with the outcome of interest to that in subjects without the outcome. By calculating odds ratios, the cross-sectional study is analysed as if it were a case–control study. However, cross-sec-

Example 10.14. *A cross-sectional survey was carried out among women attending a university health service to investigate the determinants of cervical human papillomavirus (HPV) infection. A sample of 467 women were asked to complete a self-administered questionnaire on socio-demographic variables and sexual behaviour at the time of their visit to the clinic. A polymerase chain reaction DNA amplification method was used to detect HPV infection. The prevalence of HPV infection was then examined in relation to marital status and lifetime number of male sexual partners (Ley et al., 1991). The results are shown in Table 10.5.*

Table 10.5.
Prevalence of HPV infection by marital status and lifetime number of male sexual partners.[a]

	No. of women	% positive for HPV	Prevalence ratio (95% CI)
Marital status			
Single[b]	437	47.4	1.0
Ever-married	30	20.0	0.4 (0.2–0.9)
Lifetime no. of sexual partners			
1[b]	90	21.1	1.0[c]
2–3	101	32.7	1.5 (0.9–2.4)
4–5	93	54.8	2.6 (1.7–4.0)
6–9	66	56.1	2.7 (1.7–4.3)
10+	102	68.6	3.3 (2.1–4.9)

[a] Data from Ley *et al.* (1991).

[b] Taken as the baseline category.

[c] χ^2 test for trend = 53.10, 1 d.f.; $P < 0.0001$.

(95% confidence intervals (CI) and χ^2 test for trend calculated using the formulae given in Appendix 6.1.)

The prevalence ratio for each exposure level was calculated by forming 2×2 tables as illustrated below for women with 10+ partners.

	Number of male sexual partners		Total
	10+	1	
HPV-positive	70	19	89
HPV-negative	32	71	103
Total	102	90	192

Prevalence among women with 10+ partners = 70/102 = 68.6%

Prevalence among women with one partner = 19/90 = 21.1%

Prevalence ratio = 68.6% / 21.1% = 3.3

tional studies differ from case–control studies in that the 'cases' and the 'controls' are defined *a posteriori*, i.e., during the analysis and not at the design stage. In fact, if the outcome of interest is quantitative, it is even possible to carry out several analyses using different definitions of 'cases' and 'controls' by changing the cut-off point.

Example 10.15. In the hypothetical study of Example 10.13, we can calculate the odds of having ever used oral contraceptives among women with ('cases') and without ('controls') breast cysts.

Odds of exposure to oral contraceptives among 'cases' = 124/77 = 1.61
Odds of exposure to oral contraceptives among 'controls' = 3123/2567 = 1.22
Odds ratio = 1.61 / 1.22 = 1.3

Note, however, that the odds ratio will yield a good estimate of the prevalence ratio only if the baseline prevalence of the condition is low (as in Example 10.15).

Example 10.16. Using data from Table 10.5, we can calculate the odds of having had 10 or more partners ('exposure') among HPV-positive ('cases') and HPV-negative ('controls') women as:

Odds of exposure among the cases = 70/19 = 3.68
Odds of exposure among the controls = 32/71 = 0.45
Odds ratio = 3.68/0.45 = 8.2

This odds ratio of 8.2 contrasts with the prevalence ratio of 3.3 calculated in Example 10.14.

In Example 10.16, it would be inappropriate to take the odds ratio as a measure of relative prevalence, because in this example the baseline prevalence of HPV infection is relatively high (21.1% in women who reported only one partner).

10.4 Interpretation

Cross-sectional surveys are relatively easy and economical to conduct and are particularly useful for investigating exposures that are fixed characteristics of individuals, such as ethnicity and blood group.

Cross-sectional surveys are not, however, the appropriate study design to investigate causal relationships because they are based on prevalent rather than incident cases. Studies of this type can reveal the presence or absence of a relationship between the study variables and prevalent (existing) cases. This implies a need for caution, since prevalent cases may not be representative of all cases of the disease. Cases of short duration, because of either rapid recovery or death, have a smaller chance of being detected in a one-time prevalence survey than cases of longer duration. It follows logically that cases of long duration are over-represented in a cross-sectional study. The characteristics of these long-duration cases may, on average, differ in a variety of ways from the characteristics of all cases of the disease being studied. Prevalent cases can also become unrepresentative of all cases when certain types of case leave the community. Some affected subjects may be institutionalized elsewhere or move to another city where there are special facilities for treatment.

Cross-sectional surveys are also an inadequate approach to the study of rare conditions, since it would be necessary to survey a very large population to identify enough cases. Thus, their use in cancer epidemiology has been limited to the investigation of factors associated with prevalence of precursor lesions.

Another major limitation of cross-sectional studies is their difficulty in establishing the time sequence of events. For instance, in our hypothetical example of breast cysts and oral contraceptive use, it cannot be assumed that oral contraceptive use preceded the appearance of cysts. In fact, women with benign breast disorders are sometimes prescribed oral contraceptives to improve their condition. In contrast, there would be no doubt about the time sequence of the cancer and such traits as blood type or maternal exposure to radiation.

Box 10.1. Key issues

- Cross-sectional surveys are studies in which a group of subjects (*sample*) is selected from a defined population (*source population*) and contacted at a single point in time. On the basis of the information obtained from the subjects at that point in time, they are then classified as having or not having the attribute of interest.

- Various methods may be used to select a representative sample from the source population. *Random sampling* is the best one, because it ensures that chance alone determines who is included in the sample, removing any possibility of *selection bias*. Different sampling designs may be used to select a random sample depending on the specific objectives of the study, availability of a suitable sampling frame, size and geographical spread of the source population, and costs.

- Selecting a random sample does not eliminate selection bias from the study. Selection bias may still be introduced into the study if those who participate differ in significant ways from those who refuse or cannot be traced. It is therefore important to ensure a high participation level.

- The main advantages of cross-sectional surveys are:

  1. They are easier to conduct than other individual-based studies because no follow-up is required.

  2. They provide a good picture of the health care needs of the population at a particular point in time.

  3. They can be used to investigate multiple exposures and multiple outcomes.

- The main disadvantages of cross-sectional surveys are:

  1. Being based on prevalent (existing) rather than incident (new) cases, they are of limited value to investigate etiological relationships.

  2. They are not useful to investigate rare diseases or diseases of short duration.

  3. They are not suitable to investigate rare exposures.

  4. It is difficult to establish the time sequence of events.

Further reading

* A practical book on the role, planning and conduct of surveys in developing countries is that by Casley & Lury (1987).

* Ross & Vaughan (1986) provide a methodological review of the use of cross-sectional surveys to obtain morbidity data and information on the use of health services in developing countries.

Chapter 11
Studies based on routine data

Routine-data-based studies are characterized by the fact that data on both the exposure(s) and the outcome(s) of interest are obtained from routine data-collection systems (e.g., cancer registries, hospital registries, death notification, etc.). Thus, studies of this type can be carried out relatively quickly and cheaply, without the need to contact the study subjects. Their main limitation, however, is that the number of variables available from routine surveillance systems is generally limited.

Studies based on routine data can be carried out at an *individual* or at an *aggregated* level.

11.1 Individual level

Most routine data-collection systems collect data on personal attributes such as age, sex, place of birth, place of residence, occupation, etc. Cancer occurrence can then be examined in relation to these variables, either to search for patterns that may suggest etiological hypotheses or to confirm a specific hypothesis.

11.1.1 Place of residence

Routine-data-based studies of the variability in cancer incidence across the world have given an indication of the extent to which environmental factors are implicated in the causation of each cancer type (Example 11.1).

Examination of geographical variations in cancer incidence may provide important etiological clues and stimulate further investigations. Cancer of the oesophagus is one of the cancer sites with the most striking patterns of geographical variation. Its incidence varies sharply from one area to another, with foci of very high risk completely surrounded by areas of very low risk. The remarkable geographical variation in the risk of this cancer in central Asia (Example 11.2) stimulated the conduct of a series of cross-sectional and case–control studies in northern Iran with the specific aim of investigating possible risk factors. These studies were interrupted in 1978 by the civil unrest in the area but initial results suggested a strong association with a diet poor in vegetables and with the use of opium (Joint Iran–International Agency for Research on Cancer Study Group, 1977).

Part of the international differences in cancer risks may be genetic rather than environmental. But for many cancer sites, there are still marked variations in incidence within countries, even when their populations are genetically fairly homogeneous.

The distribution shown in Example 11.3 was initially assumed to be due

Table 11.1.
International variations in recorded incidence for selected cancer sites: the highest and lowest rate among all the population-based cancer registries included in *Cancer Incidence in Five Continents*, Vol. V. Rates per 100 000 pyrs, age-standardized to the world standard population.[a]

Example 11.1. *Data from population-based cancer registries located throughout the world were used to examine international variations in cancer incidence. For most cancer sites, there was a more than ten-fold variation between the highest and the lowest recorded incidence rates (Table 11.1).*

Cancer site (ICD 9 code)	Males			Females		
	Highest rate (H)	Lowest rate (L)[b]	H:L ratio	Highest rate (H)	Lowest rate (L)[b]	H:L ratio
Lip (140)	15.1	0.1	151	1.6	0.1	16
Tongue (141)	9.4	0.4	24	3.4	0.2	17
Mouth (143–145)	13.5	0.5	27	15.7	0.2	79
Nasopharynx (147)	30.0	0.3	100	12.9	0.1	129
Pharynx (146, 148–149)	31.3	0.4	78	4.3	0.2	22
Oesophagus (150)	29.2	1.2	24	12.4	0.3	41
Stomach (151)	82.0	3.7	22	36.1	3.0	12
Colon (153)	34.1	1.8	19	29.0	1.8	16
Rectum (154)	21.5	3.0	7	13.4	1.3	10
Liver (155)	34.4	0.7	49	11.6	0.4	29
Larynx (161)	17.8	2.2	8	2.7	0.2	14
Lung (162)	110.0	5.8	19	68.1	1.2	57
Melanoma of skin (172)	30.9	0.2	155	28.5	0.2	143
Breast (174/175)	3.4	0.2	17	93.9	14.0	7
Cervix uteri (180)	–	–	–	83.2	3.0	28
Ovary (182)	–	–	–	25.8	3.3	8
Prostate (185)	91.2	1.3	70	–	–	–
Testis (186)	8.3	0.6	14	–	–	–
Bladder (188)	27.8	1.7	16	8.5	0.8	11
Nervous system (191–192)	9.7	1.1	9	10.0	0.8	13
Non-Hodgkin lymphoma (200, 202)	11.4	1.5	8	8.7	0.9	10
Hodgkin's disease (201)	4.8	0.5	10	3.9	0.3	13

[a] Data from Whelan *et al.* (1990).
[b] Rates based on less than 10 cases were excluded.

to consumption of home-produced apple cider. Normandy and Brittany are the only French provinces where apple cider is produced in considerable quantities and this beverage is largely consumed in the provinces themselves (Tuyns *et al.*, 1983). Further research has shown that all types of alcoholic beverage appear to increase the risk of oesophageal cancer.

11.1.2 Place of birth and ethnicity

People who migrate from one country to another have lifestyle characteristics that are a combination of those prevailing in the host country and those from their homeland. Thus, evidence of a gradient of increasing, or decreasing, risks between population of origin, migrants and the

Example 11.2. Data from local cancer registries were used to examine the geographical distribution of oesophageal cancer in central Asia (Muñoz & Day, 1996). The results from this analysis showed that the incidence of this cancer was extremely high in an area encompassing Kazakhstan, Uzbekistan and Turkmenistan, the north-east of Iran and northern Afghanistan (Figure 11.1).

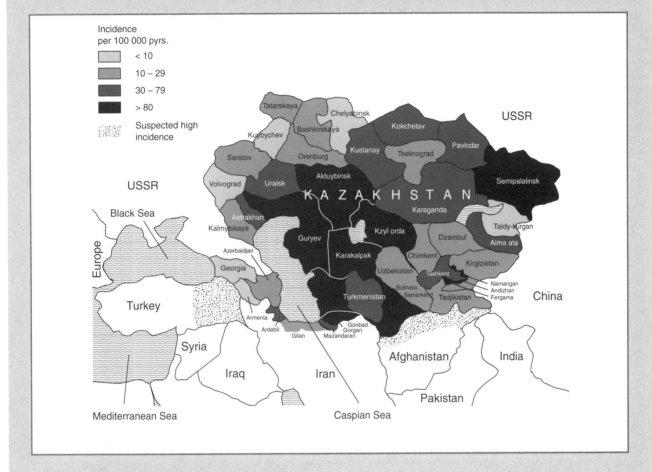

host population can suggest or confirm the importance of environmental factors over genetic factors in the etiology of a particular cancer.

This approach can be refined by adding a time component to it. The degree of cultural integration into the host country can be measured indirectly by information on age at migration and/or time since migration.

In Example 11.4, European immigrants were at lower risk of dying from melanoma than the Australian-born, particularly southern Europeans. This finding may reflect the protective effect of darker complexions. The data also suggested that migration in childhood was associated with a higher risk than migration later in life, but it is difficult to separate this effect from that of duration of stay (i.e., migration at an early age was inevitably associated with a longer stay than migration at an older age).

Figure 11.1.
Oesophageal cancer among men in central Asia. Incidence rates age-standardized to the world standard population (reproduced, by permission of Oxford University Press, from Muñoz & Day, 1996).

Figure 11.2.
Age-standardized mortality rates for cancer of the oesophagus among males, by canton in (*a*) the Normandy departments of Calvados and Orne (reproduced with permission from Tuyns & Vernhes, 1981 © Masson Editeur, 1981), and (*b*) Brittany, 1958–66 (modified from Tuyns & Massé, 1973).

Example 11.3. Routinely collected mortality data were used to examine the geographical distribution of oesophageal cancer in Brittany and the Normandy departments of Calvados and Orne (Figure 11.2). Although rates in most cantons were similar to the average rate in France, in some cantons in eastern Brittany and north-western Orne, mortality was five to ten times higher (Tuyns & Vernhes, 1981).

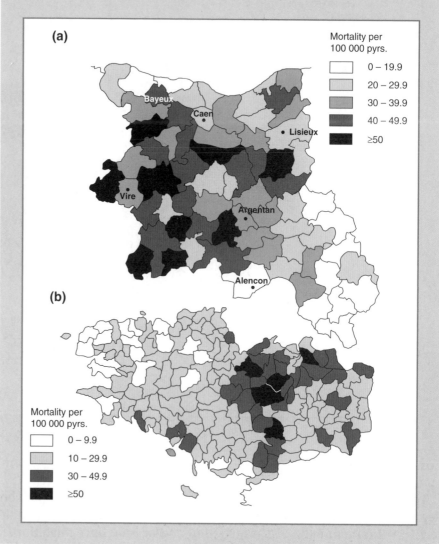

If information on both place of birth and ethnicity is available, it is possible to distinguish first-generation immigrants (born in the country of origin) from their children, often born in the host country, who are considered as second-generation immigrants. This distinction provides another useful indicator of the likely degree of assimilation by the immigrants of the lifestyle characteristics of the host country, which tends to be more marked in the second than in the first generation.

Example 11.4. Data on deaths registered in Australia during the period 1964–85 were obtained from the Australian Bureau of Statistics to examine mortality from malignant melanoma of the skin in immigrants compared with Australian-born individuals, and to investigate changes in risk with age at arrival and duration of stay. Each death record contained information on the following items: sex, country of birth, duration of stay in Australia, year of death, age at death, and cause of death (Khlat et al., 1992). Some of the results from this study are shown in Figure 11.3.

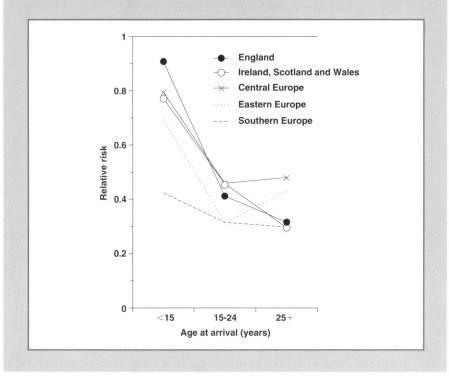

Figure 11.3.
Relative risks (RRs) of mortality from melanoma in male European immigrants to Australia, by region of birth and age at arrival compared to Australian-born (taken as the baseline group: RR=1); Australia, 1964–85 (reproduced with permission from Khlat *et al.*, 1992).

In Example 11.5, there was a consistent pattern: the risk for all four cancer sites converged towards the risk in the host country. For stomach and liver cancer, both of which were more common in Japan than among whites in the United States, men who were born in Japan but migrated to California had considerably lower risks of death than men of the same age in Japan. But risks in the second generation were still lower. In contrast, the risk of colon and prostatic cancers, which were common in California but rare in Japan, rose to approach that of white men in California with migration. These findings clearly show the importance of environmental factors over genetic factors linked to ethnicity. There was still a residual difference between rates in second-generation immigrants and rates in California. These residual differences might reflect differences in genetic susceptibility to these malignancies or, alternatively, they might indicate that second-generation immigrants maintained some of the 'traditional' Japanese lifestyle.

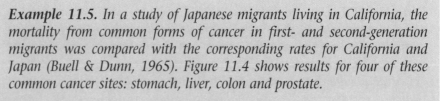

Example 11.5. *In a study of Japanese migrants living in California, the mortality from common forms of cancer in first- and second-generation migrants was compared with the corresponding rates for California and Japan (Buell & Dunn, 1965). Figure 11.4 shows results for four of these common cancer sites: stomach, liver, colon and prostate.*

Figure 11.4.
Age-adjusted mortality rate ratios (RRs) for cancer of the stomach, liver, colon and prostate among Japanese men in Japan, and first- and second-generation Japanese immigrants to California, compared with white men in California (taken as the baseline group: RR=1); Japan, 1958–59 and California, 1956–62 (data from Buell & Dunn, 1965).

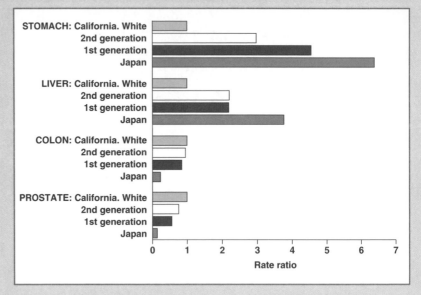

Any differences in cancer risk between migrants and those who remained in their country of origin must be interpreted cautiously, however, since migrants are usually a self-selected group not representative of the population of their country of origin. Migrants are also likely to differ from the host population in a number of demographic and socioeconomic characteristics that should be taken into account when comparing risks. In Example 11.6, most of the migrants originated from the southern part of Italy, which had lower mortality from pancreatic cancer than the country as a whole.

In routine-data-based studies, migrants are identified on the basis of place or country of birth and ethnicity and, when information on these two variables is not available, on the basis of name analysis. More rarely, information on language and religion has also been used. It should, however, be kept in mind that these approaches do not yield similar results. For instance, some of the people born in the Indian subcontinent who migrated to England and Wales are, in fact, of Caucasian ethnicity. Thus, analyses exclusively based on country of birth will include first-generation migrants regardless of their ethnicity. By contrast, analyses exclusively based on ethnicity will include migrants of a particular ethnic group regardless of whether they are of first or of subsequent generations.

Example 11.6. *Mortality from cancer of the pancreas in Italian migrant men was compared with mortality in their country of birth (Italy) and with mortality in eight host countries. Most of the Italian migrants originated from southern Italy. In order to attempt to allow for selection bias, relative risks (RR) were examined for both southern Italy and the whole country. Figure 11.5 shows that, for instance, mortality from pancreatic cancer was much lower in southern Italy (RR = 0.38) and in the whole of Italy (RR = 0.65) than in Canada (taken as the baseline: RR = 1). However, the mortality in Italian migrants to Canada was close to that of the host population (RR = 0.93) (Balzi et al., 1993).*

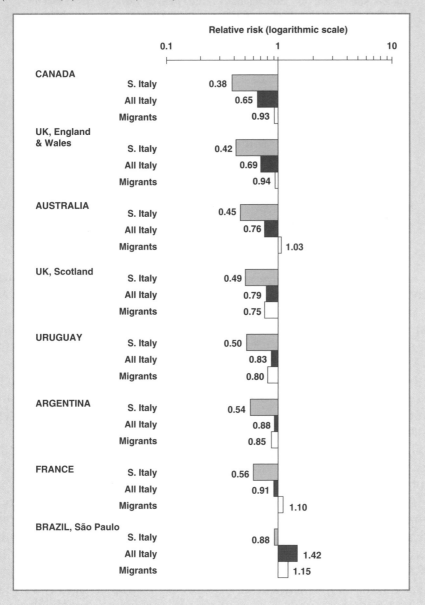

Figure 11.5.
Relative risk (RR) of mortality from pancreatic cancer in Italy (South, all Italy), and in eight male Italian immigrant populations compared with the host country populations (each taken as the baseline group: RR=1) (reproduced with permission from Balzi *et al.*, 1993).

Example 11.7. Death records from residents in São Paulo County (Brazil) during 1978–82 were examined to investigate socioeconomic differentials in cancer mortality. The death certificates contained information on sex, age, place of birth and residence, cause of death, marital status, education and last occupation of the deceased. Information on education was provided by the family of the deceased, as years of schooling, recorded in five categories: less than 1, 1 to 8, 9 to 11, 12 or more, unknown (Bouchardy et al., 1993). Table 11.2 shows educational differentials in mortality in females from cancer at selected sites.

Table 11.2.
Mortality from selected cancer sites by years of schooling, for females aged 35–64 years in São Paulo (Brazil), 1978–82.[a]

Cancer site (ICD-9 code)	No. of deaths	Educational level unknown (%)	Odds ratio by years of education[b]				χ^2 test for trend [c]
			<1[d]	1–8	9–11	>11	
Stomach (151)	691	6.2	1.0	0.7	0.3	0.3	43.5; $P<0.001$
Colon (153)	338	7.1	1.0	1.4	2.1	2.2	13.3; $P<0.001$
Breast (174)	1744	5.9	1.0	1.6	2.4	2.6	77.5; $P<0.001$
Cervix uteri (180)	645	7.2	1.0	0.7	0.4	0.2	50.2; $P<0.001$

[a] Data from Bouchardy *et al.* (1993)

[b] Controls are all cancers except the one under investigation (see Section 11.1.6 for discussion of the method of analysis). Odds ratios are adjusted for age, civil status, and country of birth.

[c] After exclusion of subjects with unknown level of education.

[d] Taken as the baseline category.

11.1.3 Socioeconomic status and occupation

Analyses of cancer risks by socioeconomic and occupational groups have also provided important insights into the epidemiology of cancer.

Example 11.7 shows marked associations between mortality and educational level. The gradient was positive for breast and colon cancers but negative for stomach and cervical cancers (Table 11.2). These gradients are similar to those found in western countries.

In Example 11.8, men engaged in outdoor occupations had the highest proportional incidence of lip cancer (Table 11.3). These findings suggest that sun exposure may be important in the etiology of this cancer.

People with different occupations tend to have different lifestyles as well as different occupational exposures. Thus, differences in their cancer risks might also give etiological clues in relation to factors that are not directly related to the occupation (as in Example 11.9).

Table 11.4 shows a strong social-class gradient in the risk of married women dying from cervical cancer in England and Wales. Wives of men in social class I (highest social class) experienced a mortality rate which was only 34% the rate for all married women. In contrast, the mortality of wives of men in social class V (lowest social class) was 81% higher than that of all married women. Within each social class, however, the highest rates were among wives of men in occupations involving travel

Example 11.8. Cancer registries in England and Wales collect data on the occupation of the cancer cases at the time of their diagnosis. These data were examined to identify occupational groups associated with high incidence of lip cancer (OPCS, 1978). The results are shown in Table 11.3.

Occupation	Observed number of cases	Proportional incidence ratio (PIR)[b]
Farmers, farm managers, market gardeners	23	2.18
Agricultural workers	35	5.26
Bricklayers, tile setters	14	2.39
Construction workers	16	2.35

[a] Data from OPCS (1978)

[b] Age-adjusted. $P < 0.01$ for all the PIRs shown.

(See Example 11.14 for illustration of calculation of proportional incidence ratios).

Table 11.3.
Lip cancer incidence in men aged 15–74 years, England and Wales, 1968–69, by occupation, for those occupations associated with statistically significant increases in proportional incidence ratios.[a]

and absence from home for long periods, a situation known to be associated with high risk of venereal diseases among men. This pattern supported the hypothesis that cervical cancer might be a sexually transmitted infection long before any infectious agent was identified (Beral, 1974).

In interpreting differences in incidence or mortality between socioeconomic groups, it must be remembered that health itself may determine entry into a specific group. For instance, people with poor health are usually forced to work in physically less demanding jobs and more demanding jobs selectively include only those in good health.

11.1.4 Time trends

Information on changes in cancer risk over time can generate etiological hypotheses or support suspected associations between risk factors and disease. Moreover, while the existence of geographical variation in incidence between populations may be explained by genetic differences, changes in incidence in single populations imply the introduction or disappearance of environmental risk factors much more clearly.

In Example 11.10 the incidence of papillary carcinoma of the thyroid increased steadily in the younger age groups in Connecticut during the 40-year study period, resulting in a peak at ages 25–44 years (Figure 11.6). This sudden increase in incidence in the USA followed the widespread use of radiation therapy for 'enlarged thymus' and other benign conditions of the head and neck among children and adolescents between the early 1920s and the late 1950s (Pottern *et al.*, 1980). No similar increase in the incidence of this cancer was observed in populations where the use of this therapy had not been common. This example provides a good illustration of a large increase in the incidence of a particular cancer due to the introduction of a specific exposure.

Table 11.4.
Cervical cancer mortality among married women by husband's social class and occupation, England and Wales, 1959–63.[a] (Only data for occupations with the lowest and highest mortality levels are shown in the table to illustrate the range of risks within each social class.)

> **Example 11.9.** *Routinely collected mortality data for England and Wales were used to examine risk of mortality from cervical cancer among married women by husband's occupation and social class (Beral, 1974). (In this country, death registrars are required to enter the husband's occupation on the death certificate of a married woman or widow; social class for married women is determined by the husband's occupation.) The results are shown in Table 11.4.*

Social class	Occupation of husband	Standardized mortality ratio (SMR, %)[b]
I	All occupations	34
	Clergymen	12
	Scientists	17
	Civil engineers	60
II	All occupations	64
	Teachers	30
	Senior government officials	40
	Publicans and innkeepers	120
	Lodging house and hotel keepers	150
III	All occupations	100
	Clerks of work	40
	Clerks	64
	Crane and hoist operators	159
	Drivers of road goods vehicles	168
IV	All occupations	116
	Shopkeepers and assistants	71
	Gardeners and groundsmen	98
	Fishermen	257
	Deck and engine-room ratings, barge and boatmen	263
V	All occupations	181
	Office and window cleaners	95
	Labourers	222

[a] Data from Beral (1974)

[b] Age-specific rates for all married women in England and Wales taken as the standard.

In Example 11.11, there was no consistent change in the risk of testicular cancer for successive generations of men born between 1880 and 1920. However, for generations born since then, the risk increased steadily, except for men born in Denmark, Norway and Sweden during 1930–45 (the years around the Second World War). The reasons for the marked increase in incidence are not known. The rise has occurred mainly in industrialized countries and in upper socioeconomic groups, suggesting that lifestyle factors associated with affluence may be responsible. Paradoxically, the small

Example 11.10. Data on all thyroid cancer cases incident between 1935 and 1975 were extracted from the Connecticut Tumor Registry (USA) to examine changes over time in the rates of this cancer and its four main histological types (Pottern et al., 1980). The temporal changes for papillary carcinoma, one of the four histological types, are shown in Figure 11.6.

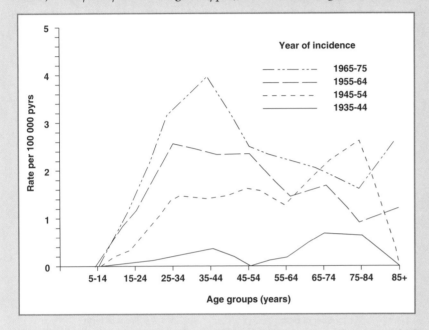

Figure 11.6.
Age-specific incidence rates for papillary carcinoma of the thyroid in women by calendar period, Connecticut (USA), 1935–75 (reproduced with permission from Pottern *et al.*, 1980).

decline in risk for generations born during the Second World War occurred in Denmark, Norway and Sweden, which were apparently less affected by the war than Poland, the former East Germany and Finland.

Time trends can also be used to assess and monitor the effectiveness of cancer control activities such as mass screening programmes. In Example 11.12, there was a close relationship between the decline in incidence of cervical cancer in each country and the degree of coverage by organized mass screening programmes. The decline in incidence was most marked in Finland and Iceland, where national screening programmes were initiated in the early 1960s. The fall was less marked in Sweden, where the programme was introduced more gradually, and in Denmark where only 40% of the population lived in areas with organized mass screening. There was no obvious decline in the incidence of cervical cancer in Norway, the only country which did not have an organized programme (except in one county).

11.1.5 Record linkage studies

Linkage of cancer registry records with records from other sources such as census data, mortality data, company records, hospital admission records, etc., has been undertaken to investigate risk factors for a large

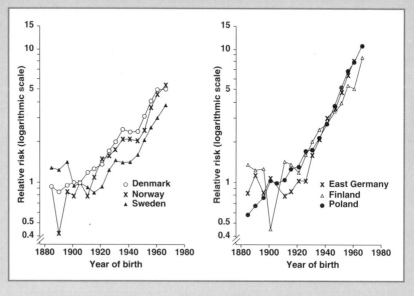

Figure 11.7.
Relative risk (RR) of developing testicular cancer by country and year of birth. (Men born in the study countries between 1900 and 1909 were taken as the baseline category: RR=1) (reproduced with permission from Bergström *et al.*, 1996).

Example 11.11. Data from six European countries (Denmark, Finland, the former German Democratic Republic, Norway, Poland and Sweden) where cancer registration dates back to the 1940s or 1950s were used to examine long-term time trends in the incidence of testicular cancer. These registries cover a total population of about 76 million people. A total of 30 908 incident cases of testicular cancer diagnosed during 1945–84 in men aged 20–84 years were identified (Bergström et al., 1996). Figure 11.7 shows cohort trends (i.e., trends by year of birth of the men) in each country.

number of cancers such as occupational and reproductive-related cancers (see Section 2.9.3).

In Example 11.13, a cohort of 73 917 men in Denmark was identified retrospectively from hospital discharge and pathology registries as having had vasectomy during 1977–89. They were passively followed from the time of their operation to 31 December 1989, when their vital and migration status was assessed by linkage with the population registry. The occurrence of cancer among cohort members was ascertained by linkage with the national cancer registry.

11.1.6 Analysis

Studies based on routine data conducted at an individual level may be regarded as cohort studies in which a group of people, or cohort, is followed up in time. For instance, comparison of cancer incidence or mortality across different occupational groups may be regarded as a study of groups of people with different occupational 'exposures' who were followed up in time and their cancer experience compared. Thus, the analysis of these studies is similar to the analysis of any other cohort study and the methods are basically those described in Chapters 4 and 8. The analysis is based on calcula-

Example 11.12. *Data from five Nordic national cancer registries were extracted to examine time trends in the incidence of cervical cancer in each country in relation to their screening activities (Hakama, 1982).*

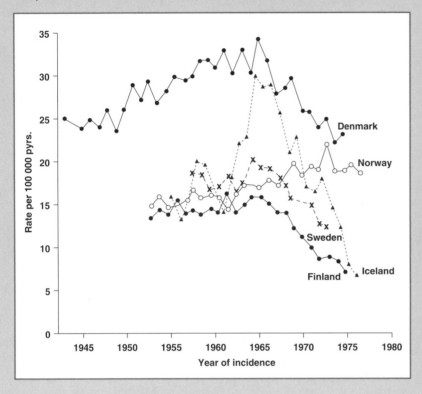

Figure 11.8.
Trends in age-adjusted incidence of cervical cancer in the five Nordic countries, 1943–78 (reproduced with permission from Hakama (1982)).

tion of *rates* as measures of disease occurrence, and of *rate ratios* and *rate differences* as measures of effect. The analysis of time trends by calendar period and birth cohort was considered in Section 4.3.2.

Calculation of rates requires information on *person-time at risk* (i.e., denominators) for each of the groups of interest. Population estimates to allow these calculations are not always available, however. For instance, although national statistical offices in many countries are able to provide population estimates for the whole country and for relatively large geographical areas, they may be unable to provide data for smaller geographical areas. Moreover, cancer registrations and death certificates may contain information on many variables for which data are not collected by the census (or any other population enumeration system). For instance, cancer registries may collect information on ethnicity, but proper denominators will not be available if information on that variable is not collected by the census. In other situations, denominators are available from the census but case-finding is so incomplete (for instance, if on a large proportion of death certificates, data on occupation of the deceased is missing) that the numerator data are not comparable with the available denominator data.

> *Example 11.13.* *A study was conducted in Denmark to assess whether vasectomy increases the risk of cancers of the testis and prostate. The study was based on a computerized record linkage between four population-based registries. The linkage was done by using the unique personal identification number allocated to every resident in Denmark.*
>
> *The Danish Hospital Discharge Registry has recorded all hospital admissions in the country since 1977, recording dates of admission and discharge, diagnosis, and operations. Some hospital departments, however, regarded vasectomy as an outpatient service and did not inform the registry.*
>
> *Pathology registries were set up in some counties to record all specimens analysed in hospital pathology departments within the county. As the tissue removed at vasectomy is routinely sent for pathological examination, in counties where pathology registries exist it is possible to identify all vasectomized men (whether treated as inpatients or as outpatients) from their files.*
>
> *The Danish Central Population Registry records information about vital status and date of emigration or death of everyone who was alive in 1968 or who was born in or immigrated into Denmark thereafter.*
>
> *The Danish Cancer Registry covers all cases of cancer in Denmark diagnosed since 1943, based on notifications from hospital departments, specialists, necropsy reports and death certificates.*
>
> *In the present study, the Hospital Discharge Registry and the Pathology Registry were searched to identify all men who underwent vasectomy from 1977 to 1989. A total of 73 917 men were identified and their records were then linked with the Central Population Registry to provide information on their vital status on 31 December 1989 and dates of emigration or death. Cancer occurrence among the cohort members was identified by record linkage with the Danish Cancer Registry (Møller et al., 1994).*

The traditional answer to situations where suitable denominators are not available has been to calculate *proportional incidence or mortality ratios* (see Section 4.3.5). This is illustrated in Example 11.14.

Proportional incidence (or mortality) ratios are usually age-adjusted by using the indirect method of standardization in a way similar to that used in the calculation of standardized incidence (or mortality) ratios, except that a set of age-specific proportions rather than age-specific rates is taken as the standard in the calculation of expected numbers (see Section 4.3.3).

It can be shown that *odds ratios* may be more appropriate than proportional incidence (or mortality) ratios in situations where no proper denominators are available (Miettinen & Wang, 1981). Odds ratios can be calculated to estimate the risk of a particular cancer ('cases') relative to other cancer sites ('controls') in a population group A ('exposed') compared with another population group B ('unexposed').

Example 11.14. Suppose that an investigator is interested in examining the incidence of lung cancer among men working in the printing industry. Information on the occupation of all new lung cancer cases that occurred in a particular region A during the years 1970–74 can be obtained from the local population-based cancer registry but no population estimates by occupational group are available from the census. In this instance, it is not possible to calculate rates since there are no denominator data. Instead, proportional incidence measures are calculated.

Suppose that a total of 10 000 male incident cancers occurred in region A during the years 1970–74, of which 2000 were lung cancers. Thus, the proportion of male lung cancers in this region was

2000/10 000 = 0.20

Suppose also that the total number of incident cancers among male printers during the same period (1970–74) was 100, of which 40 were lung cancers. The proportion of male lung cancers among printers was

40/100 = 0.40

*We can calculate the **number of lung cancer cases we would have expected (E) among the printers if they had the same proportion of lung cancers as the whole population of the region.** This would be equal to*

100 × 0.20 = 20.

*The **proportional incidence ratio (PIR)** can be obtained by dividing the observed number of lung cancers among the printers (O) by the expected number (E):*

PIR = O/E = 40/20 = 2.0

(or, equivalently, the PIR can be calculated by dividing the proportion of lung cancers among the printers by the proportion of lung cancers in the region (i.e., PIR = 0.40/0.20 = 2.0).)

Thus the number of lung cancers observed among the printers was twice the number we would expect if they had the same proportion of lung cancers (out of all cancers) as the whole region.

In Example 11.15, the mortality data were examined as a series of case–control analyses. In each of these analyses, all cancers except the particular one under investigation were taken as the 'controls' and people born in England and Wales as the 'unexposed'.

Example 11.15. In England and Wales, information on country of birth of the deceased has been entered on death certificates since 1969, and this information has been coded and included in national mortality files by the Office of Population Censuses and Surveys (OPCS). Information on ethnicity is not recorded in the death certificate but, for deaths from 1973 to 1985, OPCS undertook ethnic-origin coding for persons born in the Indian subcontinent. The coding was based on name analysis, exact place of birth and other items on the death certificate, and it separated the Indian-born into those of Indian ethnic origin, British ethnic origin and others. Data on ethnicity were not collected by the census at that time and therefore no proper denominators were available. Thus, age-adjusted odds ratios were calculated to estimate relative risks of mortality from different cancer sites in the migrants compared with people born and resident in England and Wales (Swerdlow et al., 1995). Table 11.5 shows results from this analysis for certain cancer sites.

Table 11.5.
Age-adjusted odds ratios of cancer mortality for selected sites in male migrants from the Indian subcontinent to England and Wales, by ethnic group, compared with males born and resident in England and Wales, 1973–85.[a]

Cancer site (ICD-9 code)	England and Wales born[b]		British ethnic, born in India		Indian ethnic, born in India	
	No.	Odds ratio	No.	Odds ratio (95% CI)[c]	No.	Odds ratio (95% CI)[c]
Oral (141, 143–145)	4564	1.0	24	1.7 (1.1–2.5)	30	2.2 (1.5–3.1)
Pharynx (except nasopharynx) (146, 148,149)	3440	1.0	22	2.1 (1.4–3.1)	55	5.5 (4.2–7.2)
Liver (155)	6177	1.0	33	1.7 (1.2–2.5)	88	5.0 (4.0–6.2)
Lung (163)	296 012	1.0	759	0.7 (0.7–0.8)	581	0.6 (0.6–0.7)

[a] Data from Swerdlow *et al.* (1995).
[b] Taken as the 'unexposed' baseline group.
[c] CI = confidence interval

Thus, for example, for lung cancer in Indian ethnic migrants, a 2 × 2 table was constructed as follows:

	Indian ethnic, born in India	England and Wales-born
Lung cancer ('cases')	a (581)	b (296 012)
Other cancer ('controls')	c (1737)	d (466 756)

OR = $(a/b)/(c/d)$ = (581/296 012)/(1737/466 756)=0.5

(The methods described in Chapter 14 were used to adjust for age.)

A similar approach was used in Example 11.7 to examine educational differentials in cancer mortality in São Paulo (Brazil). Although data on educational level were collected by the census, the quality of these data was likely to differ from that in the death certificates since the information on the census forms was provided by the individuals themselves, whereas that on the death certificate was given by the relatives of the deceased. To overcome the lack of comparability between numerator and denominator data, odds ratios were calculated instead of rates.

A discussion of the relative merits of odds ratios versus proportional ratios is beyond the scope of this chapter. Suffice it to say that it can be shown that the odds ratio equals the rate ratio (the measure that would have been calculated if suitable denominators had been available) provided that the total incidence rate of 'other cancers' is similar in the two population groups, in other words, that the total incidence rate of 'other cancers' in the analysis is unrelated to the 'exposure' (Miettinen & Wang, 1981). No similar relationship exists between proportional ratios and rate ratios. Despite this advantage of the odds ratios, it should be noted that the calculation of odds ratios does not solve one important problem of the proportional ratios—the 'borrowing effect' occurring in populations with high incidence of a particularly common cancer, which inevitably leads to lower proportional incidence for other cancers. In other words, the proportion (or odds) for an individual cause may be high because the incidence for that cause is high or because the incidence for other major causes is low. These two situations can be distinguished only when proper denominator data are available (see Section 4.3.5).

11.1.7 Interpretation

Routine surveillance systems usually cover large catchment populations, sometimes of millions of people followed up over long periods of time. Thus, one of the main advantages of routine-data-based studies is that they allow the study of a very large number of people at a very low cost.

A major limitation, however, is the restricted range of variables collected by these systems, that often tend to be just proxy measures of more biologically relevant exposures. For instance, country of birth may act just as marker of environmental factors (e.g., diet, reproductive variables) for which data are not available in routine data systems.

Data quality

Potential data artefacts need to be considered when interpreting results from these studies. The observation of differences in recorded cancer incidence between populations does not necessarily reflect true underlying variations in cancer risks. Differences in recorded incidence may arise because of differences in health service access (including screening), diagnosis, and registration practices. In addition, they may be due to variations in the accuracy of enumeration of the population. Some of these issues were discussed briefly in Section 2.9 and Appendix A2.2.

An example is the difficulty in assessing rising trends in the recorded incidence of prostatic cancer in many western countries due to uncertainty about the effect of changes in diagnostic and registration practices. Strong parallels have been observed in the USA between time trends in the recorded incidence of localized prostate cancer and time trends in the use of transurethral resection of the prostate (Potosky *et al.*, 1990; Severson, 1990), a surgical procedure performed to relieve commonly occurring symptoms of benign prostatic hyperplasia. An increasing use of this medical procedure seems to have led to an increased detection of clinically silent tumours that would otherwise not have been diagnosed. Inter-country variations in the use of this technique also seem to account for some of the difference between recorded incidence rates in Japan and the USA (Shimizu *et al.*, 1991).

Cancer incidence data are not available in many countries, and, if available, the registration scheme may not cover the whole population or the data collected may be incomplete. Mortality data are available for a much larger number of countries and for much longer periods. Mortality data, however, have the disadvantage of not directly reflecting incidence, particularly for cancers with a good prognosis. This is because mortality depends on both incidence and case fatality. Death rates closely parallel incidence rates only if the disease is fatal and if death occurs shortly after diagnosis. For example, death rates are a good indication of the magnitude of the incidence rates for lung cancer because this tumour has a high and early fatality, but not for testicular cancer, for which survival is relatively good. Moreover, the accuracy of the mortality data provided in death certificates is influenced by geographical differences and trends in diagnostic and certification practices as well as by changes in the frequency with which post-mortem examinations are carried out.

Routine mortality statistics in many countries are based on a single underlying cause of death. The rules for determining the underlying cause of death are primarily those of the *International Classification of Diseases* (see Appendix A.2.2), but national vital statistics offices may, on occasions, superimpose their own rules. For instance, the Office of Population Censuses and Surveys in England and Wales changed one of these rules (rule 3) in 1983, so that cancer is now more likely to be coded as the cause of death even if it is only recorded as a contributory cause in the death certificate (Ashley & Devis, 1992). This change in coding affected secular trends in recorded cancer mortality. It has been estimated that close to 50% of the increase in prostatic cancer mortality at ages 75–84 years in England and Wales from 1970 to 1990 could possibly be explained by changes in coding practices (Grulich *et al.*, 1995).

Many other factors, some of them less apparent, may affect recorded incidence and mortality data. Mortality rates for malignant neoplasms of the brain decreased greatly in England and Wales during the years 1981–82, but it is clear from examination of the data for neoplasms of unspecified nature of the brain that this decrease was largely, or entirely, an artefact. Most of the unspecified cases are allocated to malignancies of the brain after further enquiries are sent to the certifiers requesting clarification of the cause of death. The artefact shown in Figure 11.9 occurred because the number of enquiries referred to certifiers was reduced during a strike by registrars in 1981–82.

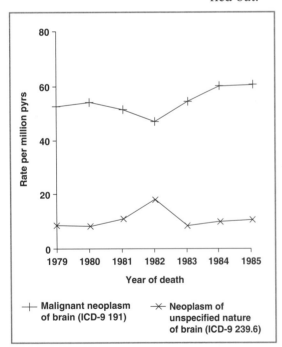

Figure 11.9.
Mortality from brain neoplasms, malignant and of unspecified nature, in males, England and Wales, 1979–85. Death rates age-standardized to the 1981 England and Wales population (reproduced by permission of Churchill Livingstone, from Swerdlow (1989)).

Comparability of the numerator and denominator data

Calculations of rates requires estimates of person-years at risk, according to the variables under study. These usually rely upon census data. It is essential that the variables in the census are defined, classified and coded in a similar way to the variables in cancer registration and mortality databases. However, even when the same criteria are used, individuals may still be classified differently in the two databases if the way the information was obtained differs. For instance, the information in the census is provided by the individuals themselves, whereas that on the death certificates is given by informants (usually relatives of the deceased). Informants may not be able to provide accurate information on many items such as occupation of the deceased, or may deliberately report a more prestigious occupation (OPCS, 1978).

Selection bias

People who migrate are not generally a representative group of their population of origin. For instance, migrants tend to be healthier than those who stay in the home country. This 'healthy migrant effect' will affect comparisons with home population risks. A similar bias may occur in analyses by occupation (the 'healthy worker effect') and this will affect comparisons with the general population (see Sections 8.2.2 and 13.1.1).

Another source of bias, that is more difficult to detect, results from changes in 'exposure' which are related to the disease event itself. For example, migrants may return to their country of origin soon before death or people move jobs as a consequence of being diagnosed with a particular condition. In these situations, risks in the host country or in the job held before diagnosis will be under-estimated.

Confounding

One of the main limitations of routine-data-based studies is that information on important confounding factors (with the exception of age and sex) is generally not available. For instance, the high risks of lung cancer found in some occupational groups are not due to occupational exposures but to high prevalence of smoking. Unfortunately, data on smoking habits are rarely collected by routine surveillance systems.

Final remarks

In summary, the study of variations in cancer incidence and mortality by place of residence and birth, ethnicity, socioeconomic status and over time is a valid and useful exercise, provided that the investigator has a thorough knowledge of the way data are collected and processed so that all possible sources of data artefacts, bias and confounding are considered in the interpretation of the findings.

11.2 Aggregated level (ecological studies)

The routine-data-based studies considered thus far share the characteristic that the observations made pertain to individual subjects. It is, however, possible to conduct research at a group level rather than at the individual level. Studies which involve investigating the frequency of disease (or of any other outcome of interest) in relation to the level of exposure in several groups of individuals (or in the same group over different periods of time) are called ecological studies. In this type of study, it is not possible to link the exposure of a particular individual with his or her outcome. Thus, the group rather than the individual is the unit of observation and analysis. The groups may be defined in a large number of ways, according to place of residence, place of birth, socioeconomic status, occupation, etc.

Ecological studies are frequently used as a first step in investigating a possible exposure–outcome relationship, because they can be performed quickly and inexpensively by using readily available information. Exposure data may be available from governmental and private organizations which routinely collect data on demographic, environmental and lifestyle variables. Disease rates may be available from vital statistics offices, surveillance programmes or disease registries (e.g., cancer registries).

In Example 11.16, it is not possible to link the ovarian cancer mortality experience of any individual woman with her family size because the only pieces of information available were an estimate of the average family size and an estimate of the average level of mortality from ovarian cancer for each country included in the analysis. Thus, the country rather than the individual was the unit of study.

Similar comparisons can be performed between changes over time in the average exposure level and changes in the disease rate for a single population (as in Example 11.17).

Ecological studies may be the most appropriate design to study exposures that are easier to define and measure at a population rather than at an individual level. This is the case with many environmental exposures such as air pollution, water quality and ultraviolet radiation (Example 11.18).

Ecological studies are also useful for monitoring the effectiveness of population interventions such as health education campaigns (e.g., anti-smoking campaigns), immunization programmes and mass screening programmes.

11.2.1 Analysis

Ecological studies differ from individual-based epidemiological studies in that the 'exposed' and 'unexposed' individuals in each of the populations are not actually identified. Thus, it is not possible to measure the strength of an association between exposure and outcome by using any of the approaches described in Chapter 5 for individual-based studies.

Moreover, in contrast to other epidemiological studies, the outcome measure in an ecological study is usually a quantitative variable (e.g., mortality rate) rather than a binary one (such as 'diseased' versus 'non-diseased'). The

Example 11.16. Routinely collected data on ovarian cancer mortality in twenty countries were examined in relation to their average family size as estimated from various demographic surveys. There was a clear inverse relationship between mortality from this tumour and average completed family size, i.e., total number of children per woman at the end of her reproductive life (Figure 11.10) (Beral et al.*, 1978). This finding suggested that pregnancy protected against ovarian cancer, a hypothesis that has been confirmed in many case–control and cohort studies.*

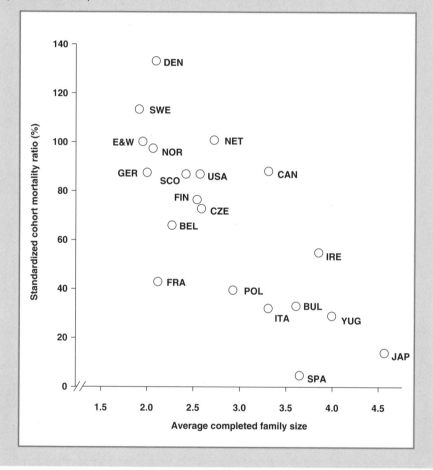

Figure 11.10.
Scattergram showing the relationship between age-standardized mortality ratios from ovarian cancer and average completed family size for women born around 1901 in 20 countries. The age-specific mortality rates in England & Wales were used as the standard, i.e. the mortality ratio for England & Wales = 100. (Reproduced with permission from Beral *et al.*, 1978. © by The Lancet Ltd, 1978). BEL=Belgium; BUL=Bulgaria; CAN=Canada; CZE=former Czechoslovakia; DEN=Denmark; E&W=England and Wales; FRA=France; FIN=Finland; GER=former West Germany; IRE=Ireland; ITA=Italy; JAP=Japan; NET=Netherlands; NOR=Norway; POL=Poland; SCO=Scotland; SPA=Spain; SWE=Sweden; USA=United States of America; YUG=former Yugoslavia.

exposure variable also tends to be measured on a quantitative scale. Even qualitative variables become quantitative when averaged for a population: sex is a binary variable, but the proportion of a population that is male (or female) is quantitative.

A statistical measure called a *correlation coefficient*, denoted by *r*, has been widely used to measure the strength of associations between exposure and outcome in ecological studies. Another, more appropriate, approach is to fit a *regression* line which predicts incidence or mortality as a function of the exposure level. These two statistical methods are briefly introduced below.

Introduction to regression and correlation

When investigating the relationship between two quantitative variables, the first step should always be to plot the data (see Section 3.3.3). The required plot is called a *scattergram* (or *scatter diagram*), in which the vertical (or *y*) axis refers to the outcome variable and the horizontal (or *x*) axis to the exposure variable (as in Figures 11.10–11.12). In such a graph, each unit under consideration is represented by a point.

> *Example 11.17.* In the study on ovarian cancer mortality and family size described in Example 11.16, it was shown that mortality from ovarian cancer among successive generations of women born in England and Wales, and in the USA was closely related to their completed family size (Figure 11.11).

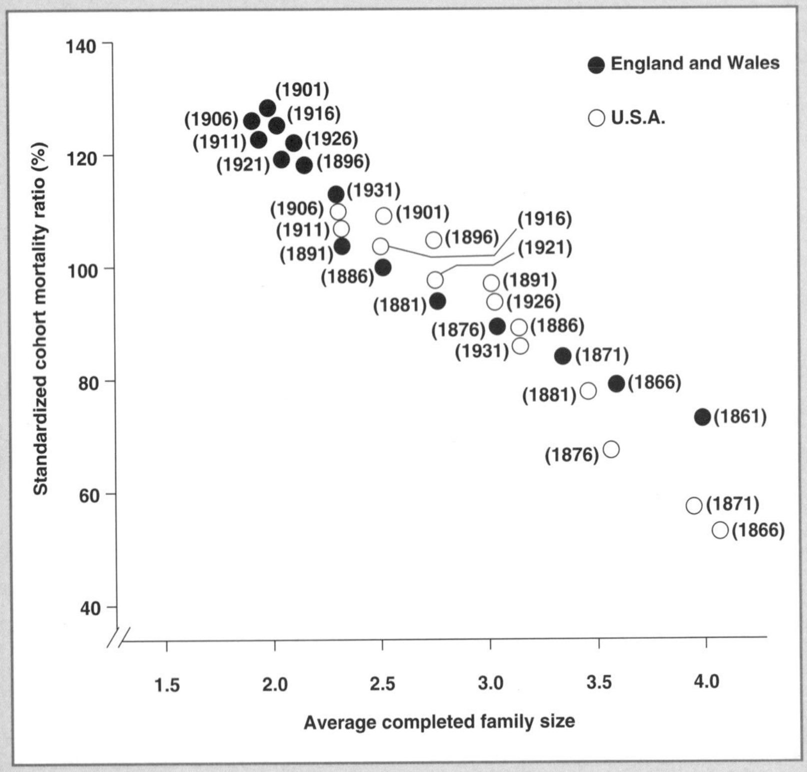

Figure 11.11.
Scattergram showing the relationship between age-standardized mortality ratios from ovarian cancer and average completed family size for different generations of women born in England and Wales and the USA. The average age-structure of the combined population of England & Wales and the USA from 1931–73 was taken as the standard. Thus, a ratio of 140 means that the ovarian cancer mortality of the cohort is 40% higher than the average for women in England & Wales and the USA. (The mid-year of birth of each generation is shown in brackets) (reproduced with permission from Beral *et al.*, 1978. © by The Lancet Ltd, 1978).

Consider the scattergram in Figure 11.13(*a*). The points on the scattergram show a clear trend, upwards and to the right; there is said to be a *positive* relationship between the two variables. High values of one variable are associated with high values of the other, and low with low. To summarize the relation between the two variables, so as to be able to predict the value of one variable when we only know the other variable, we could just draw a straight line through the scatter of points. Any straight line drawn on a graph can be represented by an equation. In the above example, this relationship could be summarized as *y* = *x*, because each

Example 11.18. Routinely collected data from a large number of population-based cancer registries and published measurements of ambient solar ultraviolet light were obtained to assess whether the geographical distribution of squamous-cell carcinoma of the eye was related to solar ultraviolet light. The analysis was based on data from 47 populations: 3 in Africa, 9 in Australasia, 20 in Europe, 12 in North America, 2 in South America and 1 in the Middle East. The study period covered by each registry varied, but most encompassed the 1980s. The results (Figure 11.12) were consistent with the hypothesis that exposure to solar ultraviolet light increases the risk of squamous-cell carcinoma of the eye (Newton et al., 1996).

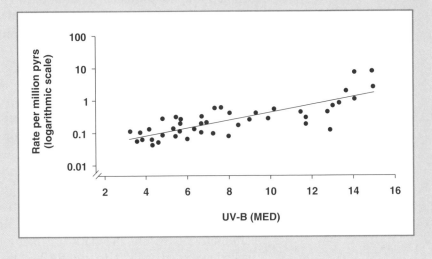

Figure 11.12.
Age- and sex-adjusted incidence rates of squamous-cell carcinoma of the eye in relation to measurements of ultraviolet B radiation expressed as minimum erythemal dose (MED), a unit which reflects more closely the biologically effective dose (reproduced with permission from Newton *et al.*, 1996. © by The Lancet, Ltd, 1996).

value of *y* is exactly equal to the corresponding value of *x*. If the value of *y* was always 0.9 times the value of *x* , we could express the relationship as $y = 0.9x$.

More generally, the equation for a straight line is expressed as

$$y = a + bx$$

where *y* refers to values of the outcome variable and *x* to values of the exposure variable, *a* is the intercept of the line on the *y* axis, and *b* is the slope of the line, the increase (or decrease) in *y* per unit increase in *x* (Figure 11.14). In the special case in which the line passes through the origin (O) of the two axes, as in Figure 11.13(*a*), and each value of *y* is exactly equal to the corresponding value of *x*, the equation reduces to $y = x$, since $a = 0$ and $b = 1$.

In Figure 11.13(*b*), there is also a perfect association between *x* and *y*, but the trend is downwards to the right; there is then said to be an *inverse*, or *negative*, relationship between the two variables. Such a relationship can also be expressed by the equation $y = a + bx$, except that in this case the coefficient *b* has a negative value, indicating that as one variable increased, the other decreased.

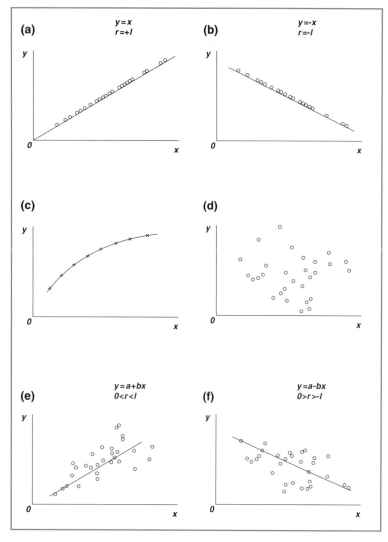

Figure 11.13.
Scattergrams, regression equations and correlation coefficients.

In Figures 11.13(*a*) and (*b*), the points on the scattergram lie on a straight line and the relationship is said to be *linear*. In Figure 11.13(*c*), there is still a clear relationship between the two variables, but it is *non-linear* in form, and the equation is more complex. Finally, in Figure 11.13(*d*), there is no apparent relationship between *x* and *y*. High values of *x* are associated with both high and low values of *y*. The points in the scattergram show no particular trend and, in the absence of any relationship between the two variables, the use of an equation is inappropriate.

The relationships illustrated in Figure 11.13(*a*), (*b*) and (*c*) are perfect, in that all the points on the scatter diagram lie on a line. In most real situations, however, the points are scattered around it (as in Figures 11.13(*e*) and (*f*). In these circumstances, we use a straight line that gives the 'best' prediction of *y* for any value of *x*. We could just draw a line 'by eye', but such a subjective method is unlikely to yield the best line. An alternative is to use the statistical method called *regression analysis*, to find the best line that *'fits'* the data. The equation of the straight line obtained by this method is called the *regression equation* (see Armitage and Berry (1994) for illustration of calculations).

This statistical method was applied to the ovarian cancer mortality data shown in Figure 11.11 (using the data from both countries) and yielded the following regression equation (Beral *et al.*, 1978):

$$y = 182 - 30x$$

This equation means that for any given value of *x* (i.e., average family size), an associated value for *y* (i.e., ovarian cancer mortality) can be calculated. Thus, the age-standardized mortality ratio from ovarian cancer in any particular birth cohort of women can be predicted from this equation. For example, the mortality ratio in a cohort with a mean family size of three children can be predicted by substituting *x* = 3 into the regression equation

$$y = 182 - 30 \times 3 = 92$$

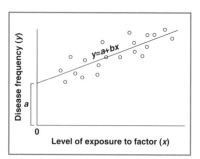

Figure 11.14.
Scattergram and regression line.

which is the value we would have estimated by examining the graph. This predicted value can be interpreted as the *average* value of y associated with a given value of x.

If all the values in the scattergram lay on the regression line, the predicted and observed values of y would be identical. The regression equation would describe exactly the relationship between average family size and ovarian cancer mortality. In other words, the variation in ovarian cancer mortality would be completely explained by the variations in family size. In practice this is not the case. Ovarian cancer mortality can vary independently of variations of family size, so that two populations with the same average family size may have different ovarian cancer mortality risks. Thus, the regression equation can only measure the *average* relationship between the two variables.

If the points on the scattergram lie close to the regression line, this suggests that the observed values for y do not differ markedly from the predicted values represented by the regression line. Thus, most of the variation in y can be explained by the variation in x. If, on the other hand, there is a wide scatter of points around the regression line, a considerable amount of the variation in y is not explained by the variation in x.

To quantify the degree of scatter around the regression line, we can calculate a measure called a correlation coefficient, r. The value of this coefficient always lies between −1 and +1:

(a) For perfect *positive* correlations (Figure 11.13(a)), r = +1.

(b) For perfect *negative* correlations (Figure 11.13(b)), r = −1.

(c) If there is some scatter about the regression line (Figure 11.13(e) and (f)), r lies between 0 and +1 (or between 0 and −1). The less the scatter, the closer r is to 1 (or −1).

(d) If there is *no linear* relationship between y and x, r is close to 0. This implies that either there is no relationship at all between the two variables (Figure 11.13(d)) or the relationship is non-linear (Figure 11.13(c)).

Use of correlation and regression in the analysis of ecological studies

The correlation coefficient is quite often used in the analysis of ecological studies as a measure of the strength of the association between exposure and disease. It is not, however, the most appropriate approach. First, its magnitude depends on the range of the exposure variable; if this is wide, the correlation will be greater than if it is narrow. Second, the value of the correlation coefficient cannot be translated into any of the conventional measures of relative effect and it is therefore difficult to interpret in epidemiological terms.

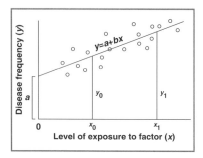

Figure 11.15.
Illustration of the association between disease frequency (y) and level of exposure (x) to the factor being studied in various populations.

A more appropriate method to quantify the effect of exposure in an ecological study is to fit a regression line to the data, which predicts incidence or mortality as a function of the level (or prevalence) of exposure. In contrast to the correlation coefficient, a regression line remains unaffected by changes in the range of the exposure variable. Moreover, a measure of relative effect can be estimated from the slope and the intercept of the regression line (Beral *et al.*, 1979).

Let us assume that in n different populations the level of disease (y) is linearly related to the average level of exposure (x) to the factor being studied. This relationship can be expressed by a regression equation fitted to the data from n populations:

$$y = a + bx$$

We can consider two of these populations with different average levels of exposure x_0 and x_1 and associated disease frequencies y_0 and y_1, respectively (Figure 11.15). The relative risk between the two populations can be defined as the frequency of disease in individuals with average exposure x_1, relative to that in individuals with average exposure x_0, or simply y_1/y_0.

Thus, if

$$y_0 = a + bx_0 \qquad \text{and} \qquad y_1 = a + bx_1$$

the relative risk estimate (RR) can be calculated as

$$RR = \frac{y_1}{y_0} = \frac{a + bx_1}{a + bx_0}$$

For instance, in our ovarian cancer mortality example, the regression equation was found to be $y = 182 - 30x$. Thus, the relative risk of ovarian cancer in a population with an average family size of two children compared to that with an average of four children can be estimated as:

$$RR = \frac{182 - 30 \times 2}{182 - 30 \times 4} = 2.0$$

If the exposure is measured in terms of the *proportion* of people in the population exposed to the factor of interest (e.g., proportion of cigarette smokers) rather than in terms of the *average level* of exposure (e.g., mean number of children) as in the above example, the relative risk can be estimated as:

$$RR = \frac{slope}{intercept} + 1 = \frac{b}{a} + 1$$

This formula is just a special case of the previous equation obtained by setting $x_0=0$, $x_1=1$, which are the range of values a proportion can take.

Certain assumptions underlie this approach. First, it assumes that the y variable (disease frequency) is linearly related to the x variable (exposure). Secondly, it presumes that the frequency of the disease in each population group is entirely determined by the level of exposure. Thirdly, it assumes that exposure is measured without error. As we shall see below, most often these assumptions are not satisfied, limiting the use and interpretation of these methods.

11.2.2 Interpretation of ecological studies
Ecological fallacy

The observation that there is a relationship at a population level between two variables does not necessary imply that the same relationship will hold at an individual level. This is known as the 'ecological fallacy'. For instance, the previous analyses on family size and ovarian cancer suggested that pregnancy might confer protection against ovarian cancer. We do not know, however, if the women who died from ovarian cancer in each population group were really those with few or no children.

Example 11.19. Approximately 500 Finnish municipalities were grouped into various categories (five or four) according to various socioeconomic indicators such as average monthly income per inhabitant in 1968, percentage of inhabitants belonging to the two highest social classes (social classes 1 and 2) in 1970, percentage of people with secondary education in 1970, number of television licences per 1000 inhabitants in 1970, percentage of people living in dwellings with more than two inhabitants per room in 1950 (crowdedness), and percentages of dwellings with running water, central heating and electricity in 1950. The incidence of breast and cervical cancers was then calculated for each of these groups of municipalities (Hakama et al., 1982). The results are shown in Figure 11.16.

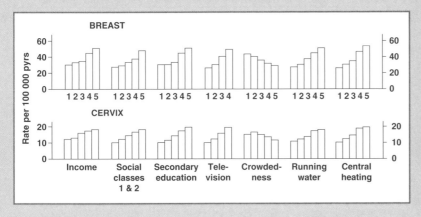

Figure 11.16.
Age-standardized incidence rates of breast and cervical cancers in groups of municipalities defined according to the levels of various socioeconomic characteristics of each municipality, Finland, 1955–74. The average Finnish population in 1955–74 was taken as the standard population. (Reproduced with permission from Hakama *et al.*, 1982).

In an ecological study, exposure levels represent the average levels for each population group. Since the true interest is in individual risk as determined by individual exposure, ecological studies are justified only in the ideal situation in which all individuals within a group have the same level of exposure. This may be the case with environmental exposures such as air pollution, natural radiation and water quality.

Most often, however, exposure is heterogeneous within a group, with some individuals not exposed at all and those exposed likely to be exposed in different levels. In such situations, the exposure–response relationship observed at the group level need not reflect the exposure–response relationship at the individual level. Thus, the finding of a linear relationship

Example 11.20. In the study described in Example 11.19, analyses were also carried out at an individual level by individually linking all breast and cervical cancer registrations with the 1970 census forms. For each cancer patient, occupational and educational data were extracted from the census tapes, and the patients were grouped into socioeconomic and educational classes on the basis of the original census codes (Hakama et al., 1982). The results of this individual analysis are shown in Table 11.6.

Table 11.6.
Age-standardized incidence ratios (SIR) of breast and cervical cancer by socioeconomic status and educational level in women aged 30–69 years. Finland, 1971–75.[a]

	Breast cancer			Cervical cancer		
	Observed (O)	Expected[b] (E)	SIR (%) (100×O/E)	Observed (O)	Expected[b] (E)	SIR (%) (100×O/E)
Socioeconomic status[c]						
Employees	172	148.9	116	24	35.0	69
Farmers	562	705.1	80	108	165.9	65
Other self-employed	127	128.2	99	26	30.2	86
Managerial	343	229.3	150	24	53.8	45
Clerical	1061	842.7	126	177	197.3	90
Skilled workers	797	890.6	90	271	208.8	130
Unskilled workers	357	412.5	87	146	96.9	151
Pensioners	1169	1228.2	95	313	299.3	105
Educational level						
Primary	3011	3356.1	90	897	797.1	113
Secondary	975	847.5	115	150	200.0	75
High school	255	186.7	137	26	44.0	59
College/ university	356	206.8	172	17	48.9	35

[a] Data from Hakama *et al.* (1982)

[b] The breast and cervical cancer age-specific rates for the whole Finnish female population aged 30–69 years were taken as the standard.

[c] In Finland, socioeconomic status is based on occupation. For economically inactive women (e.g., housewives), it was defined as that of the head of the household (usually the husband).

between average exposure and disease frequency in an ecological study does not imply that such a linear relationship will be present at the individual level.

In the ecological analysis illustrated in Example 11.19, the risk of both breast and cervical cancer increased with increasing average socioeconomic level of the municipalities. This positive gradient is what we would expect for breast cancer but not for cervical cancer (see Examples 11.7 and 11.9). When analyses were conducted at an individual level, however, the socioeconomic and educational trends in risk were different for breast and cervical cancers (Example 11.20). Women with better jobs and higher education had a higher risk of breast cancer but a lower risk of cervical cancer (Table 11.6).

The difference in the cervical cancer results between the individual and the ecological approaches may be due to the fact that, for instance, women from the poorest socioeconomic groups (e.g., prostitutes) tend to be concentrated in urban municipalities, which are also the ones with a higher proportion of residents of higher socioeconomic status. This could potentially account for the positive relationship between high socioeconomic level and cervical cancer risks observed in the ecological analysis.

Confounding

A second major limitation of ecological studies is the lack of ability to control for the effects of potential confounding factors. For example, in a study of average *per caput* daily intake of fat in 24 countries in relation to their breast cancer incidence in women aged 35–64 years, there was a positive relationship between these two variables (Armstrong & Mann, 1985), suggesting a possible association between fat intake and risk of developing breast cancer. However, increased fat consumption may merely be acting as a marker for other factors that are related to elevated risk of breast cancer, such as higher socioeconomic status, lower fertility and later age at first birth. Data on known or suspected confounders are not generally available in ecological studies and, even if available, it would be difficult to adjust for them at a population level.

It should be noted that risk factors which are independent of exposure at the individual level may become correlated with it, and therefore become confounders, when aggregated at the population level. For example, in an investigation of the relationship between the proportion of woodworkers and lung cancer across geographically defined areas, smoking will induce confounding if cigarette consumption changes with the proportion of woodworkers in each area, even if the two factors in ques-

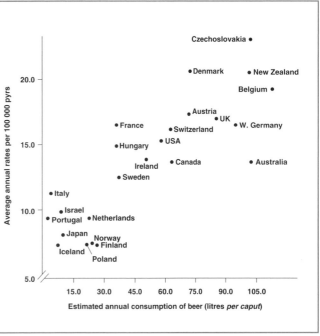

Figure 11.17.
Scattergram showing relationship between estimated average annual age-adjusted incidence rates for rectal cancer among males in 24 countries and *per caput* beer consumption, 1960–62 (approx.) (reproduced, by permission of Oxford University Press, from Breslow & Enstrom, 1974).

tion are independent at the individual level. Conversely, a confounding variable at the individual level may not be a confounder at the ecological level. For example, although the risk of lung cancer is much greater for men than women, sex, as an ecological variable (e.g., percent male), will not be associated with disease rate across geographically defined groups if the proportion of males is similar in all groups.

Measurement errors

Exposure is most often estimated from data collected for other reasons, which generally provide only an indirect measure of possible risk factors. For example, data on smoking and alcohol are often based on sales, which only partially reflect consumption, because losses and unregistered imports are not taken into account. Moreover, since the data are not collected by the investigators themselves, it may be difficult to assess their quality adequately.

Measurement of cancer incidence and mortality can also be affected by errors, as discussed in Section 11.1.7.

Latent period

Most ecological studies compare exposure measured at one point in time with disease measured at another (or the same) point in time. This is illustrated in Figure 11.17, where data on both the disease rate and the exposure of interest (*per caput* beer consumption) refer to approximately the same period (1960–62).

Ideally, an appropriate time-lag period should be incorporated into the analysis, so that exposure data refer to the relevant etiological period (e.g., 10–20 years before the development of cancer). Data on past exposures are not always available and, quite often, we are forced to rely on data from a period far too recent. This constitutes a serious problem when exposures are likely to have changed markedly over time (e.g., smoking and alcohol consumption), particularly if the rate of change has been different in the different groups. Even when relevant past exposure data are available, the populations on which exposure and outcome are measured may not be the same, as a result of dynamic changes introduced by births, deaths and migrations.

A special situation arises when birth cohort changes in exposure are related to birth cohort changes in disease risk or when both the exposure and the disease data refer to a specific birth cohort of individuals. Examples 11.16 and 11.17 illustrate this point. The average family size summarized the reproductive experience of each generation of women, that is the total number of children achieved by the end of their reproductive lives. The ovarian cancer cohort risks used in these examples also summarized the mortality experience of each generation of women (see Beral *et al.* (1978) for details of the calculations). In such situations, there is no need to build any time lag into the analysis.

Final remarks

Despite their limitations, ecological studies have been useful in describing differences in populations. Even if confounded by unknown or uncontrollable factors, such differences at least signal the presence of effects worthy of further investigation.

Ecological studies are particularly helpful in identifying factors responsible for risk differences *between* populations rather than risk variations *within* the same population. For instance, international comparisons have shown a strong relationship between fat intake and breast cancer risks. However, most individual-based studies conducted within populations have failed to observe such a relationship. It has been suggested that a possible reason for this difference in results is that between-population variability in levels of fat intake is much higher than the inter-individual variation within populations.

Box 11.1. Key issues

• Routine-data-based studies make use of routine surveillance systems to obtain data on both the exposure(s) and outcome(s) of interest. Thus, this type of study can be conducted without establishing contact with any of the study subjects.

• Routine-data-based studies can be carried out at an *individual* level (if the individual is the unit of study) or at an *ecological (aggregated)* level (if the group is the unit of study).

• The main advantages of routine-data-based studies are:

For individual level and ecological studies

1. They are very economical and rapid, since they generally use existing data on exposure and outcome, with no costs involved in collection.

2. They allow the study of very large numbers of people and, therefore, small increases in risk can be investigated.

3. They may include populations with a very wide range of exposure levels (more than can be found in a single population used for conventional cohort or case–control studies).

For ecological studies

4. They may be the only practical method if exposure level is relatively homogeneous in a population, but differs between populations (e.g., water quality), or when individual measurements of exposure are impossible (e.g., air pollution).

Further reading

* The book by Estève *et al.* (1994) gives a comprehensive (although statistically elaborate) review of methods used in the analysis of routine-data-based studies.

* A fuller discussion on ecological studies can be also found in papers by Greenland & Morgenstern (1989), Walter (1991a, b) and Greenland & Robins (1994).

* A discussion of the rationale and methodology of migrant studies in cancer epidemiology is also given in Parkin & Khlat (1996).

Box 11.1. (Contd) Key issues

• The main disadvantages of routine-data-based studies are:

For individual level and ecological studies

1. The number of variables on which data are available is limited.

2. It is difficult to assess errors in the measurement of exposure and outcome variables, since the data are not collected by the investigators themselves.

3. Data on potential confounding variables (except sex and age) are rarely available.

For ecological studies

4. They are prone to the *ecological fallacy*.

5. It is difficult to control for confounding even when data on potential confounders are available.

6. It is usually difficult to incorporate an appropriate time-lag period.

Chapter 12
Introduction to survival analysis

12.1 Introduction

In this chapter we examine another method used in the analysis of intervention trials, cohort studies and data routinely collected by hospital and
population-based cancer registries. Consider the following example:

> *Example 12.1*. *A cohort of 40 women diagnosed with breast cancer in a
> particular hospital during the years 1989–93 were followed up from diagno-
> sis to the end of 1995 to assess their survival experience. Table 12.1 gives the
> dates of diagnosis and death (or of last contact) for each of the study sub-
> jects.*

In Example 12.1, the patients entered and left the study at different points
in time (Table 12.1). We discussed in previous chapters (Chapters 4, 7 and 8)
one way of analysing data of this type which takes into account the varying
individual lengths of follow-up. That approach involves the calculation of
rates based on *person-time at risk*. These calculations are based on the assumption that the rate under consideration remains approximately constant over
time, so that 100 person-years of observation are treated identically, whether
they involve 100 subjects followed over one year or 50 subjects followed over
two years.

In many situations, however, the rate of occurrence of the event under
study does not remain constant over time. For instance, the probability of
dying may rise suddenly with the onset of disease and then decline gradually as time since diagnosis increases. The most appropriate approach in these
situations is to conduct *survival analysis*.

12.2 Estimation of survival

The first requirement for the estimation of survival is a *clear and well
defined case definition*. For cancer patients, this should specify the site of the
cancer, histology, stage, and the sex of the patients. In Example 12.1, all histologically confirmed female breast cancer cases were included in the analysis.

The second requirement is a *clear and well defined starting point*. The dates
of the first diagnosis, the initiation of therapy, or the admission to a hospital
are frequently used. Although date of onset of the clinical phase of the disease would seem more appropriate, this is generally difficult to define. In
clinical trials, the appropriate starting point is the time of randomization,

Table 12.1.
Follow-up of 40 women diagnosed with breast cancer in a certain hospital during the years 1989–93: hypothetical data.

Patient study number	Age (years)	Stage[a]	Date of diagnosis	Date of last contact or death	Vital status at last contact[b]	Cause of death[c]	No. of complete years of observation from diagnosis to last contact or death	No. of days from diagnosis to last contact or death
1	39	1	01/02/1989	23/10/1992	A	–	3	1360
2	55	1	22/03/1989	12/02/1995	A	–	5	2153
3	56	2	16/04/1989	05/09/1989	D	BC	0	142
4	63	1	23/05/1989	20/12/1992	D	BC	3	1307
5	62	2	12/06/1989	28/12/1995	A	–	6	2390
6	42	2	05/09/1989	17/12/1990	A	–	1	468
7	45	1	05/10/1989	04/08/1995	A	–	5	2129
8	38	2	30/11/1989	11/10/1991	D	BC	1	680
9	53	2	07/01/1990	25/10/1990	D	BC	0	291
10	55	1	03/02/1990	31/01/1991	D	BC	0	362
11	49	2	23/03/1990	29/08/1992	A	–	2	890
12	61	1	28/04/1990	13/05/1994	A	–	4	1476
13	58	1	14/05/1990	01/06/1990	A	–	1	383
14	45	2	15/07/1990	10/09/1993	D	BC	3	1153
15	60	2	03/08/1990	27/11/1994	A	–	4	1577
16	69	1	31/08/1990	06/10/1995	D	O	5	1862
17	58	2	18/09/1990	02/01/1993	D	BC	2	837
18	54	2	09/11/1990	18/06/1995	A	–	4	1682
19	56	2	28/11/1990	27/06/1995	D	BC	4	1702
20	52	1	12/12/1990	13/05/1995	D	O	4	1613
21	67	2	24/01/1991	23/12/1994	D	BC	3	1429
22	64	2	17/02/1991	06/09/1994	D	O	3	1297
23	73	1	21/04/1991	24/12/1993	A	–	2	978
24	48	2	09/06/1991	26/06/1994	A	–	3	1113
25	42	2	20/06/1991	15/03/1992	D	BC	0	269
26	56	2	25/08/1991	19/08/1994	A	–	2	1090
27	43	1	01/03/1992	06/06/1994	D	BC	2	827
28	64	2	12/04/1992	13/02/1995	D	O	2	1037
29	35	2	13/04/1992	15/04/1994	D	BC	2	732
30	77	1	05/05/1992	10/05/1995	A	–	3	1100
31	59	2	10/08/1992	08/11/1992	D	BC	0	90
32	68	1	13/10/1992	21/10/1993	D	BC	1	373
33	70	1	19/11/1992	20/12/1995	A	–	3	1126
34	58	1	17/01/1993	29/10/1994	A	–	1	650
35	75	2	02/02/1993	10/03/1994	D	BC	1	401
36	55	2	02/05/1993	29/09/1993	D	BC	0	150
37	45	1	11/05/1993	07/02/1994	D	BC	0	272
38	69	1	09/11/1993	26/05/1995	A	–	1	563
39	70	1	07/12/1993	27/05/1995	A	–	1	536
40	27	1	31/12/1993	03/06/1995	A	–	1	519

[a] Stage: 1 = absence of regional lymph node involvement and metastases

2 = involvement of regional lymph node and/or presence of regional or distant metastases

[b] A=alive; D=dead

[c] BC=breast cancer; O=causes other than breast cancer

because this is the point when the treatment groups are comparable. In Example 12.1, the date of diagnosis was taken as the starting point.

The third requirement is a *clear and well defined outcome*. Often the outcome of interest is death, but it need not be so. It can be recurrence of

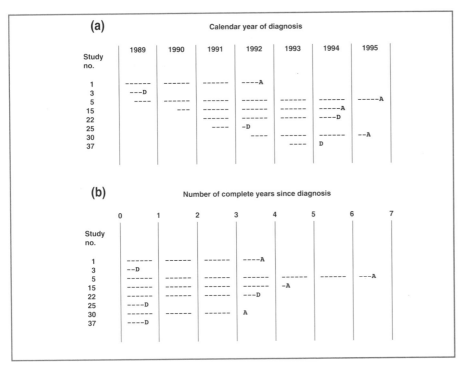

Figure 12.1.
Diagram illustrating how follow-up data from 8 of the 40 women with breast cancer (see Table 12.1) can be presented (*a*) by calendar year of diagnosis and (*b*) by time since entry into the study (A=alive; D=dead).

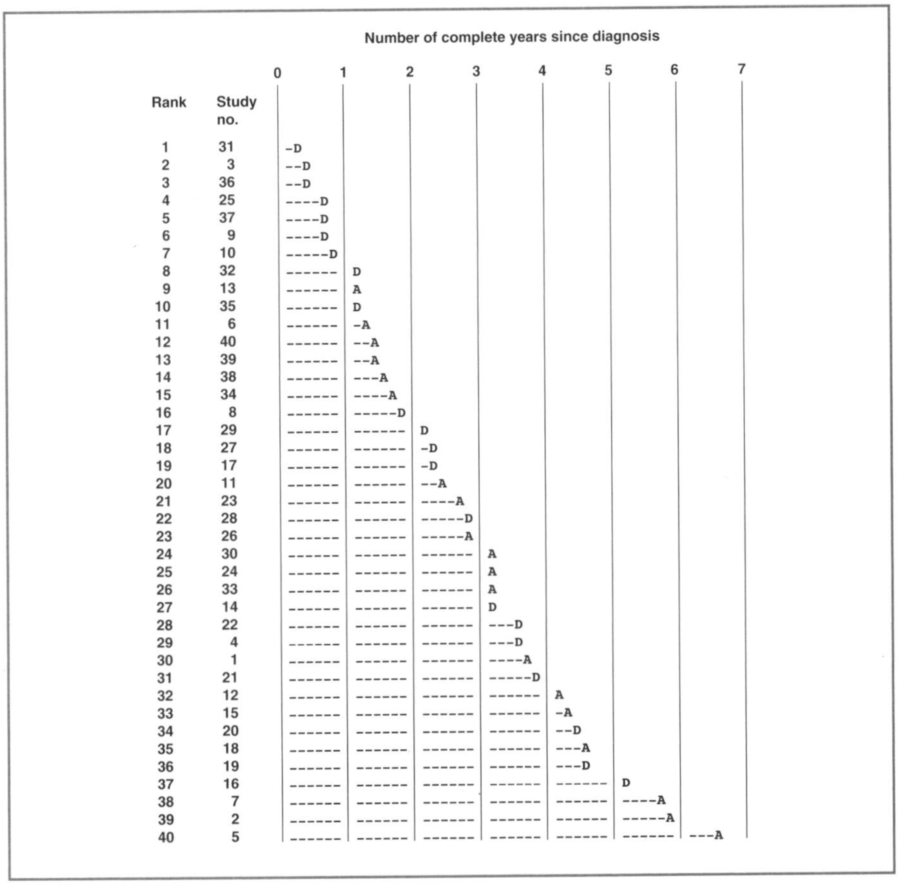

Figure 12.2.
The data of Table 12.1 ordered by length of observed survival time, with (D) representing dead and (A) alive at the end of the follow-up period.

tumour, first occurrence of a particular complication, etc. The only requirement is that the endpoint is a binary variable (e.g., being alive versus being dead) and that each subject can have one and only one endpoint. In our example (12.1), death was considered the outcome of interest.

The time between the starting point and the occurrence of the outcome of interest (or the date of the last contact) is known as *survival time*. The calculation of survival time for some of the patients in Table 12.1 is illustrated in Figure 12.1(*b*). Note that subjects may have different dates of diagnosis but still have the same survival time. For instance, patients No. 25 and 37 had similar survival time, despite differing dates of entry (20/06/1991 and 11/05/1993, respectively; Figure 12.1(*a*); Table 12.1). Figure 12.2 shows the individual survival times for the 40 breast cancer women of Example 12.1 ranked by increasing duration.

The interpretation of the results of a survival study depends greatly upon the length of time each person was followed up. A typical survival study involves a patient accrual period during which patients are recruited and their follow-up is initiated, a follow-up period during which patients are followed up but no further recruitments are made, and a closing date for the analysis. In Example 12.1, the recruitment period was from the start of 1989 until the end of 1993, the follow-up period continued from the beginning of 1994 to the end of 1995, and the closing date for the present analysis was the end of 1995.

One way of summarizing survival data is to report the proportion of patients still alive at a fixed point in time. In Example 12.1, we might initially restrict our analysis to patients for whom we have complete information on the first two years of follow-up. Figure 12.2 shows that six women (Nos 13, 6, 40, 39, 38 and 34) were lost to follow-up before completing a two-year period and should therefore be excluded from the analysis.

In summary, 34 patients completed a two-year follow-up, of whom 10 died and 24 were still alive (Figure 12.2). These results can be presented in a tree diagram (Figure 12.3), in which the upper branch of the tree corresponds to deaths and the lower branch to survivors.

On the basis of these results, we might estimate the *probability (or risk) of dying* in the first two years as 10/34 = 0.29 = 29%.

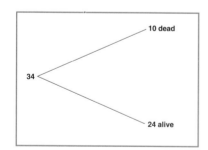

Figure 12.3.
Tree diagram illustrating the two possible outcomes for the 34 patients who completed a two-year follow-up period.

12.3 Censored observations

A closed group consists of a group of individuals in which there are only complete observations. In practice, it is rare to find a closed group, because there are almost always some subjects whose follow-up is incomplete. This occurs because they join the cohort too late to complete the appropriate follow-up before the study ends or because they are lost to follow-up (because of, for example, change of address or migration). Early termination of follow-up for any such reason is called *censoring*.

Our previous calculation of the probability of dying in the first two years excluded censored observations. However, the fact that censored subjects did not die during the time they were in the study provides some information about the probability of dying. Suppose we do not know the exact dates when censoring occurred and all we know is the number of patients who were unable to complete the defined follow-up period. If the time-interval is relatively short, we can make a simple estimate by assuming that on average we observed each censored patient for half the follow-up period without observing any deaths among them. Thus, for a cohort of size N with D observed deaths and L losses due to censoring, we estimate the probability of dying in the interval as

$D/(N - 0.5L)$

Thus censoring reduces the effective size of the cohort by half the size of the group lost to follow-up ($0.5L$). This rather crude way of taking account of censoring works adequately provided L is small compared with N.

We can now re-calculate the probability of dying in the first two years in Example 12.1. Thus, of the 40 breast cancer patients recruited into the study

10 died during the two-year follow-up period ($D = 10$)

24 were still alive at the end of the follow-up ($A = 24$)

6 survived but were lost to follow-up ($L = 6$)

These results can be presented in a tree diagram similar to the one shown in Figure 12.3, except that there is now an additional middle branch corresponding to the censored observations (Figure 12.4).

We have now included all 40 patients in our calculations. However, the effective size of the cohort is no longer 40 but 37 due to the six censored observations ($= 40 - 0.5 \times 6$). The probability of dying is estimated as 10 / 37 = 0.27 = 27%.

Similarly, we can calculate the probability of dying during the first three years of diagnosis. Since the last attempt to contact patients was made in 1995, patients diagnosed after 31 December 1992 entered the study too late to have been able to complete a three-year follow-up. Thus, the observations for four patients (Nos 34, 38–40) were censored (Table 12.1). Five other women (Nos 13, 6, 11, 23, 26) did not complete the three-year observation period because they were lost to follow-up (Figure 12.2). Thus, of the 40 breast cancer patients recruited into the study:

14 died during the three-year follow-up period

17 were still alive at the end of the follow-up

9 were lost to follow-up or joined the cohort too late to complete three years of observation.

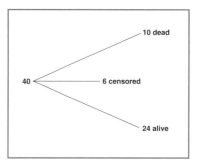

Figure 12.4.
Tree diagram illustrating the outcome of the 40 breast cancer patients from Example 12.1 at the end of a two-year follow-up period.

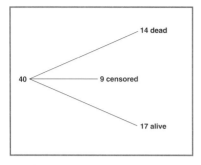

Figure 12.5.
Tree diagram illustrating the outcome of the 40 breast cancer patients from Example 12.1 at the end of a three-year follow-up period.

The corresponding tree diagram is shown in Figure 12.5. The probability of dying in the first three years after a diagnosis of breast cancer can be estimated as $14 / (40 - 0.5 \times 9) = 39\%$.

12.4 Consecutive follow-up intervals

The use of a single interval of follow-up has several limitations. Firstly, it is a very crude way of summarizing the survival experience of a cohort, since it ignores any information about when the deaths and censoring took place. Only the total number of deaths and the total number of censored observations that occurred during the defined interval is required for the calculations. Secondly, it is possible to compare the survival experience of different cohorts only if the same follow-up interval is used. For instance, it is not possible to compare the survival experiences of two cohorts of breast cancer patients if the experience of one cohort is summarized as the probability of dying in the first two years after diagnosis and that of the second as the probability of dying in the first five years.

One way of overcoming these limitations is to use a number of shorter consecutive intervals of time, rather than just one long interval. The experience of the cohort during each of these intervals can then be used to build up the experience over the entire period. Instead of a single calculation of the probability of dying, there will be a sequence of calculations, one for each interval.

Consider again the three-year follow-up shown in Figure 12.5. This period can be divided into three one-year intervals. We can use the data shown in Figure 12.2 to present the number of patients who contribute to each of the three possible outcomes (i.e., death, censoring and survival) in each of the three consecutive years of follow-up. The resulting tree diagram is shown in Figure 12.6.

In this tree diagram, the survivors from one year go on to the start of the next year. In the first year, there were 40 breast cancer patients of whom seven died and none were censored, leaving 33 patients at the start of the second year. Of these 33 patients, three died and six were censored during the second year, leaving 24 at the beginning of the third year. During the third year, four women died, three were censored and 17 were known to be alive.

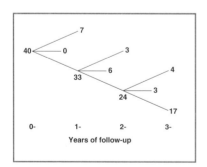

Figure 12.6.
Tree diagram showing the number of breast cancer patients from Example 12.1 who contributed to the different outcomes in each of the first three years of follow-up.

12.5 Estimation of probabilities

We can now replace the numbers of patients on our tree by the probabilities of dying and surviving in each of the intervals. The probability of dying in each interval can be calculated as before, taking account of the censored observations in that interval. The *probability of survival* in the interval is just one minus the probability of dying in the interval.

In the *first year* there were no censored observations, thus

the probability of dying in the year is $7/40 = 0.175$;
the probability of surviving the year is $1 - 0.175 = 0.825$.

In the *second year*, six women were censored. The effective size of the cohort in this year can then be estimated as $33 - (0.5 \times 6) = 30$. Thus

> the probability of a subject dying during the second year, given that the subject was alive at the start of the year, is estimated to be $3/30 = 0.10$;
> the probability of surviving the year is estimated to be $1 - 0.10 = 0.90$.

In the *third year*, three women were censored. The effective size of the cohort is $24 - (0.5 \times 3) = 22.5$. Thus

> the probability of a subject dying during the third year, given that the subject was alive at the start of the year, is estimated to be $4/22.5 = 0.178$;
> the probability of surviving the year is estimated to be $1 - 0.178 = 0.822$.

The full tree with the branch (conditional) probabilities of dying in each year given that the subject survived the previous years is shown in Figure 12.7.

There are now four possible outcomes of interest, corresponding to the tips of the tree. The probability of each outcome can be calculated by multiplying down the branches of the tree. Therefore the probabilities for each outcome are:

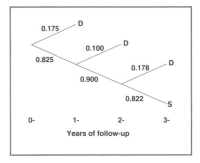

Figure 12.7.
Tree diagram showing the probabilities of each possible outcome in each of the first three years of follow-up (D = death; S = survival).

1. Probability of dying during the first year = 0.175
2. Probability of dying during the second year (i.e., probability of surviving in year 1 × probability of dying in year 2) = $0.825 \times 0.10 = 0.083$
3. Probability of dying during the third year = $0.825 \times 0.90 \times 0.178 = 0.132$
4. Probability of being alive by the end of the three years = $0.825 \times 0.90 \times 0.822 = 0.610$

These probabilities will always add up to 1, since there are no other possible outcomes. The probability of dying at *some point* during the three-year interval is equal to $0.175 + 0.083 + 0.132 = 0.390$. This probability can be found more conveniently by subtracting the probability of surviving the whole three-year period from 1, giving $1 - 0.610 = 0.390$.

The final probability of surviving (0.610) is an example of a *cumulative survival probability* for the cohort, i.e., the probability of surviving three consecutive years.

12.6 Actuarial life-table

The data from the previous calculations are often presented in the form of an actuarial life table, which shows the numbers of deaths and censorings occurring in each consecutive interval. A life table for the 40 breast cancer patients from Example 12.1 is shown in Table 12.2.

In this table, the probability of dying during each year is calculated as $D/(N - 0.5L)$. Thus, the probability of surviving the year is equal to $1 - D/(N - 0.5L)$. The cumulative survival is found by multiplying the survival probabilities for each of the consecutive years to obtain the cumulative

Table 12.2.
Actuarial life table for the 40 breast cancer patients of Example 12.1.

Year	No. at start of interval (N)	No. of deaths (D)	No. of losses (L)	Effective denominator (N–0.5L)	Probability of dying during the year	Probability of surviving the year	Cumulative survival
0–	40	7	0	40	0.175	0.825	0.825
1–	33	3	6	30.0	0.100	0.900	0.743
2–	24	4	3	22.5	0.178	0.822	0.610
3–	17	4	4	15.0	0.267	0.733	0.447
4–	9	2	3	7.5	0.267	0.733	0.328
5–	4	1	2	3.0	0.333	0.667	0.219
6–	1	0	1	0.5	0.0	1.00	0.219
Total		21	19				

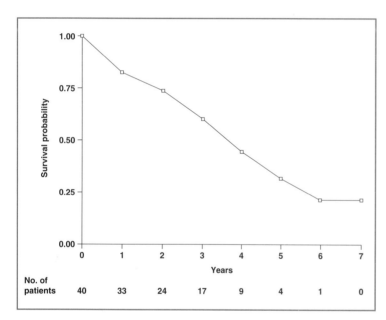

Figure 12.8.
Life-table (actuarial) survival curve for the 40 breast cancer patients of Example 12.1.

probabilities of surviving 1, 2, ..., 6 years. For example, the probability of surviving three years without dying is $0.825 \times 0.90 \times 0.822 = 0.610$ (the same value we calculated before). The life table is therefore just a convenient way of displaying these probabilities which are derived in the same way as those on the tree diagram. Life-tables are useful to examine whether the probability of dying changes with follow-up time, and for presenting concisely summary measures for different intervals of follow-up.

The cumulative survival probabilities can also be displayed graphically as in Figure 12.8. This plot is called a *survival curve*. The curve starts at 1 (all patients alive) and with time progressively declines towards 0 (all patients have died).

12.7   Kaplan–Meier method

The actuarial life-table method described in Section 12.6 does not require information on the exact time when deaths or censoring occur. Only knowledge of the subjects' vital status at each of the limits of the intervals is required. If the *exact times* when deaths occur are known, survival probabilities can be estimated immediately after each individual death without any need to aggregate the data into intervals of one year (or of any other length). This method of estimating the cumulative survival probabilities is called the *Kaplan–Meier method* and it is the preferred approach whenever event and censoring times are available (see Estève *et al.* (1994) for a full description of the calculations).

Similarly to the life-table survival curve, the Kaplan–Meier estimates can be used to plot cumulative survival probabilities. In this instance, however, the plot is in the form of a *stepped line*, rather than a smooth curve, since the cumulative survival drops at the precise time that a death occurs and remains at a plateau between successive death times. For instance, the curve for the 40 breast cancer patients of Example 12.1 shown in Figure 12.9 starts at 1 and continues horizontally until the first death (patient number 31) at day 90; at this time it drops by a function of the estimated probability of dying. It then continues horizontally until the next death (patient 3) at day 142, and so on. The graph will reach zero only if the patient with the longest observed survival time has died. If this patient is still alive at the end of the follow-up period, the Kaplan–Meier curve has a plateau commencing at the time of the last death and continuing until the censored survival time of this longest surviving patient. In Figure 12.9, the survival time of each censored observation is marked in the curve by a cross. After the last death (patient 16, at day 1862 (5.1 years)), the curve remains flat until the longest censored survival time (patient 5, at day 2390 (6.5 years)).

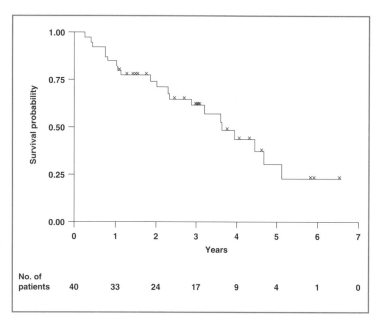

Figure 12.9.
Survival curve produced by the Kaplan–Meier method for the 40 breast cancer patients of Example 12.1 (x indicates censoring times).

It is useful to give the number of patients at risk at selected time points (for example, at the start of each year) under the graph and/or to present confidence intervals around the survival probability estimates. This information is crucial for a sensible interpretation of any survival curve.

12.8   Comparison of survival curves

In many situations, the primary objective of the study is to compare the survival experience of different groups of patients. These groups may be defined according to sex, stage of the tumour at the time of diagnosis (as in Example 12.2), histological type, etc. In clinical trials, the groups will be defined on the basis of the treatment given. Cumulative survival probabilities are calculated separately for each group and the two curves plotted on the same graph for comparison (Figure 12.10).

A visual comparison of survival curves is extremely useful. Consider the graphs presented in Figure 12.11. In graph (a), the two curves overlap in the first two years of follow-up but diverge thereafter. In graph (b), group A initially has better survival than group B, but the curves cross after four years of follow-up and ultimately group A does worse than group B.

These patterns would be missed if the comparison was restricted to a specific follow-up period. For instance, if only two-year survival probabilities were calculated, they would indicate that there was no clear difference between the treatments in graph (a) and that treatment A was much superior to treatment B in graph (b). These two examples clearly illustrate that comparison of survival experiences should always be based on survival curves. Statistical tests for the formal comparison of two survival curves, such as the *logrank test*, can then be used to assess the statistical significance of any observed differences (see Estève *et al.*, 1994).

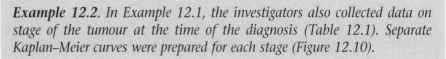

Example 12.2. In Example 12.1, the investigators also collected data on stage of the tumour at the time of the diagnosis (Table 12.1). Separate Kaplan–Meier curves were prepared for each stage (Figure 12.10).

Figure 12.10.
Kaplan–Meier survival curves for patients with breast cancer by stage of the tumour at the time of diagnosis (group 1 = tumour without lymph node involvement or metastasis; group 2 = tumour with lymph node involvement and/or regional or distant metastasis). The numbers on the survival curves represent censored observations.

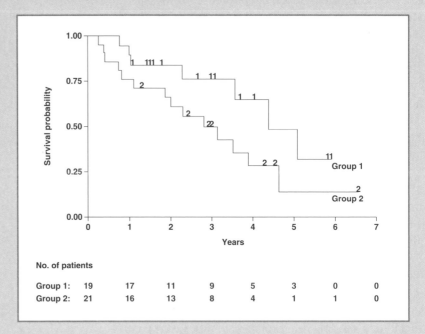

Figure 12.11.
Two examples of comparative survival curves (reproduced by permission of the BMJ Publishing Group, from Gore, 1981).

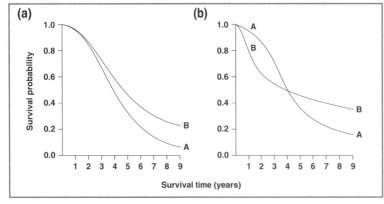

When comparing survival curves in relation to a particular prognostic (or therapeutic) factor, it is important to ensure that the groups are similar in relation to other prognostic factors. In Example 12.2, for instance, other characteristics such as age should have been taken into account. In randomized trials this is accomplished by the random allocation of the subjects to the various arms of the trial (provided the sample size is large). In observational studies, it is possible to obtain Kaplan–Meier curves adjusted for confounders such as age, sex, stage of the tumour, etc. (see Estève *et al.*, 1994) provided data on these variables are collected.

12.9 Overall survival and cause-specific survival

The first step in the analysis of the survival experience of a group of patients should be to examine their *overall survival*. In our breast cancer example, no distinction was made between deaths from breast cancer and deaths from other causes. However, a subject who dies in a traffic accident is no longer at risk of dying from breast cancer. One way of adjust-

Year	No. at start of interval (N)	No. of deaths (D)	No. of losses (L)	Effective denominator (N–0.5L)	Probability of dying during the year	Probability of surviving the year	Cumulative survival
0–	40	7	0	40	0.175	0.825	0.825
1–	33	3	6	30.0	0.100	0.900	0.743
2–	24	3	4	22.0	0.136	0.864	0.641
3–	17	3	5	14.5	0.207	0.793	0.509
4–	9	1	4	7.0	0.143	0.857	0.436
5–	4	0	3	2.5	0.0	1.0	0.436
6–	1	0	1	0.5	0.0	1.0	0.436
Total		17	23				

Table 12.3.
Life-table probabilities of dying from breast cancer for the 40 breast cancer patients of Example 12.1. In this table, deaths from causes other than breast cancer were considered as censored observations.

ing for these 'competing' causes of death is to treat patients who died from other causes as if they had been withdrawn alive (i.e., censored at the time of their death) and then carry out the life-table calculations as described above. The survival probabilities obtained by this method are *cause-specific survival probabilities*, since they take into account deaths due to causes other than the disease under study.

In Example 12.1, four patients died from causes other than breast cancer (see Table 12.1). A new actuarial life-table can then be constructed by considering these deaths as censored observations (Table 12.3). The total number of deaths is decreased by 4 (17 instead of 21) and the number of losses increased by 4 (23 instead of 19). Similarly, when the exact dates at which deaths occur are known, it is possible to use the Kaplan–Meier method to estimate these cause-specific survival probabilities (Figure 12.12).

The calculation of cause-specific survival probabilities requires information on cause-specific mortality. This information may not be easy to obtain. Deaths from other causes tend to be under-reported in cancer patients, as many of them will be entered in the death certificate simply as deaths from cancer. Even when other causes apart from cancer are reported, it is difficult to establish whether the cause of death was unrelated to the cancer of interest (e.g., cancer in adjacent organs).

If accurate cause-specific mortality data are not available, this method cannot be used. It may be possible, however, to compare the *observed survival* with what would have been *expected* for a group of people in the general population similar to the patient group with respect to race, sex, age and calendar period of observation. This expect-

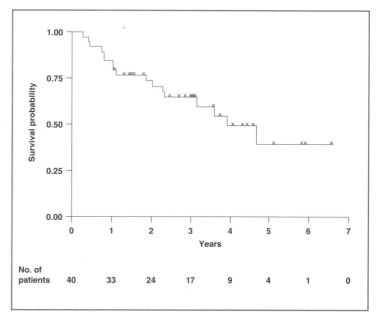

No. of patients: 40, 33, 24, 17, 9, 4, 1, 0

Figure 12.12.
Kaplan–Meier breast cancer-specific survival curve for the 40 breast cancer patients of Table 12.1.

ed survival can be derived from published demographic life tables (see below). The comparison yields *relative survival ratios* which are adjusted for the patients' probability of dying from a cause other than the one under study (see Parkin & Hakulinen (1991) for an illustration of these calculations). Thus, the relative survival ratios represent the survival experience of a group of patients adjusted for their probability of dying from causes other than the one under investigation. In practice, the 'all causes' and 'all causes minus cancer' demographic life tables are very similar and since the former are more readily available, these are generally used in the calculations.

12.10 Demographic life tables

All the above discussion of life tables relates to data derived from real cohorts, i.e., from groups of people who were actually followed up in time.

Demographic life tables, computed on the basis of national (or regional or specific for a particular ethnic or socioeconomic group) mortality data, can be obtained by applying the currently observed mortality risks at various ages to an imaginary cohort. Thus the life expectancy of women at birth in England and Wales, which was 77 years in 1981 (Bone *et al.*, 1995), depends on the assumption that baby girls born in 1981 will be exposed to 1981 age-specific risks of dying as they go through life (e.g., when they are age 30 in the year 2011, they will experience the 1981 mortality risks for 30-year-olds). Although taken literally, this assumption is unrealistic, demographic life tables are a good way of summarizing current mortality risks. These demographic life tables are usually prepared and published by governmental statistical offices.

12.11 Other outcomes

The methods described in this chapter are part of a group of statistical techniques used in 'survival analysis'. The term 'survival' comes from the fact that the first use of such techniques arose in the insurance industry, which was particularly interested in developing methods of costing insurance premiums. For this purpose, they needed to know the average life expectancy for different types of customer.

The use of survival analysis techniques is, however, by no means restricted to studies where death is the outcome of interest. It has also been widely used to study other outcomes such as fertility, compliance with treatment, recurrence of disease, occurrence of complications, etc.

The trial described in Example 12.3 had more than one outcome of interest. The results in Figure 12.13 show little evidence of a difference in overall survival ($P = 0.5$) or survival free from regional or distant recurrence ($P = 0.19$). However, the trial provided moderate evidence in favour of the hypothesis that women who received radiation had a lower risk of developing local recurrences ($P = 0.06$).

Example 12.3. *A total of 381 women with invasive breast cancer in histopathological stage I had sector resection with meticulous control for complete excision of local disease plus axillary dissection. After this surgery, 187 were randomized to receive postoperative radiotherapy to the breast and 194 women to receive no further treatment. The outcomes of interest were overall survival and time from treatment to local recurrence and to regional or distant metastasis. The Kaplan–Meier method was used in the analysis (Uppsala-Örebro Breast Cancer Study Group, 1990). The main results from this trial are shown in Figure 12.13.*

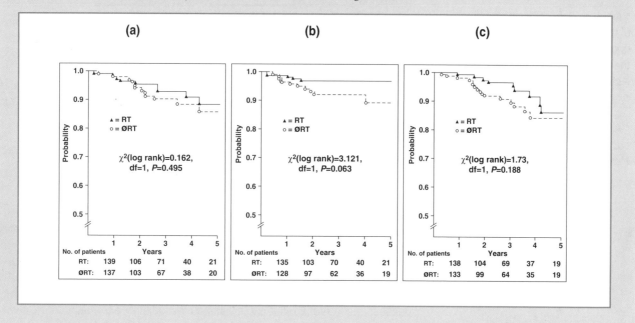

12.12 Final notes

Survival analysis can be carried out easily with many statistical computer packages such as STATA, EGRET, SAS or SPSS. Unfortunately, it is not possible to conduct this type of analysis in EPI INFO.

The application of survival analysis to data collected by cancer registries is discussed in Section 17.6.2.

Figure 12.13.
Probability of (*a*) overall survival; (*b*) of remaining free from local recurrence; and (*c*) of remaining free from regional or distant metastasis for 381 breast cancer patients according to type of postoperative treatment (RT = postoperative radiotherapy to the breast; ØRT = no further treatment) (reproduced, by permission of Oxford University Press, from Uppsala-Örebro Breast Cancer Study Group, 1990).

Further reading

* The use of probability trees in this chapter was based on the approach suggested by Clayton & Hills (1993).

* A more elaborate presentation of the general statistical concepts underlying survival analysis and their application to routinely collected data is given in Estève *et al.* (1994).

* A guide to the use of survival curves in cancer trials is given by Peto *et al.* (1976, 1977).

Box 12.1. Key issues

• Survival analysis is another method used in the analysis of data from intervention trials, cohort studies and data routinely collected by cancer registries. It is particularly useful when the probability of occurrence of the event under study changes with time since entry into the study.

• The survival experience of a group of people may be summarized by reporting the proportion still alive at a particular point in time (e.g., at the end of a two-year follow-up). This approach has several limitations, however. First, no account is taken of the time when deaths and censoring took place. Second, it is possible to compare the survival experience between groups of people only if the same follow-up period is used. Third, it does not provide any indication of changes in survival with follow-up time.

• All the above limitations can be overcome by calculating *cumulative survival probabilities* for consecutive follow-up intervals. These probabilities can then be displayed graphically in a plot called a *survival curve.*

• Cumulative survival probabilities can be calculated by using either the *actuarial life-table* method or the *Kaplan–Meier* method. The two methods are basically similar, but the shape of the resulting survival curve is slightly different. The actuarial life-table method produces a smooth curve because cumulative survival probabilities are calculated only at the end of each of the consecutive follow-up intervals, whereas the Kaplan–Meier method produces a stepped line because these probabilities are calculated immediately after each death takes place.

• The first step in survival analysis should be to estimate the *overall survival* experience of the entire cohort. Sometimes it may be useful to proceed to estimate *cause-specific survival.* This can be easily done if accurate cause-specific mortality data are available for the study subjects. If these data are not available, it is still possible to look at cause-specific survival by using information from demographic life-tables.

Chapter 13
Interpretation of epidemiological studies

In epidemiology, studies are carried out to identify exposures that may affect the risk of developing a certain disease or other health-related outcome and to estimate quantitatively their effect. Unfortunately, errors are inevitable in almost any epidemiological study, even in the best conducted randomized trial. Thus, when interpreting findings from an epidemiological study, it is essential to consider how much the observed association between an exposure and an outcome may have been affected by errors in the design, conduct and analysis. Even if errors do not seem to be an obvious explanation for the observed effect, it is still necessary to assess the likelihood that the observed association is a causal one. The following questions should be addressed before it is concluded that the observed association between exposure and outcome is a true cause–effect relationship:

(1) Could the observed association be due to systematic errors (*bias*) in the way subjects were selected and followed up or in the way information was obtained from them?
(2) Could it be due to differences between the groups in the distribution of another variable (*confounder*) that was not measured or taken into account in the analyses?
(3) Could it be due to *chance*?
(4) Finally, is the observed association likely to be *causal*?

Most of these issues were already raised in Chapters 7–11 in relation to each specific study design. In this chapter, we will consider them in a more structured way.

13.1 Could the observed effect be due to bias?

Bias tends to lead to an incorrect estimate of the effect of an exposure on the development of a disease or other outcome of interest. The observed estimate may be either above or below the true value, depending on the nature of the error.

Many types of bias in epidemiology have been identified (Sackett, 1979) but, for simplicity, they can be grouped into two major types: *selection bias* and *measurement bias*.

13.1.1 Selection bias

Selection bias occurs when there is a difference between the characteristics of the people selected for the study and the characteristics of those who were not. In all instances where selection bias occurs, the result is a difference in the relation between exposure and outcome between those who entered the study and those who would have been eligible but did not participate. For instance, selection bias will occur with volunteers (self-selection bias). People who volunteer to participate in a study tend to be different from the rest of the population in a number of demographic and lifestyle variables (usually being more health-conscious, better educated, etc.), some of which may also be risk factors for the outcome of interest.

Selection bias can be a major problem in case–control studies, although it can also affect cross-sectional studies and, to a lesser extent, cohort studies and randomized trials.

The selection of an appropriate sample for a *cross-sectional survey* does not necessarily guarantee that the participants are representative of the target population, because some of the selected subjects may fail to participate. This can introduce selection bias if non-participants differ from participants in relation to the factors under study.

In Example 13.1, the prevalence of alcohol-related problems rose with increasing effort to recruit subjects, suggesting that those who completed the interview only after a large number of contact attempts were different from those who required less recruitment effort. Constraints of time and money usually limit the recruitment efforts to relatively few contact attempts. This may bias the prevalence estimates derived from a cross-sectional study.

In *case–control studies*, controls should represent the source population from which the cases were drawn, i.e. they should provide an estimate of the exposure prevalence in the general population from which the cases come. This is relatively straightforward to accomplish in a *nested case–control study*, in which the cases and the controls arise from a clearly defined population—the cohort. In a *population-based case–control study*, a source population can also be defined from which all cases (or a random sample) are obtained; controls will be randomly selected from the disease-free members of the same population.

The sampling method used to select the controls should ensure that they are a representative sample of the population from which the cases originated. If they are not, selection bias will be introduced. For instance, the method used to select controls in Example 13.2 excluded women who were part of the study population but did not have a telephone. Thus, control selection bias might have been introduced if women with and without a telephone differed with respect to the exposure(s) of interest. This bias could be overcome by excluding cases who did not have a telephone, that is, by redefining the study population as women living in households with a telephone, aged 20–54 years, who resided in the eight selected areas. Moreover, the ultimate objective of the random-digit dialling method was not merely to provide a random sample of households with telephone but a random sample of *all* women aged 20–54 years living in these households during the study period. This depended on the extent to which people

Example 13.1. *A cross-sectional study was conducted in St Louis, Missouri (USA) to assess the prevalence of psychiatric disorders. This study is quite unusual in that great efforts were made to recruit as many eligible subjects as possible. Subjects were chosen according to a five-stage probability sampling plan which gave each household a known probability of being selected. Once the household was selected, the residents were enumerated by age and sex, and one resident over age 18 years was randomly chosen to enter the study. Replacement was not allowed. Enumeration of residents was completed in 91% of the eligible households. Of the 3778 selected subjects, 3004 (80%) were successfully interviewed. Figure 13.1 shows that 32% of the respondents were interviewed after two contact attempts and 66% after five. Not until the 14th attempt were 95% of the interviews completed. The maximum number of attempts that resulted in an interview was 57. The mean for the 3004 responders was 5.3; the median, 4. Being young, male, black, a non-rural resident, well educated, and full-time employed were the demographic characteristics associated with increased contact efforts (Cottler et al., 1987). Table 13.1 shows prevalence estimates for alcohol-related problems by number of attempts made to obtain an interview.*

Interview completed within this number of contact attempts	Cumulative sample (n)	Estimated prevalence of current alcohol abuse and dependence disorder (%)
5	1943	3.89
7	2285	3.98
8	2415	4.22
9	2511	4.26
57	2928[b]	4.61

[a] Data from Cottler *et al.* (1987).

[b] This number is slightly lower than the number of subjects for whom the interview was completed (3004) because questionnaires with missing data were excluded from this analysis.

Table 13.1.
Prevalence estimates for current alcohol abuse and dependence disorder by number of contact attempts necessary to complete interview, St Louis Epidemiologic Catchment Area project, 1981–82.[a]

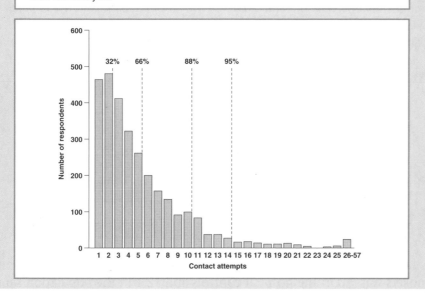

Figure 13.1.
Number of contact attempts necessary to complete interview for the St Louis Epidemiologic Catchment Area project, 1981–82 (reproduced with permission from Cottler *et al.*, 1987).

Example 13.2. The effect of oral contraceptive use on the risk of breast, endometrial and ovarian cancers was investigated in the Cancer and Steroid Hormone Study. The study population was women aged 20–54 years who resided in eight selected areas in the USA during the study period. Attempts were made to identify all incident cases of breast, ovarian and endometrial cancer that occurred in the study population during the study period through local population-based cancer registries. Controls were selected by random-digit dialling of households in the eight locations. A random sample of household telephone numbers were called; information on the age and sex of all household members was requested and controls were selected among female members aged 20–54 years according to strict rules (Stadel et al., 1985).

answering the telephone numbers selected were willing to provide accurate information on the age and sex of all individuals living in the household.

Sometimes, it is not possible to define the population from which the cases arise. In these circumstances, *hospital-based controls* may be used, because the source population can then be re-defined as 'hospital users'. Hospital controls may also be preferable for logistic reasons (easier and cheaper to identify and recruit) and because of lower potential for recall bias (see below). But selection bias may be introduced if admission to hospital for other conditions is related to exposure status.

Example 13.3. A classic case–control study was conducted in England in 1948–52 to examine the relationship between cigarette smoking and lung cancer. The cases were 1488 patients admitted for lung cancer to the participating hospitals, 70% of which were located in London. A similar number of controls were selected from patients who were admitted to the same hospitals with other conditions (except diseases thought at that time to be related to smoking). The smoking habits of the hospital controls were compared with those of a random sample of all residents in London (Table 13.2). These comparisons showed that, among men of similar ages, smoking was more common in the hospital controls than in the population sample (Doll & Hill, 1952).

Table 13.2.
Age-adjusted distribution of male hospital controls without lung cancer and of a random sample of men from the general population from which the lung cancer cases originated according to their smoking habits.[a]

Subjects	Percentage of subjects					Number (%) interviewed
	Non-smokers	Most recent number of cigarettes smoked per day				
		1–4	5–14	15–24	25+	
Hospital controls	7.0	4.2	43.3	32.1	13.4	1390 (100)
Sample of general population	12.1	7.0	44.2	28.1	8.5	199 (100)
[a] Data from Doll & Hill (1952).						

Table 13.2 shows that among men of similar age, the percentage of non-smokers was 7.0 in the hospital controls and 12.1 in the population sam-

ple. The percentage smoking at least 25 cigarettes per day was 13.4 in the hospital controls but only 8.5 in the population sample. The investigators stated that this difference in smoking habits between the hospital controls and the population random sample might be explained by previously unknown associations between smoking and several diseases. Thus, the strength of the association between lung cancer and cigarette smoking was *underestimated* in the case–control study, because the prevalence of smoking in the hospital controls was higher than in the general population from which the cases of lung cancer were drawn.

A hospital control series may fail to reflect the population at risk because it includes people admitted to the hospital for conditions caused (or prevented) by the exposures of interest. Individuals hospitalized for diseases related to the exposure under investigation should be excluded in order to eliminate this type of selection bias. However, this exclusion should not be extended to hospital patients with a history of exposure-related diseases, since no such restriction is imposed on the cases. Thus, patients admitted to hospital because of a smoking-related disorder (e.g., chronic bronchitis) should be excluded from the control series in a case–control study looking at the relationship between smoking and lung cancer, whereas those admitted for other conditions (e.g., accidents) but with a history of chronic bronchitis should be included.

Selection bias is less of a problem in *cohort studies*, because the enrolment of exposed and unexposed individuals is done before the development of any outcome of interest. This is also true in *historical cohort studies*, because the ascertainment of the exposure status was made some time in the past, before the outcome was known. However, bias may still be introduced in the selection of the 'unexposed' group. For instance, in occupational cohort studies where the general population is used as the comparison group, it is usual to find that the overall morbidity and mortality of the workers is lower than that of the general population. This is because only relatively healthy people are able to remain in employment, while the general population comprises a wider range of people including those who are too ill to be employed. This type of selection bias is called

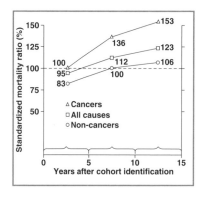

Figure 13.2.
Decline in the healthy worker effect with passage of time after initial identification of a cohort of active workers. Graph based on mortality data among a cohort of asbestos product workers (Enterline, 1965) (reproduced with permission from McMichael, 1976). © American College of Occupational and Environmental Medicine, 1976).

Example 13.4. Suppose that a particular cohort was defined as workers who were in active employment at a particular point in time and that no new members were allowed to join the cohort later. If all the cohort members are followed up, including those who leave or retire for health reasons, the healthy worker effect will decline with time, because the initial healthy selection process at the time of recruitment into the workforce will become weaker with the passage of time. Note that employed people are not only generally healthier but also, if unhealthy, less likely to suffer from long-term and easy-to-detect diseases (e.g., cardiovascular conditions) than from diseases which remain asymptomatic for long periods (e.g., many cancers) (McMichael, 1976).

the *healthy worker effect*. It may be minimized by restricting the analysis to people from the same factory who went through the same healthy selection process but have a different job (see Section 8.2.2).

Example 13.4 shows that the healthy selection bias varies with type of disease, being less marked for cancer than for non-cancer conditions (mainly cardiovascular disorders), and it tends to decline with time since recruitment into the workforce.

Incompleteness of follow-up due to non-response, refusal to participate and withdrawals may also be a major source of selection bias in cohort studies in which people have to be followed up for long periods of time. However, this will introduce bias only if the degree of incompleteness is different for different exposure categories. For example, subjects may be more inclined to return for a follow-up examination if they have developed symptoms of the disease. This tendency may be different in the exposed and unexposed, resulting in an over- or under-estimation of the effect. Definitions of individual follow-up periods may conceal this source of bias. For example, if subjects with a certain occupation tend to leave their job when they develop symptoms of disease, exposed cases may not be identified if follow-up terminates at the time subjects change to another job. A similar selection bias may occur in migrant studies if people who become ill return to their countries of origin before their condition is properly diagnosed in the host country.

Randomized intervention trials are less likely to be affected by selection bias since subjects are randomized to the exposure groups to be compared. However, refusals to participate after randomization and withdrawals from the study may affect the results if their occurrence is related to exposure status. To minimize selection bias, allocation to the various study groups should be conducted only after having assessed that subjects are both eligible and willing to participate (see Section 7.9). The data should also be analysed according to 'intention to treat' regardless of whether or not the subjects complied with their allocated intervention (see Section 7.12).

13.1.2 Measurement bias

Measurement (or information) bias occurs when measurements or classifications of disease or exposure are not valid (i.e., when they do not measure correctly what they are supposed to measure). Errors in measurement may be introduced by the observer (*observer bias*), by the study individual (*responder bias*), or by the instruments (e.g., questionnaire or sphygmomanometer or laboratory assays) used to make the measurements (see Chapter 2).

Misclassification of a single attribute (exposure or outcome) and observed prevalence

Suppose that a cross-sectional survey was conducted to assess the prevalence of a particular attribute in a certain study population. A questionnaire was administered to all eligible participants; there were no refusals. Let us denote the observed proportion in the population classified as having the attribute by p^* and the true prevalence by p. p^* has two components. One component comes from those individuals with the attribute that are correctly classified by the questionnaire as having it (true positives). The other component comes from those individuals that actually do not have the attribute but erroneously have been classified (that is, misclassified) as having it (false positives). The proportion of individuals that is classified by the questionnaire as having the attribute (p^*) is then:

$$p^* = p \times \text{sensitivity} + (1 - p) \times (1 - \text{specificity})$$

and thus depends on the true prevalence of the attribute (p) and on the sensitivity and specificity of the measurement method. For example, if p = 0.1%, sensitivity = 90% and specificity = 90%, then p^* = 10.1%. This means that if the prevalence were estimated by the proportion that is classified as having the attribute by the questionnaire, the estimate would be 10.1%, compared with a true prevalence of only 0.1%. This misclassification corresponds to a 100-fold overestimation.

It is possible to obtain a corrected estimate of the true prevalence in situations where the sensitivity and the specificity of the measurement procedure are both known, or may be estimated, by re-arranging the above formula as follows:

$$p = \frac{p^* + \text{specificity} - 1}{\text{sensitivity} + \text{specificity} - 1}$$

True prevalence (%)	Specificity (%)	Sensitivity (%)		
		99	90	80
0.1	99	1.1	1.1	1.1
	90	10.1	10.1	10.1
	80	20.1	20.1	20.1
0.5	99	1.5	1.4	1.4
	90	10.4	10.4	10.4
	80	20.4	20.4	20.3
2.5	99	3.5	3.2	3.0
	90	12.2	12.0	11.8
	80	22.0	21.8	21.5
12.5	99	13.3	12.1	10.9
	90	21.1	20.0	18.8
	80	29.9	28.8	27.5
50.0	99	50.0	45.5	40.5
	90	54.5	50.0	45.0
	80	59.5	55.0	50.0
62.5	99	62.3	56.6	50.4
	90	65.6	60.0	53.8
	80	69.4	63.8	57.5

Table 13.3.
Observed prevalence (p^*) (%) of an attribute in a population for different levels of the true prevalence (p), and different values of sensitivity and specificity of the measurement procedure.

Table 13.3 shows the effects of different levels of sensitivity and specificity of a measurement procedure on the observed prevalence of a particular attribute. In most cases, the observed prevalence is a gross overestimation of the true prevalence. For instance, the observed prevalence at 90% sensitivity and 90% specificity assuming a true prevalence of 0.1% is only about one half of that which would be obtainable if the true prevalence were 12.5% (i.e., 10% versus 20%). The bias in overestimation is severely influenced by losses in specificity (particularly when the true prevalence is less than 50%). In contrast, losses in sensitivity have, at most, moderate effects on the observed prevalence.

Misclassification and exposure–outcome relationships

Two main types of misclassification may affect the interpretation of exposure–outcome relationships: nondifferential and differential. *Nondifferential misclassification* occurs when an exposure or outcome classification is incorrect for equal proportions of subjects in the compared groups. In other words, nondifferential misclassification refers to errors in classification of outcome that are unrelated to exposure status, or misclassification of exposure unrelated to the individual's outcome status. In these circumstances, all individuals (regardless of their exposure/outcome status) have the same probability of being misclassified. In contrast, *differential misclassification* occurs when errors in classification of outcome status are dependent upon exposure status or when errors in classification of exposure depend on outcome status.

These two types of misclassification affect results from epidemiological studies in different ways. Their implications also depend on whether the misclassification relates to the exposure or the outcome status.

Nondifferential exposure misclassification

Nondifferential exposure misclassification occurs when all individuals (regardless of their current or future outcome status) have the same probability of being misclassified in relation to their exposure status. Usually, this type of misclassification gives rise to an underestimation of the strength of the association between exposure and outcome, that is, it '*dilutes*' the effect of the exposure.

In the case–control study illustrated in Example 13.5, nondifferential exposure misclassification introduced a bias towards an underestimation of the true exposure effect.

Nondifferential misclassification of exposure will also affect the results from studies of other types. For instance, historical occupational cohort studies rely upon records of exposure of individuals from the past. However, there often were no specific environmental exposure measurements that would allow accurate classification of individuals. This means that individuals were classified as 'exposed' or 'unexposed' by the job they did or by membership of a union. These proxy variables are very crude markers of the true exposure levels and their validity is limited. It is, however, unlikely that the validity of

Example 13.5. *A case–control study was conducted to assess whether coffee intake increased the risk of pancreatic cancer. Subjects were classified as "ever" or "never" drinkers. The true results of this study in the absence of exposure misclassification (i.e., exposure measurement with sensitivity = 100%; specificity = 100%) are shown in Table 13.4.*

	Coffee intake		Total
	Ever	Never	
Pancreatic cancer cases	200	100	300
Controls	150	150	300
Total	**350**	**250**	**600**
True odds ratio = (200/100) / (150/150) = 2.00.			

Table 13.4.
Results from a hypothetical case–control study: true exposure status (sensitivity = 100% and specificity =100% for both cases and controls).

Suppose that the information on coffee intake was obtained through a self-administered questionnaire and that only 80% of study subjects who usually drank coffee (regardless of whether or not they had pancreatic cancer) reported this in the questionnaire (sensitivity = 80%). Similarly, only 90% of those who never drank coffee correctly mentioned this in the questionnaire (specificity = 90%).

	Coffee intake		Total
	Ever	Never	
Pancreatic cancer cases	(200×0.8)+(100×0.1) = 170	(100×0.9)+(200×0.2) = 130	300
Controls	(150×0.8)+(150×0.1) = 135	(150×0.9)+(150×0.2) = 165	300
Total	**305**	**295**	**600**
Observed odds ratio = (170/130) / (135/165) = 1.60			

Table 13.5.
Bias due to nondifferential exposure misclassification: observed exposure status (sensitivity = 80% and specificity = 90% for both cases and controls).

these records would be different for those who later developed the outcome of interest and those who did not. As long as the misclassification is nondifferential, it will generally dilute any true association between the exposure and the outcome.

The implications of nondifferential exposure misclassification depend heavily on whether the study is perceived as 'positive' or 'negative'. This bias is a greater concern in interpreting studies that seem to indicate the absence of an effect. In these circumstances, it is crucial that the researchers consider the problem of nondifferential exposure misclassification in order to determine the probability that a real effect was missed. On the other hand, it is incorrect to dismiss a study reporting an effect simply because there is substantial nondifferential misclassification, since an estimate of effect without the misclassification would generally be even greater.

It should be noted that nondifferential exposure misclassification leads to an underestimation of the relative risk (bias towards relative effect of 1) only if the exposure is classified as a binary variable (e.g., 'exposed' versus 'unexposed'). When there are three or more exposure categories, nondifferential exposure misclassification can result in either over- or under-estimation of the effect (Flegal *et al.*, 1986). For example, in a study of the effect of different levels of coffee intake (classified as 'never', 'low' and 'high') on the risk of pancreatic cancer, the relative risk associated with low levels of coffee intake will be overestimated if there is a general tendency for subjects with a true high intake to underreport it (but not so extreme as to report themselves as non-drinkers). On the other hand, if some people with a true high intake are classified as never-drinkers, the relative risk associated with low levels of coffee intake would be underestimated or even reversed (as in Example 13.6).

Example 13.6. *Table 13.6 shows results from a hypothetical case–control study with a positive exposure–response trend. Suppose that both cases and controls were classified correctly in relation to exposure, except that 60% of subjects who were truly in the 'none' exposure group were misclassified into the 'high' exposure group, and 60% of those truly in the 'high' group were misclassified into the 'none' exposure group. While the odds ratios in the original data were 2.00 and 8.00 for the low and high exposure categories, respectively, they were 0.90 and 0.73 in the misclassified data. This misclassification led to the creation of an inverse exposure–response trend.*

Table 13.6.
Nondifferential exposure misclassification involving more than two exposure categories.[a]

Disease status	True exposure status		
	None[b]	Low	High
Cases	53	40	60
Controls	424	160	60
True odds ratio	1.00	2.00	8.00
	Misclassified exposure status (60% misclassification)		
	None[b]	Low	High
Cases	53−(53×0.6)+(60×0.6)=57	40	60−(60×0.6)+(53×0.6)=56
Controls	424−(424×0.6)+(60×0.6)=206	160	60−(60×0.6)+(424×0.6)=278
Observed odds ratio	1.00	0.90	0.73

[a] Data from Dosemeci *et al.* (1990).
[b] Taken as the baseline category

In this discussion, we have assumed that the misclassification occurs between 'exposure' and 'no exposure' or between different levels of exposure. Obviously, one exposure may be misclassified as another. For example, when studying the effect of oral contraceptive pills on the risk of breast cancer, women may confuse them with other drugs that they might have taken in the past.

Differential exposure misclassification

This type of misclassification can *bias the estimates of the association in either direction* and, hence, it can be responsible for associations which prove to be spurious.

Example 13.7. *Consider the example of a case–control study on oral contraceptive use and breast cancer. The results of this study in the absence of misclassification are shown in Table 13.7.*

	Oral contraceptive use		Total
	Ever	**Never**	
Breast cancer cases	150	200	350
Controls	150	200	350
Total	**300**	**400**	**700**

True odds ratio = (150/200) / (150/200) = 1.00

Suppose now that 20% of the cases who had never used oral contraceptives incorrectly reported having done so, whereas all case users correctly reported their habits (sensitivity = 100%; specificity = 80%). The controls correctly reported their use (sensitivity = 100%; specificity = 100%).

	Oral contraceptive use		Total
	Ever	**Never**	
Breast cancer cases	150+(200×0.20)=190	200−(200×0.20)=160	350
Controls	150	200	350
Total	**340**	**360**	**700**

Observed odds ratio = (190/160) / (150/200) = 1.58

Table 13.7.
Data from a hypothetical case–control study: true exposure status (sensitivity = 100% and specificity =100% for both cases and controls).

Table 13.8.
Bias due to differential exposure misclassification: observed exposure status (sensitivity = 100% and specificity = 80% among cases; sensitivity = 100% and specificity = 100% among controls).

In Example 13.7, patients with breast cancer were more likely to incorrectly report having ever used oral contraceptives than healthy controls, resulting in a spurious association between oral contraceptives and breast cancer. This is a particular type of differential misclassification called *recall bias*. One way of minimizing recall bias is to use hospital controls, because then the controls would generally have the same incentive as the cases to remember events in the past. Subjects should also be unaware of the specific study hypothesis.

In Example 13.8, there is no biological evidence to suggest that the effect of vasectomy would be different between Catholic and Protestant men. Thus, the most likely explanation for the observed findings is that Catholic controls were less likely to report that they had had a vasectomy than Catholic men with testicular cancer. This differential exposure misclassification biased the exposure effect upwards among Catholic men.

Sometimes, it is possible to obtain direct evidence of the presence and magnitude of differential misclassification. In Example 13.9, cases, but not controls, considerably overreported their inability to tan after being diagnosed with skin melanoma: the proportion of cases reporting inability to tan was 26% (=9/34) in 1982 before skin cancer was diagnosed but 44% (=15/34) after the diagnosis.

Table 13.9.
History of vasectomy in testicular cancer cases and controls by religious background.[a]

Example 13.8. A case–control study was conducted in western Washington state (USA) to assess the effect of vasectomy (surgical sterilization) on the risk of testicular cancer. Exposure information was obtained by telephone interview. The results showed a 50% excess risk associated with vasectomy: odds ratio (OR) = 1.5 (95% CI: 1.0–2.2). However, further analyses showed that the effect of vasectomy was considerably different for Catholic and Protestant men: OR = 8.7 for Catholic, and OR = 1.0 for Protestant background. Whereas a history of vasectomy was reported with approximately equal frequency by Catholic and non-Catholic cases, only 6.2% of Catholic controls reported such a history in contrast to 19.7% of other controls (Strader et al., 1988).

Religious background	Cases		Controls		Age-adjusted odds ratio (95% CI[c])
	No.	% with vasectomy[b]	No.	% with vasectomy	
Protestant	129	18.0	295	19.0	1.0 (0.6–1.7)
Catholic	42	24.4	96	6.2	8.7 (2.8–27.1)
Other	57	32.3	122	21.0	1.3 (0.6–3.0)

[a] Data from Strader *et al.* (1988).

[b] Adjusted to age distribution of all controls.

[c] CI = confidence interval.

Example 13.9. The Nurses' Health Study is an on-going cohort study of 121 700 female nurses who were aged 30–55 years when the cohort was assembled in 1976. These women have been sent postal questionnaires biennially since then. The 1982 questionnaire included questions on risk factors for skin melanoma. A nested case–control study was conducted in 1984, which included 34 skin melanoma cases diagnosed after the return of the 1982 questionnaire and 234 controls randomly selected from cohort members without a history of cancer who responded to the same mailed questionnaire. Two questions from the 1982 questionnaire were asked again in the case–control questionnaire. These related to hair colour and ability to tan (Weinstock et al., 1991). The responses given in the two questionnaires are shown in Table 13.10.

Table 13.10.
Self-reported hair colour and tanning ability before and after the diagnosis of skin melanoma in a nested case–control study.[a]

	1982 questionnaire		Case–control questionnaire	
	Cases	Controls	Cases	Controls
Hair colour				
Red or blond	11	37	11	41
Brown or black[b]	23	197	23	193
	OR=2.5 (95% CI=1.1–5.7)		OR=2.3 (95% CI=1.0–5.0)	
Tanning ability				
No tan or light tan	9	79	15	77
Medium, deep or dark[b]	25	155	19	157
	OR=0.7 (95% CI=0.3–1.5)		OR=1.6 (95% CI=0.8–3.5)	

[a] Adapted from Weinstock *et al.* (1991).

[b] Baseline category.

Similarly, observers who know the outcome status of an individual may be consciously or unconsciously predisposed to assess exposure variables according to the hypothesis under study. This type of bias is known as *observer bias*. One way of minimizing this type of bias is to keep the observers *blind* to the outcome status of the study subjects. For many diseases/conditions this is clearly impossible.

Example 13.10. Consider a hypothetical trial in which 20 000 men were randomly allocated to receive a new intervention or placebo. They were then followed up for five years to assess whether the intervention could prevent lung cancer. There were no losses to follow-up. A total of 75 lung cancer cases occurred during the follow-up period. With no outcome misclassification (i.e., outcome measurement method with sensitivity = 100% and specificity = 100%), the results would be as shown in Table 13.11.

	Intervention		Total
	New	Placebo	
Cases	25	50	75
Non-cases	9 975	9 950	19 925
Total	**10 000**	**10 000**	**20 000**

True risk in the new intervention group (r_1) = 25/10 000 = 25 per 10 000

True risk in the placebo group (r_0) = 50/10 000 = 50 per 10 000

True risk ratio = r_1/r_0 = 0.50

True risk difference = $r_0 - r_1$ = 25 per 10 000

True prevented fraction = $(r_0 - r_1)/r_0$ = 25 per 10 000 / 50 per 10 000 = 0.50 = 50%

Table 13.11.
Results from a hypothetical intervention trial: true outcome status (sensitivity = 100% and specificity = 100% for both the new intervention and placebo groups).

Suppose that only 80% of the cases of lung cancer were correctly identified (sensitivity = 0.80) among both those who received and those who did not receive the new intervention. This would give the results presented in Table 13.12.

	Intervention		Total
	New	Placebo	
Cases	25×0.80 = 20	50×0.80=40	60
Non-cases	9 975+(25×0.20) = 9 980	9 950+(50×0.20)=9 960	19 940
Total	**10 000**	**10 000**	**20 000**

Observed r_1 = 20 per 10 000

Observed r_0 = 40 per 10 000

Observed risk ratio = r_1/r_0 = 0.50

Observed risk difference = $r_0 - r_1$ = 20 per 10 000

Observed prevented fraction = $(r_0 - r_1)/r_0$ = 20 per 10 000 / 40 per 10 000 = 0.50 = 50%

Table 13.12.
Bias due to nondifferential outcome misclassification: observed outcome status (sensitivity = 80% and specificity = 100% for both the new intervention and placebo groups).

Nondifferential outcome misclassification

Misclassification of the outcome is nondifferential if it is similar for those exposed and those unexposed. This type of misclassification either does not affect the estimates of relative effect (if specificity = 100% and sensitivity < 100%), or it introduces a bias towards a relative effect of 1 (if specificity < 100% and sensitivity ≤ 100%).

When specificity = 100%, as in Example 13.10, a lack of sensitivity does not result in a bias in the estimate of the risk ratio or prevented fraction. The estimate of the risk difference is, however, biased.

Example 13.11. Consider again the hypothetical trial described in Table 13.11. Suppose now that all cases of lung cancer were correctly identified (sensitivity = 100%), but that 10% of the subjects without lung cancer in each study group were misclassified as being lung cancer cases (specificity = 90%). The results would now be as shown in Table 13.13.

Table 13.13.
Bias due to nondifferential outcome misclassification: observed outcome status (sensitivity = 100%; specificity = 90% for both the new intervention and placebo groups).

	Intervention		Total
	New	**Placebo**	
Cases	25 + (9 975×0.10) = 1 022	50 + (9 950×0.10) = 1 045	2 067
Non-cases	9 975 × 0.90 = 8 978	9 950 × 0.90 = 8 955	17 933
Total	**10 000**	**10 000**	**20 000**

Observed r_1 = 1022 per 10 000

Observed r_0 = 1045 per 10 000

Observed risk ratio = r_1 / r_0 = 0.98

Observed risk difference = $r_0 - r_1$ = 23 per 10 000

Observed prevented fraction = $(r_0 - r_1) / r_0$ = 23 per 10 000 / 1045 per 10 000 = 0.022 = 2.2%

In Example 13.11, a decline in specificity resulted in a risk ratio close to unity and in marked underestimation of the prevented fraction.

Differential outcome misclassification

Outcome misclassification is *differential* if the misclassification differs between the exposed and unexposed subjects. Differential disease misclassification introduces a bias towards an under- or over-estimation of the true exposure effect.

Differential disease misclassification is introduced if the exposure influences the follow-up and identification of cases. For example, exposed subjects may be more (or less) likely than unexposed subjects to report symptoms of disease or to visit a doctor. Similarly, the staff involved in the follow-up and diagnosis of disease may be influenced by awareness of the exposure status of subjects (*observer bias*). One way of minimizing this type of bias is to keep the observers blind to the exposure status of the individuals. But for certain exposures (e.g. surgical procedures, interventions with typical secondary effects), this is clearly not feasible.

> *Example 13.12.* *A historical cohort study was conducted in England and Wales to examine the relationship between occupational exposure to asbestos and mortality from lung cancer. Information on cause of death was obtained from death certificates supplemented by autopsy reports. A total of 11 lung cancer deaths were observed among asbestos workers compared with only 0.8 expected on the basis of the mortality of men in the general population of England and Wales (SMR (O/E) = 14). However, autopsies among asbestos workers were likely to have been much more frequent than in the general population since asbestosis is an occupational disease for which people are entitled to compensation (Doll, 1955).*

In Example 13.12, the risk of lung cancer among asbestos workers may have been slightly overestimated because the cause of death is likely to have been ascertained more carefully among asbestos workers than among the general population.

13.1.3 How can we identify bias in epidemiological studies?

Bias is a consequence of defects in the design or execution of an epidemiological study. Bias cannot be controlled for in the analysis of a study, and it cannot be eliminated by increasing the sample size, except for those introduced by non-differential misclassification of exposure or outcome. Ways of minimizing bias in different types of epidemiological study were discussed in previous chapters (see Chapters 7–11). Box 13.1 highlights some of the questions that help to identify bias in epidemiological studies.

In addition to identifying potential sources of bias in a particular study, we also need to estimate their most likely direction and magnitude. Some procedures can be introduced deliberately into the study to assess the effect of a potential bias. For instance, in a mortality study, the vital status of people who were lost to follow-up may be ascertained from routine vital statistics registries and their mortality compared with that of the people who did participate in the study. Again, it is essential that the same sort of procedures will be applied to any subject irrespective of his/her exposure or disease status.

13.2 Could the observed effect be due to confounding?

Confounding occurs when an estimate of the association between an exposure and an outcome is mixed up with the real effect of another exposure on the same outcome, the two exposures being correlated.

For example, tobacco smoking may confound estimates of the association between work in a particular occupation and the risk of lung cancer. If death rates for lung cancer in the occupational group are compared with those for the general population (of a similar sex and age composition), it might appear that the occupational group has an

Box 13.1. How to check for bias in epidemiological studies

- Selection bias
    - Was the study population clearly defined?
    - What were the inclusion and exclusion criteria?
    - Were refusals, losses to follow-up, etc. kept to a minimum?

    In cohort and intervention studies:
    - Were the groups similar except for the exposure/intervention status?
    - Was the follow-up adequate? Was it similar for all groups?

    In case–control studies:
    - Did the controls represent the population from which the cases arose?
    - Was the identification and selection of cases and controls influenced by their exposure status?

- Measurement bias
    - Were the exposures and outcomes of interest clearly defined using standard criteria?
    - Were the measurements as objective as possible?
    - Were the subjects and observers blind?
    - Were the observers and interviewers rigorously trained?
    - Were clearly written protocols used to standardize procedures in data collection?
    - Were the study subjects randomized to observers or interviewers?
    - Was information provided by the patient validated against any existing records?
    - Were the methods used for measuring the exposure(s) and outcome(s) of interest (e.g.; questionnaires, laboratory assays) validated?

- Were strategies built into the study design to allow assessment of the likely direction and magnitude of the bias?

increased risk of lung cancer. This might lead to the inference that the occupation is a direct cause of lung cancer. However, without further analysis, this inference would be invalid if those people employed in the occupation smoked more heavily than members of the general population.

For a variable to be a *confounder*, it must be associated with the exposure under study and it must also be an independent risk factor for the disease. In Figure 13.3, confounding occurs only in example I—smoking is associated with the particular occupation under study and it is on its own a risk factor for lung cancer. In example II, alcoholic cirrhosis of the liver is an intermediate factor in the causal path between the exposure (alcohol intake) and the disease (liver cancer). In example III, alcohol intake is associated with the exposure under study (smoking) but is not a risk factor for the disease (lung cancer).

A potential confounder is any factor which is believed to have a real effect on the risk of the disease under investigation. This includes both factors that have a direct causal link with the disease (e.g., smoking and lung cancer), and factors that are good proxy measures of more direct unknown causes (e.g., age and social class).

Confounding can be dealt with at the study design level or, provided the relevant data have been collected, in the analysis. Three approaches may be used to control for confounding in the design of an epidemiological study:

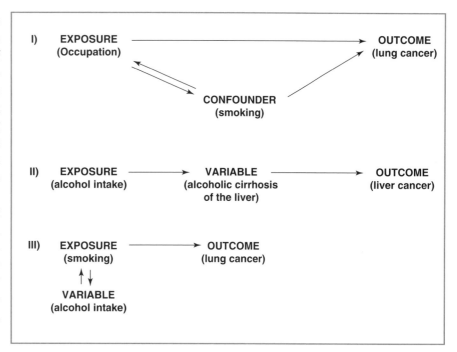

Figure 13.3.
Diagram illustrating the relationship between exposure, outcome and potential confounding variables.

Randomization—this is the ideal method of controlling for confounders because it ensures that the distribution of known and, more importantly, unknown confounding variables will be similar in the groups to be compared, provided that the sample size is relatively large. But this method can be used only in experimental studies.

Restriction—a procedure that limits participation in the study to people who are similar in relation to the confounder. For instance, if participation in a study is restricted to non-smokers, any potential confounding effect of smoking will be removed.

Matching—a procedure whereby controls are selected in such a way that the distribution of potential confounders (e.g., age, sex, race or place of residence) among them will be identical to those of the cases. This can be accomplished by selecting for each case one or more controls with similar characteristics (e.g., of the same age, sex) (individual matching) or by ensuring that as a group the controls have similar characteristics to the cases (frequency matching). In practice, matching is mainly used in case–control studies (see Section 9.3.4.), because it would be too costly to match subjects in large cohort studies and unnecessary to do so in large intervention studies. However, in small intervention studies, particularly in community trials, matching is frequently used (see Section 7.9.2.)

Confounding can also be controlled for in the analysis by using:

> *Stratification*—a technique in which the strength of the association is measured separately within each well defined and homogeneous category (*stratum*) of the confounding variable. For instance, if age is a confounder, the association is estimated separately in each age-group; the results can then be pooled using a suitable weighting to obtain an overall summary measure of the association, which is *adjusted* or *controlled* for the effects of the confounder (that is, that takes into account differences between the groups in the distribution of confounders; see Chapter 14). It should be noted that standardization, a technique mentioned in Chapter 4, is an example of stratification.

> *Statistical modelling*—sophisticated statistical methods, such as regression modelling, are available to control for confounding. They are particularly useful when it is necessary to adjust simultaneously for various confounders. These techniques are briefly introduced in Chapter 14.

It is possible to control for confounders in the analysis only if data on them were collected; the extent to which confounding can be controlled for will depend on the accuracy of these data. For instance, nondifferential (random) misclassification of exposure to a confounder will lead to underestimation of the effect of the confounder and consequently, will attenuate the degree to which confounding can be controlled. The association will persist even after the adjustment because of *residual confounding*. But in contrast to *non-differential misclassification of exposure or outcome, non-differential misclassification of a confounder will cause a bias in either direction*, depending on the direction of the confounding. For example, in a study of risk factors for cervical cancer, the association between cigarette smoking and cervical cancer persisted even after controlling in the analysis for the number of sexual partners. This might be due, at least in part, to residual confounding because 'number of sexual partners' is an inaccurate measure of sexual behaviour, including infection by human papillomavirus.

13.3 Could the observed effect be due to chance?

The assessment of the role of chance in the interpretation of results from epidemiological studies was discussed in Chapter 6. In summary, the role of chance can be assessed by performing appropriate statistical significance tests and by calculating confidence intervals.

A statistical significance test for the effect of an exposure on an outcome yields the probability (P or P-value) that a result as extreme as or more extreme than the one observed could have occurred by chance alone, i.e., if there were no true relationship between the exposure and the outcome.

If this probability is very small, it is usual to declare that chance is an unlikely explanation for the observed association and consequently, that there is a *'statistically significant'* association between exposure and outcome. If the *P*-value is large (usually greater than 0.05), it is conventionally thought that chance cannot be excluded as an explanation for the observed association.

A number of issues should be kept in mind when interpreting results from statistical tests. Firstly, the value of *P* depends both on the magnitude of the association and on the study size. It is therefore possible with small studies to obtain a *P*-value which is not statistically significant, despite the fact that the true population exposure effect is large. Conversely, with a large sample, small effects, which may be clinically and epidemiologically irrelevant, may easily achieve statistical significance. Confidence intervals are more informative than *P*-values because they provide a range of values for the exposure–outcome association, which is likely to include the true population effect (usually with a probability of 0.95, i.e. 95%). They also indicate whether a non-significant result is or is not compatible with a true effect that was not detected because the sample size was too small (see Chapter 6). Sample size calculations should always be done at the design stage to ensure that the study will have enough power (i.e., its sample size will be large enough) to detect the hypothetical effect or enough precision to quantify it (see Chapter 15).

Secondly, investigators tend to collect data on many potential risk factors and to perform multiple statistical tests to determine whether any of these variables is significantly associated with the disease or outcome of interest. However, the probability of obtaining a statistically significant *P*-value just by chance increases with the number of tests performed. It is particularly important to keep this in mind when the data are interpreted, particularly if an unexpected association is found that was not hypothesized at the beginning of the study. Such an unexpected association would have to be reproduced in studies specifically designed to test it before it could be accepted as real.

Finally, statistical methods assess only the effects of sampling variation and cannot control for non-sampling errors such as confounding or bias in the design, conduct or analysis of a study.

13.4 Could the observed effect be causal?

If bias, confounding and chance do not seem to explain an observed association, can we conclude that the association is likely to be causal? Since we can never be sure that the study was not affected by any of these factors, we need to consider the findings in the context of all available evidence. In a paper published in 1965, Bradford Hill mentioned aspects that need to considered when assessing whether an association is likely to be causal (Hill, 1965). We will consider each of these aspects below. As an illustration, we show how these aspects were applied to evaluate the association between smoking and lung cancer.

Temporal relationship

This is an essential aspect. For an exposure to be the cause of a disease, it has to precede its biological onset. This is generally easier to establish from intervention or cohort studies than from cross-sectional or case–control studies in which measurements of the exposure and the outcome are made at the same time.

"The criterion of temporality requires that cigarette smoking antedate the onset of cancer. Support for this criterion is provided by all the major prospective [cohort] studies in which an enormous number of initially disease-free subjects were followed over varying time intervals." (US Surgeon General, 1982)

Biological plausibility

The association is more likely to be causal if consistent with other biological knowledge (e.g., animal experiments, biological mechanisms). However, this aspect should not be taken too seriously, because lack of plausibility may simply reflect lack of scientific knowledge or the fact that human beings are biologically different from animals.

"Benign and malignant tumours have been induced in the larynx of hamsters by long-term exposure to diluted cigarette smoke. Attempts to induce significant numbers of bronchogenic carcinoma [lung cancer] in laboratory animals were negative in spite of major efforts with several species and strains. Neither rats nor hamsters nor baboons inhale cigarette smoke as deeply and as intensely as the cigarette smokers who have provided the data with the consequences of their 'experiment' in the form of clinical evidence gathered by epidemiologists." (US Surgeon General, 1982)

Consistency

If similar results have been found in different populations using different study designs, the association is more likely to be causal, since it is unlikely that all studies were subject to the same type of bias and/or confounding. However, a lack of consistency does not exclude a causal association, since different intensity levels and other conditions may reduce the impact of the exposure in certain studies.

"More than 50 retrospective [case–control] studies have reported smoking patterns (by type and quantity of tobacco smoked, duration of smoking, and inhalational practice) in a variety of subjects with lung cancer (e.g., males and females, different occupational groups, hospitalized patients, autopsy cases, all individuals who died from lung cancer in an area, nationwide sample of individuals who died from lung cancer, and different races and ethnic groups).

Many of these subjects have been compared with matched controls also drawn from a variety of groups (e.g., healthy individuals, patients hospitalized for cancer or other diseases, deaths from cancers of other sites, and samplings of the general population). Regardless of the method, these studies have consistently found an association between smoking and lung cancer. Relative risks for smokers are consistently greater than for nonsmokers. (...)
Eight major prospective [cohort] studies have examined the relationship between smoking and lung cancer mortality in a large number of subjects, in different countries, and in different time periods. The results of these studies (...) are consistent with each other as well as with the retrospective [case–control] studies." (US Surgeon General, 1982)

Strength

The strength of an association is measured by the magnitude of the relative measure of effect. A strong association is not easily explained by potential sources of bias or confounding and hence it is more likely to be causal than is a weak association, which could more easily be the result of confounding or bias. For example, a relative risk of magnitude 10 is more likely to reflect a true causal association than one of 1.5.

"Prospective [cohort] studies have shown that the death rate from lung cancer among cigarette smokers is approximately 10 times the rate in non-smokers (...). To account for such a high relative risk in terms of an indirect association would require that an unknown causal factor be present at least 10 times more frequently among smokers (...) than among non-smokers. Such a confounding factor should be easily detectable, and if it cannot be detected or reasonably inferred, the finding of such a strong association makes a conclusion concerning causality more probable." (US Surgeon General, 1982)

Exposure–response relationship

Further evidence of a causal relationship is provided if increasing levels of exposure are associated with increasing incidence of disease.

"The strongest exposure-relationship measured in most epidemiological studies was for the number of cigarettes smoked per day at the time of entry into the study. However, other important measures of dosage include the age at which smoking began, the duration of smoking, and inhalation practice. (...) The data (...) indicate that as the number of cigarettes smoked per day increases there is a gradient of risk for lung cancer mortality. (...) Male smokers who smoked more than 20 cigarettes daily had lung cancer mortality ratios 15 to 25 times greater than nonsmokers. Similar findings were observed among female smokers (...).

Four prospective [cohort] studies which examined lung cancer mortality by age began smoking (...) show a strong inverse relationship (...), i.e., the younger the age one began smoking, the greater the lung cancer mortality rate." (US Surgeon General, 1982)

Specificity

If a particular exposure increases the risk of a certain disease but not the risk of other diseases, this provides evidence in favour of a cause–effect relationship. However, one-to-one relationships between exposure and disease are rare and lack of specificity should not be used to refute a causal relationship.

"Tobacco smoke is a complex mixture consisting of several thousand chemical substances. These diverse substances are capable of producing more than a single biological response. The specificity of the association between smoking and lung cancer is evidenced by comparison of the magnitude of lung cancer mortality ratios to those of other cancers, as has been done in most of the prospective [cohort] studies. The mortality ratios for lung cancer are very high when compared with those of other cancers." (US Surgeon General, 1982)

Reversibility

When the removal of a possible cause results in a reduced incidence of the disease, the likelihood of the association being causal is strengthened. Ideally, this should be assessed by conducting a randomized intervention trial, but for many exposures–disease associations, such randomized trials are impossible in practice.

"Since cigarette smoking is significantly associated with lung cancer, it is logical to expect that cessation of smoking would lead to a decrease in mortality rates from lung cancer among quitters compared to persons who continue to smoke cigarettes. In fact, all of the major studies which examined cessation showed this decrease in lung cancer risk. (...) After 15 to 20 years, the ex-smoker's risk of dying from lung cancer gradually decreases to a point where it more closely approximates the risk of the non-smoker (...). The magnitude of the residual risk that ex-smokers experience is largely determined by the cumulative exposure to tobacco prior to smoking cessation (i.e., total amount the individual smoked, age when smoking began, and degree of inhalation), and varies with number of years since quitting smoking, as well as with the reasons for quitting smoking (e.g., quitting due to symptoms of disease)." (US Surgeon General, 1982)

Coherence

The putative cause–effect relationship should not seriously conflict with the natural history and biology of the disease.

"The final criterion is the coherence of the association between smoking and lung cancer with known facts in the biology and natural history of lung cancer. Coherence of the association has been noted in the following facts: 1) Sex differences in lung cancer mortality correlate well with sex differences in smoking patterns; 2) Population differences in lung cancer mortality correlate well with differences in tobacco consumption; 3) Time trends in lung cancer mortality correlate with time trends in prevalence of cigarette smoking." (US Surgeon General, 1982)

Although these aspects are often referred to as 'criteria' (as in the report of the US Surgeon General (1982)), They should not be regarded as necessary conditions to established causality. The only exception is temporality—for an exposure to be a cause of a disease it clearly has to precede its biological onset.

13.5 General comments

In epidemiology, it is rare that one study alone will provide enough 'proof' that a certain exposure affects the risk of a particular disease. However, our degree of belief in the association will depend on the type of study design. Ecological studies *per se* can show associations, but because of their great potential for confounding they can never be used to establish causation at an individual level. Well conducted randomized trials are the best tools to assess causality, but their findings should always be interpreted in the context of all other available evidence, including evidence from other areas of research. However, for some exposure–disease relationships, such randomized interventions are not possible or are unethical.

Probability of:	Ecological	Cross-sectional	Case–control	Cohort	Randomized trial
Selection bias					
Selection of subjects	N/A	medium	high	low	low
Loss to follow-up	N/A	N/A	low	high	medium
Recall bias	N/A	high	high	low	low
Confounding	high	medium	medium	low	very low

a Modified from Beaglehole *et al.* (1993)
N/A = Not applicable.

Table 13.14.
Probability of selection bias, recall bias and confounding for the different study designs.*a*

Table 13.14 gives an idea of how much the results from different types of study may be affected by bias and confounding.

Data from various studies that have addressed the same question may be pooled together and *re-analysed* by using special techniques that take into account the fact that the original studies may differ in a large number of respects (e.g., characteristics of the study subjects, methods of data collection). This approach is particularly useful when the effect of the exposure is likely to be small, so that a very large sample size will be necessary to detect and quantify it precisely (as in Example 13.13).

Meta-analysis is another technique used to combine results from various studies. It differs from a *re-analysis* in that there is no access to the raw data from each individual study. Only the published estimates of exposure effect from each study are available and can be used to generate a pooled overall result.

It is essential to ensure that practically all studies (published and unpublished) are included in any re-analysis or meta-analysis. This is because published studies tend to be a biased sample with an overrepresentation of those which showed 'positive' findings.

Example 13.13. A large number of cohort and case–control studies were conducted in recent decades to examine the relationship of oral contraceptive use and breast cancer. Their results were largely inconsistent. To clarify this issue, data from most of these studies were brought together and re-analysed. The 54 studies included in this re-analysis were conducted in 25 countries in Europe, North America, Asia, Australasia, Africa and Latin America. Together they included 53 297 women with invasive breast cancer and 100 239 without breast cancer. Figure 13.4 shows relative risks of breast cancer in ever-users versus never-users of combined oral contraceptives (the most widely used type). The risk estimates varied substantially from study to study, but most confidence intervals were wide and included the null hypothesis value of 1. The pooled estimate was slightly above 1 (1.07) and its confidence interval did not include the null hypothesis value. Current users of combined oral contraceptives or those who stopped less than 10 years previously appeared to have a small increase in the risk of having breast cancer diagnosed relative to never-users, but this excess in risk disappeared 10 or more years after stopping use (Figure 13.5d) (Collaborative Group on Hormonal Factors in Breast Cancer, 1996).

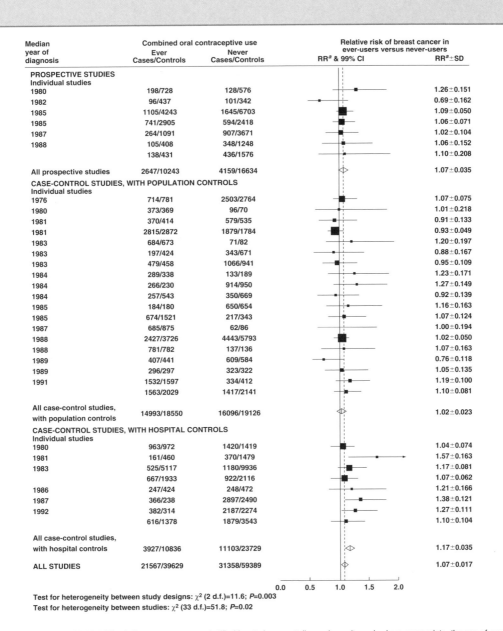

Median year of diagnosis	Combined oral contraceptive use		Relative risk of breast cancer in ever-users versus never-users	
	Ever Cases/Controls	Never Cases/Controls	RR[a] & 99% CI	RR[a] ± SD
PROSPECTIVE STUDIES				
Individual studies				
1980	198/728	128/576		1.26±0.151
1982	96/437	101/342		0.69±0.162
1985	1105/4243	1645/6703		1.09±0.050
1985	741/2905	594/2418		1.06±0.071
1987	264/1091	907/3671		1.02±0.104
1988	105/408	348/1248		1.06±0.152
	138/431	436/1576		1.10±0.208
All prospective studies	2647/10243	4159/16634		1.07±0.035
CASE-CONTROL STUDIES, WITH POPULATION CONTROLS				
Individual studies				
1976	714/781	2503/2764		1.07±0.075
1980	373/369	96/70		1.01±0.218
1981	370/414	579/535		0.91±0.133
1981	2815/2872	1879/1784		0.93±0.049
1983	684/673	71/82		1.20±0.197
1983	197/424	343/671		0.88±0.167
1983	479/458	1066/941		0.95±0.109
1984	289/338	133/189		1.23±0.171
1984	266/230	914/950		1.27±0.149
1984	257/543	350/669		0.92±0.139
1985	184/180	650/654		1.16±0.163
1985	674/1521	217/343		1.07±0.124
1987	685/875	62/86		1.00±0.194
1988	2427/3726	4443/5793		1.02±0.050
1988	781/782	137/136		1.07±0.163
1989	407/441	609/584		0.76±0.118
1989	296/297	323/322		1.05±0.135
1991	1532/1597	334/412		1.19±0.100
	1563/2029	1417/2141		1.10±0.081
All case-control studies, with population controls	14993/18550	16096/19126		1.02±0.023
CASE-CONTROL STUDIES, WITH HOSPITAL CONTROLS				
Individual studies				
1980	963/972	1420/1419		1.04±0.074
1981	161/460	370/1479		1.57±0.163
1983	525/5117	1180/9936		1.17±0.081
	667/1933	922/2116		1.07±0.062
1986	247/424	248/472		1.21±0.166
1987	366/238	2897/2490		1.38±0.121
1992	382/314	2187/2274		1.27±0.111
	616/1378	1879/3543		1.10±0.104
All case-control studies, with hospital controls	3927/10836	11103/23729		1.17±0.035
ALL STUDIES	21567/39629	31358/59389		1.07±0.017

0.0   0.5   1.0   1.5   2.0

Test for heterogeneity between study designs: χ^2 (2 d.f.)=11.6; P=0.003
Test for heterogeneity between studies: χ^2 (33 d.f.)=51.8; P=0.02

a Relative risk (given with 99% CI) relative to never-users, stratified by study, age at diagnosis, parity and, where appropriate, the age of a woman at the birth of her first child and the age when her risk of conception ceased. Separate results are given for individual studies. Each relative risk and its 99% CI is plotted as a black square and a line. The area of the square is proportional to the amount of statistical information (i.e., to the inverse of the variance of the logarithm of the relative risk). Diamonds indicate 99% CI for totals. The solid vertical line represents a relative risk of 1.0 and the broken vertical line indicates the overall relative risk for all studies combined.

Figure 13.4.
Relative risk of breast cancer in ever-users compared with never-users of combined oral contraceptives (reproduced with permission from Collaborative Group on Hormonal Factors in Breast Cancer, 1996, © by The Lancet Ltd, 1996; see this paper for full discussion of the methods and full reference to individual studies).

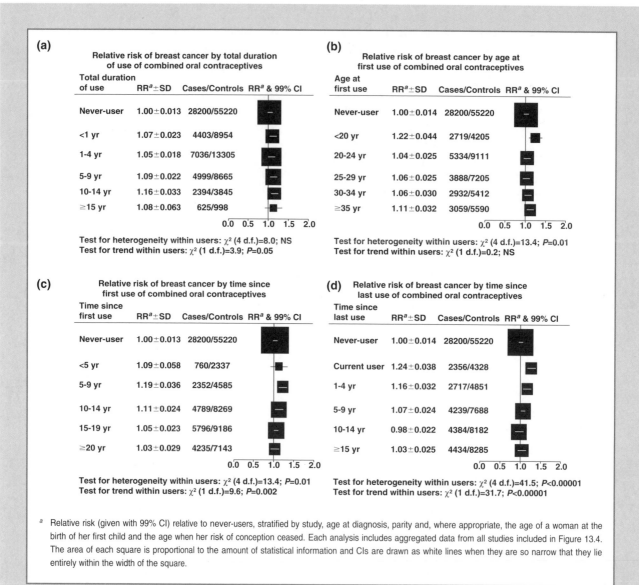

(a)

Relative risk of breast cancer by total duration of use of combined oral contraceptives

Total duration of use	RR[a]±SD	Cases/Controls	RR[a] & 99% CI
Never-user	1.00±0.013	28200/55220	
<1 yr	1.07±0.023	4403/8954	
1-4 yr	1.05±0.018	7036/13305	
5-9 yr	1.09±0.022	4999/8665	
10-14 yr	1.16±0.033	2394/3845	
≥15 yr	1.08±0.063	625/998	

Test for heterogeneity within users: χ^2 (4 d.f.)=8.0; NS
Test for trend within users: χ^2 (1 d.f.)=3.9; P=0.05

(b)

Relative risk of breast cancer by age at first use of combined oral contraceptives

Age at first use	RR[a]±SD	Cases/Controls	RR[a] & 99% CI
Never-user	1.00±0.014	28200/55220	
<20 yr	1.22±0.044	2719/4205	
20-24 yr	1.04±0.025	5334/9111	
25-29 yr	1.06±0.025	3888/7205	
30-34 yr	1.06±0.030	2932/5412	
≥35 yr	1.11±0.032	3059/5590	

Test for heterogeneity within users: χ^2 (4 d.f.)=13.4; P=0.01
Test for trend within users: χ^2 (1 d.f.)=0.2; NS

(c)

Relative risk of breast cancer by time since first use of combined oral contraceptives

Time since first use	RR[a]±SD	Cases/Controls	RR[a] & 99% CI
Never-user	1.00±0.013	28200/55220	
<5 yr	1.09±0.058	760/2337	
5-9 yr	1.19±0.036	2352/4585	
10-14 yr	1.11±0.024	4789/8269	
15-19 yr	1.05±0.023	5796/9186	
≥20 yr	1.03±0.029	4235/7143	

Test for heterogeneity within users: χ^2 (4 d.f.)=13.4; P=0.01
Test for trend within users: χ^2 (1 d.f.)=9.6; P=0.002

(d)

Relative risk of breast cancer by time since last use of combined oral contraceptives

Time since last use	RR[a]±SD	Cases/Controls	RR[a] & 99% CI
Never-user	1.00±0.014	28200/55220	
Current user	1.24±0.038	2356/4328	
1-4 yr	1.16±0.032	2717/4851	
5-9 yr	1.07±0.024	4239/7688	
10-14 yr	0.98±0.022	4384/8182	
≥15 yr	1.03±0.025	4434/8285	

Test for heterogeneity within users: χ^2 (4 d.f.)=41.5; P<0.00001
Test for trend within users: χ^2 (1 d.f.)=31.7; P<0.00001

[a] Relative risk (given with 99% CI) relative to never-users, stratified by study, age at diagnosis, parity and, where appropriate, the age of a woman at the birth of her first child and the age when her risk of conception ceased. Each analysis includes aggregated data from all studies included in Figure 13.4. The area of each square is proportional to the amount of statistical information and CIs are drawn as white lines when they are so narrow that they lie entirely within the width of the square.

Figure 13.5.
Relative risk of breast cancer for various indices of timing of use of combined oral contraceptives (reproduced with permission from Collaborative Group on Hormonal Factors in Breast Cancer, 1996, © by The Lancet Ltd, 1996; see this paper for full discussion of the methods and full reference to individual studies).

Box 13.2. Key issues

• The interpretation of findings from any epidemiological study requires consideration of bias, confounding and chance.

• *Bias* tends to lead to an incorrect estimate of the effect of an exposure on the outcome of interest. There are two main types of bias:

  Selection bias occurs when there is a difference between the characteristics of the people who participated in the study and the characteristics of those who did not. Selection bias can be a major problem in case–control studies, but can also affect cross-sectional studies and, to a lesser extent, cohort studies and randomized trials.

  Measurement bias occurs when measurements or classifications of outcome or exposure are not valid. The consequences of measurement bias depend on the type of measurement error (differential or nondifferential) and on whether it affects the exposure or the outcome.

• *Confounding* occurs when an estimate of the association between an exposure and an outcome is mixed up with the real effect of another exposure on the same outcome, the two exposures being correlated. There are various ways of dealing with confounding at the design stage (randomization, restriction, matching) and in the analysis (stratification and statistical modelling).

• The role of *chance* is assessed by performing statistical tests and, more importantly, calculating confidence intervals.

• Even if bias, confounding and chance do not seem to explain the observed association, we should assess the likelihood of an association being causal by using as guidelines the aspects suggested by Hill (1965).

Further reading

* The aspects that need to be considered when assessing whether a particular exposure–outcome relationship is likely to be causal were presented by Bradford Hill in a paper published in 1965.

Chapter 14
Dealing with confounding in the analysis

In the previous chapter we discussed briefly how confounding could be dealt with at both the design stage of a study and during the analysis of the results. We then mentioned that there are two main statistical procedures that we can use in the analysis: *stratification* and *regression modelling*. In this chapter we will discuss these two approaches in more detail. Obviously, these techniques can be applied only if data on potential confounding factors are available. Thus, potential confounding variables have to be identified at the design stage of the study to ensure that valid information on them is collected.

14.1 Introduction to stratification

A confounding factor is one that is related to both the exposure and the outcome variables and that does not lie on the causal pathway between them (see Section 13.2). Ignoring confounding when assessing the association between an exposure and an outcome variable can lead to an overestimate or underestimate of the true association between exposure and outcome and can even change the direction of the observed effect.

Example 14.1. In a hypothetical case–control study to examine the relationship between smoking and ovarian cancer among nulliparous women, the results shown in Table 14.1 were obtained.

	Smoking		Total
	Yes	**No**	
Ovarian cancer cases	24 (*a*)	36 (*b*)	60 (n_1)
Controls	58 (*c*)	40 (*d*)	98 (n_0)
Total	**82 (m_1)**	**76 (m_0)**	**158 (*N*)**
Crude odds ratio = (24/36) / (58/40)=0.46			
95% confidence interval = 0.23–0.93			
χ^2 = 5.45 on 1d.f.; *P* = 0.02			

Table 14.1.
Results of a case–control study on smoking and ovarian cancer: hypothetical data.

In Example 14.1, women with ovarian cancer had a much lower prevalence of smoking (24/60 = 40%) compared with the controls (58/98 = 59%). This suggests that smoking protects against ovarian cancer (odds ratio (OR) = 0.46). As discussed in the previous chapter, there are several possible explanations for this finding:

(i) *Bias*: the observed odds ratio of 0.46 does not accurately represent the true odds ratio because of either selection or measurement bias.

(ii) *Chance*: the observed association between smoking and ovarian cancer arose by chance. The 95% confidence interval around the observed odds ratio is equal to 0.23–0.93 and the χ^2 test yields $P=0.02$. Thus, chance is an unlikely explanation for the finding.

(iii) *Confounding*: the observed odds ratio of 0.46 is due to the effect of another variable. For example, it may be that women who smoked were different in other respects from non-smokers and less likely to develop ovarian cancer because of this, rather than because of smoking.

(iv) *Causation*: smoking reduces the risk of ovarian cancer and the 95% confidence interval indicates how precisely the sample estimate corresponds to the true effect in the population.

In Example 14.1, it is possible that the association between smoking and ovarian cancer arose because of the confounding effect of other factors such as oral contraceptive use. The results shown in Table 14.1 are for all women combined regardless of their history of oral contraceptive use. To assess whether oral contraceptive use is a confounder, we need to look at the association between smoking and ovarian cancer separately for oral contraceptive users and never-users. This is shown in Table 14.2.

Table 14.2.
Hypothetical case–control study on smoking and ovarian cancer described in Example 14.1: results presented separately for never-users and ever-users of oral contraceptives.

Never-users of oral contraceptives

	Smoking		Total
	Yes	**No**	
Ovarian cancer cases	9 (a_1)	32 (b_1)	41 (n_{11})
Controls	8 (c_1)	28 (d_1)	36 (n_{01})
Total	17 (m_{11})	60 (m_{01})	77 (N_1)

Odds ratio = 0.98 (95% confidence interval = 0.30–3.37)

Ever-users of oral contraceptives

	Smoking		Total
	Yes	**No**	
Ovarian cancer cases	15 (a_2)	4 (b_2)	19 (n_{12})
Controls	50 (c_2)	12 (d_2)	62 (n_{02})
Total	65 (m_{12})	16 (m_{02})	81 (N_2)

Odds ratio = 0.90 (95% confidence interval = 0.23–4.40)

In each category (or *stratum*) of oral contraceptive use, the prevalence of smoking was similar in women with and without ovarian cancer (22% versus 22% among never-users and 79% versus 81% among users). However, when both oral contraceptive users and never-users were combined (Table 14.1), there was a marked difference in the prevalence of smoking between cases and controls (40% versus 59%). Two factors were responsible for this finding:

1. Among the controls, smokers had a much higher prevalence of oral contraceptive use (50/58 = 86%) than non-smokers (12/40 = 30%), that is there was an association between these two variables (Table 14.3).

		Oral contraceptive use		Total
		Ever	Never	
	Yes	50	8	58
Smoking	No	12	28	40
	Total	**62**	**36**	**98**

Table 14.3.
Hypothetical case–control study described in Example 14.1: distribution of controls by smoking habits and oral contraceptive use.

Note that the association between smoking and oral contraceptive use was examined among the controls rather than the cases, or the two groups taken together. This is because controls should represent the population from which the cases were drawn and we need to assess that association in the general population. In a cohort or intervention study, the association would be looked at by constructing a similar table, replacing the number of controls with person-years at risk if the appropriate measure of effect was a rate ratio or numbers of persons at risk at the start of the follow-up if the measure of effect was a risk ratio.

2. Oral contraceptive use is considerably lower among ovarian cancer cases than among controls. The data from Table 14.2 can be rearranged so that smoking is ignored (Table 14.4).

	Oral contraceptive use		Total
	Ever	Never	
Ovarian cancer cases	19	41	60
Controls	62	36	98
Total	**81**	**77**	**158**

Table 14.4.
Hypothetical case–control study described in Example 14.1: distribution of cases and controls by oral contraceptive use.

Only 32% (=19/60) of the women with ovarian cancer were oral contraceptive users, whereas 63% (=62/98) of the controls were users.

Since oral contraceptive use in these data was associated with *both* the exposure (smoking) and the outcome of interest (ovarian cancer), it acted as a confounding factor. As a result, when the data for both users and never-users were combined, the result suggested an association between smoking and ovarian cancer far stronger than really existed (*positive confounding*). In other situations (as in Example 14.2 ; see next section), combining strata in the presence of a confounder may mask an effect that really exists (*negative confounding*), or even show an effect in the opposite direction to the true one.

14.2 The Mantel–Haenszel summary measures of effect

When we analyse the results of a study to look for evidence of a particular exposure–outcome association, we usually start by including in the analysis all the subjects in our study sample. This analysis provides a crude estimate of the effect of the exposure on the outcome of interest. The next logical step is to divide our study sample into several subgroups or strata, defined by a potential confounding variable, to see if the results are consistent across the strata. This approach is very informative, as it describes how the effect of the exposure on the outcome of interest varies across subgroups of subjects with different characteristics. We can simply report the stratum-specific effect estimates and their confidence intervals. Each of these stratum-specific estimates is supposed to be homogeneous in relation to the potential confounding variable and therefore they are unconfounded.

Usually, however, we are not much interested in the stratum-specific results *per se* and would rather have a single overall estimate. In other words, we would like to be able to calculate a summary effect estimate which, in contrast to the *crude* estimate, would take into account the confounding effect of the stratifying variable. Such *adjusted* estimates can be calculated by *pooling* results across strata. But even if the true effect is the same in all strata, we would expect our estimates to differ because of random variation. Pooling takes this into account by giving greater weight to effect estimates from larger strata. It involves calculating a *weighted average* of the individual stratum-specific estimates by choosing a set of weights that maximizes the statistical precision of the adjusted effect estimate. There are several alternative weighting procedures which achieve precise summary effect estimates. In this section, we concentrate on a procedure derived by Mantel and Haenszel which is widely used and relatively simple to apply.

14.2.1 Mantel–Haenszel odds ratio

Let us consider again Example 14.1. Since oral contraceptive use is a confounder of the relationship between smoking and ovarian cancer, we should not combine the data from ever-users and never-users for the analysis. Thus, the crude odds ratio of 0.46 obtained from Table 14.1 is not appropriate. We could just calculate separate odds ratios and their 95% confidence intervals for each group of oral contraceptive users, as shown in Table 14.2. But we would like to be able to summarize the overall results of the study in a way that removes the confounding effect of oral contraceptive use. The Mantel–Haenszel odds ratio, denoted OR_{MH}, gives a *weighted average of the odds ratios in the different strata*, where those from larger strata are given more weight.

To calculate the OR_{MH}, we start by constructing 2×2 tables of exposure by outcome for the separate strata of the confounder, as illustrated in Table 14.2. The OR_{MH} can then be obtained by applying the following formula:

$$OR_{MH} = \frac{a_1 d_1 / N_1 + a_2 d_2 / N_2}{b_1 c_1 / N_1 + b_2 c_2 / N_2}$$

If we apply this formula to the data from our ovarian cancer case–control study (Table 14.2), we obtain

$$OR_{MH} = \frac{(9 \times 28)/77 + (15 \times 12)/81}{(32 \times 8)/77 + (4 \times 50)/81} = \frac{5.49}{5.79} = 0.95$$

Thus, the *odds ratio for smoking adjusted for oral contraceptive use* is 0.95. This adjusted odds ratio contrasts with the *crude odds ratio* of 0.46 obtained from Table 14.1. Adjusting for oral contraceptive use gives an odds ratio much closer to unity, which means that the protection afforded by smoking, if any, is far less strong than the initial result led us to think.

The above formula can easily be extended to more than two strata, by summing both the numerator and the denominator over all strata:

$$OR_{MH} = \frac{\Sigma a_i d_i / N_i}{\Sigma b_i c_i / N_i}$$

In this formula, Σ means sum and the subscript i stands for the subscripts 1, 2, 3, ..., which represent each of the strata.

We can calculate a confidence interval around the OR_{MH} and a Mantel–Haenszel χ^2 test by using the formulae given in Section A14.1.1. In our ovarian cancer example, the 95% confidence interval is 0.42–2.16. The χ^2 is equal to 0.016 with one degree of freedom, which corresponds to $P = 0.93$. Thus, after adjusting for oral contraceptive use, the effect of smoking on ovarian cancer is no longer 'statistically significant'.

14.2.2 Mantel–Haenszel risk ratio

The Mantel–Haenszel method can also be used to obtain an *adjusted risk ratio*. In Example 14.2, the crude analysis shows that workers exposed to the particular chemical substance had a 52% higher risk of developing lung cancer than those not exposed (Table 14.5). Before concluding that the chemical substance is associated with an increased risk of lung cancer, we need to exclude the possibility that smoking, rather than the occupational exposure, is the explanation for the observed association. To do this, we need to examine the data separately for smokers and non-smokers.

Table 14.6 shows that the stratum-specific risk ratios are higher than the crude risk ratio (2.0 versus 1.52). This is an example of *negative confounding*. It arose because the prevalence of smoking, an important risk factor for lung cancer, was much lower among workers exposed to the chemical substance (4000/84 000=5%) than among those not exposed (16 000/96 000=17%) (Table 14.7).

Example 14.2. *Suppose that a cohort study was set up to investigate whether occupational exposure to a particular chemical substance was associated with an increased risk of lung cancer. All study subjects were followed up for five years after entry into the study (or until diagnosis of lung cancer if earlier). The results of this study are shown in Table 14.5.*

Table 14.5.
Results from a cohort study on occupational exposure to a particular chemical substance and lung cancer: hypothetical data.

		Exposure to chemical substance		Total
		Yes	No	
Lung cancer	Yes	480 (a)	360 (b)	840 (n_1)
	No	83 520 (c)	95 640 (d)	179 160 (n_0)
	Total	84 000 (m_1)	96 000 (m_0)	180 000 (N)

Crude risk ratio = (480/84 000)/(360/96 000) = 5.71 per 1000/3.75 per 1000 = 1.52
95% confidence interval = 1.33–1.75
χ^2 = 37.21 on 1 d.f.; $P < 0.0001$

Table 14.6.
Hypothetical cohort study on occupational exposure to a particular chemical substance and lung cancer described in Example 14.2: results presented separately for smokers and non-smokers.

Smokers

		Exposure to chemical substance		Total
		Yes	No	
Lung cancer	Yes	80 (a_1)	160 (b_1)	240 (n_{11})
	No	3920 (c_1)	15 840 (d_1)	19 760 (n_{01})
	Total	4000 (m_{11})	16 000 (m_{01})	20 000 (N_1)

Risk ratio = (80/4000)/(160/16 000) = 20 per 1000 / 10 per 1000 = 2.0
95% confidence interval = 1.53–2.61

Non-smokers

		Exposure to chemical substance		Total
		Yes	No	
Lung cancer	Yes	400 (a_2)	200 (b_2)	600 (n_{12})
	No	79 600 (c_2)	79 800 (d_2)	159 400 (n_{02})
	Total	80 000 (m_{12})	80 000 (m_{02})	160 000 (N_2)

Risk ratio = (400/80 000)/(200/80 000) = 5.0 per 1000 / 2.5 per 1000 = 2.0
95% confidence interval = 1.69–2.37

Table 14.7.
Hypothetical cohort study described in Example 14.2: distribution of study subjects by occupational exposure and smoking habits.

		Exposure to chemical substance		Total
		Yes	No	
Smoking	Yes	4000	16 000	20 000
	No	80 000	80 000	160 000
	Total	84 000	96 000	180 000

We can obtain a Mantel–Haenszel summary estimate of the common risk ratio (R_{MH}) by applying the following formula to our data

$$R_{MH} = \frac{\Sigma a_i m_{0i}/N_i}{\Sigma b_i m_{1i}/N_i}$$

Thus,

$$R_{MH} = \frac{(80 \times 16\ 000)/20\ 000 + (400 \times 80\ 000)/160\ 000}{(160 \times 4\ 000)/20\ 000 + (200 \times 80\ 000)/160\ 000} = \frac{264}{132} = 2.0$$

The calculation of confidence intervals around R_{MH} and of the Mantel-Haenszel χ^2 is presented in Section A14.1.2. In our example, the 95% confidence interval is 1.73 to 2.30. The χ^2 is equal to 92.99 with one degree of freedom, which gives $P < 0.0001$. Thus, there is strong evidence that the occupational exposure was associated with an increased risk of lung cancer and this effect was even stronger when differences in smoking habits between exposed and unexposed workers were taken into account.

14.2.3 Mantel–Haenszel rate ratio

The Mantel–Haenszel method can also be applied when the appropriate measure of effect is the rate ratio rather than the risk ratio. It gives an *adjusted rate ratio* (denoted RR_{MH}) by calculating a weighted average of the rate ratios in the different strata.

Example 14.3. Suppose that a cohort of healthy women aged 45–50 years was followed up to examine risk factors for various female cancers. At the time of entry into the study, the women completed a questionnaire on sociodemographic variables and gynaecological and reproductive history. A total of 1141 cervical cancer cases occurred during the follow-up period. The relationship between cervical cancer and having ever had a Pap smear test (as reported in the initial questionnaire) is shown in Table 14.8.

	Pap smear		Total
	Ever	Never	
Cases	17 (a)	1124 (b)	1141 (n)
Person-years at risk	71 184 (y_1)	1 518 701 (y_0)	1 589 885 (y)
Rate per 100 000 pyrs	23.9 (r_1)	74.0 (r_0)	71.8 (r)

Crude rate ratio = (17/71 184)/(1 124/1 518 701) = 0.32
95% confidence interval = 0.20 – 0.52
χ^2 = 23.69 on 1d.f.; $P < 0.001$

Table 14.8.
Results from a cohort study on Pap smear testing and cervical cancer: hypothetical data.

In Example 14.3, the crude rate ratio and its confidence interval are consistent with a decrease in the incidence of cervical cancer among women who reported in the initial questionnaire having ever had a Pap smear test. Other studies have shown that there is a socioeconomic gradient in the incidence of cervical cancer, with women from poor socioeconomic backgrounds being at higher risk. Thus, socioeconomic factors might have confounded the association between Pap smear testing and cervical cancer if, for instance, women from a high social background were more likely to visit their doctors and had a Pap smear as part of their regular medical examination. To clarify this issue, we need to examine the relationship between Pap smear testing and cervical cancer separately for women from different socioeconomic backgrounds. This is shown in Table 14.9, where a woman's educational level is used as a marker of socioeconomic status.

Table 14.9.
Hypothetical cohort study on Pap smear testing and cervical cancer described in Example 14.3: results stratified by women's educational level.

High educational level

	Pap smear		Total
	Ever	Never	
Cases	13 (a_1)	697 (b_1)	710 (n_1)
Person-years at risk	38 346 (y_{11})	828 149 (y_{01})	866 495 (y_1)
Rate per 100 000 pyrs	33.9 (r_{11})	84.2 (r_{01})	81.9 (r_1)

Rate ratio = 0.40; 95% confidence interval = 0.23–0.69

Low educational level

	Pap smear		Total
	Ever	Never	
Cases	4 (a_2)	427 (b_2)	431 (n_2)
Person-years at risk	32 838 (y_{12})	690 552 (y_{02})	723 390 (y_2)
Rate per 100 000 pyrs	12.2 (r_{12})	61.8 (r_{02})	59.6 (r_2)

Rate ratio = 0.20; 95% confidence interval = 0.08–0.54

The formula for the Mantel–Haenszel summary estimate of the common rate ratio is

$$\text{RR}_{\text{MH}} = \frac{\Sigma a_i y_{0i}/y_i}{\Sigma b_i y_{1i}/y_i}$$

Thus, in our example,

$$\text{RR}_{\text{MH}} = \frac{(13 \times 828\ 149)/866\ 495 + (4 \times 690\ 552)/723\ 390}{(697 \times 38\ 346)/866\ 495 + (427 \times 32\ 838)/723\ 390} = \frac{16.24}{50.23} = 0.32$$

Thus, educational level was not a confounder of the effect of Pap smear on cervical cancer in these data, since the crude and the adjusted rate ratios have exactly the same value (0.32).

By applying the formulae given in the Appendix (see Section A14.1.3), we obtain a Mantel–Haenszel χ^2 of 23.73 with one degree of freedom, corresponding to $P < 0.001$. The 95% confidence interval is 0.20 to 0.52. Thus, chance is an unlikely explanation of this finding.

Note that the Mantel–Haenszel method of controlling for confounding is similar to the method of standardization used to calculate age-adjusted rates in Chapter 4. Both these methods are referred to as *stratified analyses*, because we look at an exposure by a response for the different *strata* (levels) of a confounder. They differ, however, in the set of weights used to calculate the weighted average of the rate ratios in the different strata (see Section 4.3.3).

14.3 How to identify confounders

In order to be able to examine the effect of potential confounding variables in an analysis, we need to identify them at the design stage of the study. This should be done by taking into account findings from previous epidemiological studies and what is known about the possible etiological mechanisms of the disease under study. Age and gender are obvious potential confounders in practically all studies. Smoking will also be a potential confounder in any study examining the relationship between a particular exposure and lung cancer. It would be necessary to exclude the possibility that smoking rather than the exposure under study is responsible for any association that may be found. Potential confounding variables should also include factors such as socioeconomic status or place of residence, which are just proxy measures of more direct but unknown causes of disease.

Not all factors suspected of being potential confounding factors will actually lead to confounding of the exposure–outcome relationship in a particular study. But how do we know if a particular variable really is a confounder? We defined a confounder as a factor that is associated with both exposure and disease (and is not on the causal pathway). However, this may be difficult to assess in practice. For instance, with a large sample, small but statistically significant associations could be found between the confounder and the exposure, and between the confounder and the disease; however, they may not be strong enough to lead to confounding. Thus, the presence of or absence of confounding should not be assessed by using a statistical test of significance. The magnitude of confounding in any study should be evaluated by observing the degree of discrepancy between the crude and adjusted estimates. If there is no difference between these two estimates, the observed exposure–outcome effect was not confounded by the potential confounding variable. A large difference, as seen in Example 14.1, indicates the presence of confounding and implies that the *adjusted* summary measure is a better estimate of the effect of the exposure on the outcome of interest than the *crude* summary measure, since it removes the effect of the confounder.

Two other aspects of stratification should be noted. First, factors that are on the causal pathway between an exposure and a disease should not be regarded as confounding the association between the exposure and the outcome. Controlling for a factor that is on the causal pathway leads to underestimation of the strength of the effect of the exposure on the outcome under study. Occasionally, a variable that lies on the causal pathway may be adjusted for in the analysis if we want to assess whether the effect of the exposure on the outcome under study is entirely mediated through that intermediate variable or whether there may be other independent biological mechanisms. For instance, if we believe that human papillomavirus infection is on the causal pathway between number of sexual partners and cervical cancer, the association with number of sexual partners should disappear after adjusting for HPV infection. If the effect does not disappear completely, it would suggest that the effect of number of sexual partners on cervical cancer may be mediated through other biological mechanisms not directly related to HPV infection. In practice, this reasoning may not be so straightforward because of errors in the measurement of the intermediate variable.

Secondly, it is important to note that stratification assumes that each stratum is homogeneous in relation to the confounding variable. This assumption depends on both the validity of the data on the confounding variable (see Section 13.2) and the way strata are defined. For instance, if we control for age through stratification, this is better achieved if the strata are relatively narrow. Stratification into very broad age groups (e.g., 0–45 and 46+ years) is unlikely to be fully effective since, within each stratum, there are likely to be substantial differences in the age distribution of cases and controls (in a case–control study) or exposed and unexposed (in a cohort or intervention study).

14.4 Confounding and interaction

An underlying assumption in the calculation of a summary effect estimate is that the true effect is the same across strata and that any departures from this uniform effect are assumed to be due to random sampling variation. If there is substantial variation between the stratum-specific estimates of effect, this indicates the presence of *interaction* (also called *effect modification*) between the exposure of interest and the so-called confounding factor.

If there is interaction between the exposures under study and the confounder, a Mantel–Haenszel summary estimate of effect will be misleading, as it does not convey the full form of the exposure–outcome association, that is, that it varies according to the level of the stratifying variable. Thus, only if we are satisfied that the stratum-specific effect measures do not vary between themselves (i.e., there is no interaction), should we calculate an adjusted summary estimate of effect by taking a weighted mean of stratum-specific estimates. This concept is

Example 14.4. *Suppose we are interested in examining the relationship between an exposure A and a certain outcome B in a cohort study. We start by calculating the crude rate ratio, which gives a value of 2.0. We then decide to examine the relationship between A and B separately for those who were exposed to a third variable C (stratum 1) and those who were not (stratum 2). Table 14.10 shows three possible results of this study and how they should be interpreted. In situation I, there is no confounding, because the crude and adjusted rate ratios are similar, and no interaction, because the rate ratios are similar for both strata. In situation II, there is confounding, because the crude and the adjusted rate ratios differ, but no interaction, because the effect is similar in the two strata. In situation III, there is strong interaction between A and C because the stratum-specific rate ratios are markedly different for those exposed and those not exposed to C.*

	Crude rate ratio	Rate ratio in stratum 1	Rate ratio in stratum 2	Adjusted rate ratio	
Situation I	2.0	2.0	2.0	2.0	No confounding No interaction
Situation II	2.0	3.0	3.0	3.0	Confounding present No interaction
Situation III	2.0	4.0	0.5	–	Strong interaction

Table 14.10.
Example of confounding and interaction.

not new. We discussed it briefly in Section 4.3.3 when we mentioned that age-standardized rates were an appropriate summary of the data only if the effect was homogeneous across the age-strata.

The first step in any stratified analysis is to assess whether interaction is present (Example 14.4). In most circumstances, this decision should be based on visual inspection of the data to examine the observed patterns of variation in the stratum-specific estimates. If they are the same, there is no interaction. In this situation, however, confounding may occur if the stratum-specific effects differ from the crude effect. If the stratum-specific estimates differ from each other, interaction is present and the emphasis in the analysis should be on describing how the association of interest is modified by the stratifying factor and all stratum-specific estimates of effect, and their confidence intervals, should be reported separately.

Deciding whether interaction exists or not in any particular analysis is often difficult, since the stratum-specific estimates are likely to vary because of random variation, even if the true effect is similar. For instance, the effect of Pap smear testing on cervical cancer in Example 14.3 was more marked for women of low educational level (RR = 0.20; 95% CI = 0.08–0.54) than for women of high educational level (RR = 0.40; 95% CI = 0.23–0.69), suggesting a weak interaction between Pap smear and educational level. However, this difference between the stratum-specific rate ratios may just reflect random variation. A variety of χ^2 tests of heterogeneity are available to test the null hypothesis that the degree of variability in the series of stratum-specific estimates is consistent with random variation. In practice, however, these tests are not very powerful. Epidemiological studies, unless they are specifically designed to do this, rarely have enough statistical power to detect interactions (see Section 15.4.4). Thus, more is usually gained by visual inspection of the size and pattern of the effect estimates across strata than from tests for interaction (effect modification).

14.5 Using the Mantel–Haenszel method to adjust for several confounders

In practice, it is frequently necessary to examine and possibly adjust for several confounders. This can be achieved by using the Mantel–Haenszel method, although, as the number of confounders increases, this method becomes impractical because most strata will have very sparse data. As we shall see later in this chapter, regression modelling techniques are more efficient methods in these circumstances.

Example 14.5. Assume that a case–control study was carried out to examine risk factors for human papillomavirus (HPV) infection of the cervix uteri. A standard questionnaire was used to collect detailed information on sociodemographic variables and sexual behaviour from 188 HPV-positive female cases and 571 HPV-negative female controls. Table 14.11 shows the distribution of cases and controls by smoking and HPV infection.

Table 14.11.
Results from a case-control study on smoking and HPV infection: hypothetical data.

	Smoking		Total
	Yes	**No**	
HPV-positive	42 (a)	146 (b)	188 (n_1)
HPV-negative	90 (c)	481 (d)	571 (n_0)
Total	**132 (m_1)**	**627 (m_0)**	**759 (N)**

Crude odds ratio = (42/146) / (90/481) = 1.54

95% confidence interval = 1.02–2.32

$\chi^2 = 4.25$ on 1d.f.; $P = 0.039$

In Example 14.5, the *crude odds ratio* is 1.54. The 95% confidence interval and the *P*-value suggest that chance is an unlikely explanation of this finding. Thus, women who smoked were more likely to be HPV-positive than those who did not.

Number of sexual partners is a well known risk factor for HPV infection and it may have confounded the association between smoking and HPV infection. Table 14.12 shows the association found between smoking and HPV stratified by reported number of lifetime sexual partners (categorized as < 2 partners and ≥ 2 partners).

Examination of the stratum-specific odds ratios (and their confidence intervals) suggests that the effect of smoking on HPV infection in women who reported less than two sexual partners is similar to the

< 2 sexual partners

	Smoking		Total
	Yes	No	
HPV-positive	31 (a_1)	124 (b_1)	155 (n_{11})
HPV-negative	78 (c_1)	437 (d_1)	515 (n_{01})
Total	109 (m_{11})	561 (m_{01})	670 (N_1)

Odds ratio = 1.40

95% confidence interval = 0.88–2.22

≥ 2 sexual partners

	Smoking		Total
	Yes	No	
HPV-positive	11 (a_2)	22 (b_2)	33 (n_{12})
HPV-negative	12 (c_2)	44 (d_2)	56 (n_{02})
Total	23 (m_{12})	66 (m_{02})	89 (N_2)

Odds ratio = 1.83

95% confidence interval = 0.70–4.80

χ^2 test for heterogeneity = 0.24 on 1 d.f.; P = 0.63

$$OR_{MH} = \frac{\Sigma a_i d_i / N_i}{\Sigma b_i c_i / N_i} \quad \frac{(31 \times 437)/670 + (11 \times 44)/89}{(124 \times 78)/670 + (22 \times 12)/89} = \frac{25.66}{17.40} = 1.47$$

95% confidence interval = 0.95–2.26

χ^2 = 2.97 on 1 d.f.; P = 0.09

Table 14.12.
Hypothetical case–control study on smoking and HPV infection described in Example 14.5: results stratified by number of lifetime sexual partners.

effect in those who reported two or more. This is confirmed by the χ^2 test for heterogeneity. Since the effect of smoking on HPV infection is uniform across the two strata, it is appropriate to calculate a pooled adjusted odds ratio. Thus, after adjusting for number of sexual partners, the odds ratio of smoking is reduced a little from 1.54 to 1.47. This result suggests that this variable was a weak confounder of the association between smoking and HPV infection. But even after adjusting for number of sexual partners, the 95% confidence interval is still consistent with an effect of smoking on HPV infection. Thus, these results suggest that smoking increased the risk of HPV infection, but this risk was marginally weaker after allowing for the confounding effect of number of sexual partners.

The same technique can be used to obtain an odds ratio adjusted for age. In this hypothetical study, age (in years) was categorized into six groups (< 20, 20–24, 25–29, 30–34, 35–44, ≥ 45). Thus, we need to construct six 2 × 2 tables of smoking and HPV infection, one for each age-group. The cells of these 2 × 2 tables are shown in Table 14.13.

The OR_{MH} adjusted for age is slightly lower than the crude odds ratio (1.47 versus 1.54), suggesting that age was also a weak confounder of the association between smoking and HPV infection.

Table 14.13.
Hypothetical case–control study on smoking and HPV infection described in Example 14.5: results stratified by age-group.

Stratum	Age (years)	a_i	b_i	c_i	d_i	N_i	$a_i d_i/N_i$	$b_i c_i/N_i$
1	<20	3	10	16	79	108	2.19	1.48
2	20–24	13	44	16	92	165	7.25	4.27
3	25–29	6	33	22	62	123	3.02	5.90
4	30–34	8	25	10	75	118	5.08	2.12
5	35–44	8	22	18	89	137	5.20	2.89
6	≥45	4	12	8	84	108	3.11	0.89
All strata		42	146	90	481	759	25.85	17.55

χ^2 test for heterogeneity = 7.37 on 5 d.f.; $P = 0.20$

$$OR_{MH} = \frac{\Sigma a_i d_i/N_i}{\Sigma b_i c_i/N_i} = \frac{25.85}{17.55} = 1.47$$

95% confidence interval = 0.96–2.32
$\chi^2 = 3.06$ on 1d.f.; $P = 0.08$

Thus, so far, we have estimated the effect of smoking on HPV infection adjusted for number of sexual partners and the effect of smoking adjusted for age. We could estimate the effect of smoking on HPV infection adjusted *simultaneously* for number of partners and age using the Mantel–Haenzsel method. To do this, we need to construct a 2×2 table of smoking by HPV infection for every possible combination of number of partners and age-group. Since number of partners forms two strata (<2 and ≥2) and age forms six strata (< 20, 20–24, 25–29, 30–34, 35–44, ≥ 45), we need to construct $2 \times 6 = 12$ such 2×2 tables. The cells of the 2×2 tables for smoking for these 12 strata are shown in Table 14.14. Thus, after adjusting for the confounding effects of number of partners and age, the effect of smoking on HPV infection is even smaller ($OR_{MH} = 1.41$).

The Mantel–Haenszel method can be extended to adjust simultaneously for more than two confounders. For example, to estimate the effect of smoking on HPV infection, allowing for number of sexual partners (two strata), age (six strata), marital status (three strata: married, single, widowed/divorced) and educational level (three strata), we would construct $2\times6\times3\times3=108$ 2×2 tables. Clearly, in 108 tables formed from a data-set of 188 cases and 571 controls, some strata will have very small numbers of observations, if any.

A further problem with the Mantel–Haenszel method is that each explanatory variable included in the analysis has to be classified as either an exposure or a confounder, and there may be only one exposure. For example, smoking was our exposure, and number of partners and age were our confounders. We therefore obtained an odds ratio for smoking adjusted for number of partners and age. These results did not give us the odds ratio for number of partners adjusted for smoking and age, or the odds ratios for age adjusted for smoking and number of partners. These would have required further Mantel–Haenszel analyses.

Stratum	Age (yrs)	Number of partners	a_i	b_i	c_i	d_i	N_i	a_id_i/N_i	b_ic_i/N_i
1	<20	<2	2	8	11	67	88	1.52	1.00
2	20–24	<2	10	36	14	85	145	5.86	3.48
3	25–29	<2	3	28	19	59	109	1.62	4.88
4	30–34	<2	5	21	10	65	101	3.22	2.08
5	35–44	<2	7	19	17	78	121	4.51	2.67
6	≥45	<2	4	12	7	83	106	3.13	0.79
7	<20	≥2	1	2	5	12	20	0.60	0.50
8	20–24	≥2	3	8	2	7	20	1.05	0.80
9	25–29	≥2	3	5	3	3	14	0.64	1.07
10	30–34	≥2	3	4	0	10	17	1.76	0.00
11	35–44	≥2	1	3	1	11	16	0.69	0.19
12	≥45	≥2	0	0	1	1	2	0.00	0.00
All strata			42	146	90	481	759	24.60	17.46

χ^2 test for heterogeneity = 12.44 on 10 d.f.; $P = 0.26$

$$OR_{MH} = \frac{\Sigma a_id_i/N_i}{\Sigma b_ic_i/N_i} = \frac{24.60}{17.46} = 1.41$$

95% confidence interval = 0.91–2.24
$\chi^2 = 2.62$ on 1 d.f.; $P = 0.132$

Table 14.14.
Hypothetical case–control study on smoking and HPV infection described in Example 14.5: results stratified by age and lifetime number of sexual partners.

14.6 Using regression modelling to adjust for the effect of confounders

Regression models summarize the relationship between an outcome (also called dependent) variable and several explanatory (independent) variables as a mathematical equation. The general form of this equation is

Outcome variable = function (explanatory variables)

There are many types of regression model. The choice of any particular model depends on the characteristics of the outcome variable (i.e., continuous or categorical) and on the way it is mathematically related to the explanatory variables. The simplest mathematical model we could use has already been introduced in Section 11.2.1 to describe the relationship between two quantitative variables.

A discussion of these models and the assumptions underlying them is beyond the scope of this chapter. However, these modelling techniques are commonly used in epidemiological studies and, therefore, in the rest of this chapter we will try to illustrate how these techniques relate to the Mantel–Haenszel method, to allow the reader to understand and interpret results from published work where they have been used.

Let us consider again the hypothetical case–control study described in Example 14.5. We can use a particular regression technique, called *logistic regression*, to analyse data from unmatched case–control studies. In this analysis, we start by using a logistic regression model which includes as explanatory variables only the exposure under study–smoking. The results are shown in Table 14.15 (model 1). The odds ratio estimated by this logistic regression model is the same as the crude odds ratio we obtained in Table 14.11.

Table 14.15.
Hypothetical case–control study on risk factors for HPV cervical infection described in Example 14.5. Results obtained from logistic regression models which included an increasing number of explanatory variables: smoking, lifetime number of sexual partners and age. (The values underlined correspond to those obtained earlier with the Mantel–Haenszel technique shown in Table 14.11, 14.12 and 14.14.)

Variable	Odds ratio	95% confidence interval
Model 1		
smoking[a]	<u>1.54</u>	1.02–2.32
Model 2		
smoking[a]	<u>1.47</u>	0.97–2.23
partners[b]	1.90	1.19–3.03
Model 3		
smoking[a]	<u>1.43</u>	0.93–2.19
partners[b]	1.95	1.19–3.17
age 2[c]	4.14	2.12–8.12
age 3	3.58	1.77–7.24
age 4	3.01	1.47–6.15
age 5	2.18	1.07–4.46
age 6	1.49	0.67–3.33

[a] Categorized as 'non-smokers' (baseline) and 'smokers'.

[b] Categorized as '< 2 partners' (baseline) and '≥ 2 partners'

[c] Categorized as age1 = <20 (baseline); age2 = 20–24; age3 = 25–29; age4 = 30–34; age5 = 35–44; age6 = 45+ years.

We then move on to use a model which includes both smoking and number of sexual partners as explanatory variables (model 2 in Table 14.15). This model gives

Odds ratio for smoking versus non-smoking adjusted for number of sexual partners = 1.47 (95% CI = 0.97–2.23)

Thus, after adjusting for number of sexual partners, the effect of smoking on HPV infection became smaller (1.47 versus 1.54). This result is similar to that obtained earlier when we used the Mantel–Haenszel technique to control for the effect of number of sexual partners (Table 14.12). But in contrast to this technique, this regression model also gives us the odds ratio for number of sexual partners adjusted for smoking:

Odds ratio for ≥2 sexual partners versus <2, adjusted for smoking = 1.90 (95% CI = 1.19–3.03)

Thus, there is a statistically significant increased risk of HPV infection associated with two or more sexual partners, even after taking differences in smoking into account.

We can use a more complex model which includes smoking, number of sexual partners and age (model 3, Table 14.15). This model gives us an estimate of the effect of smoking on HPV infection adjusted for number of sexual partners and age of 1.43 (95% CI = 0.93–2.19), which is similar to that obtained before with the Mantel–Haenszel method (OR_{MH} = 1.41; 95% CI = 0.91–2.24) (see Table 14.14). However, unlike the Mantel–Haenszel analysis, the logistic regression analysis also gives the following extra odds ratios:

Odds ratio for ≥ 2 sexual partners versus < 2, adjusted for smoking and age = 1.95 (95% CI = 1.19–3.17)

Odds ratio for age 20–24 versus age <20, adjusted for smoking and partners = 4.14 (95% CI = 2.12–8.12)

Odds ratio for age 25–29 versus age <20, adjusted for smoking and partners = 3.58 (95% CI = 1.77–7.24)

Odds ratio for age 30–34 versus age <20, adjusted for smoking and partners = 3.01 (95% CI = 1.47–6.15)

Odds ratio for age 35–44 versus age <20, adjusted for smoking and partners = 2.18 (95% CI = 1.07–4.46)

Odds ratio for age 45+ versus age <20, adjusted for smoking and partners = 1.49 (95% CI = 0.67–3.33)

One of the main advantages of regression modelling is that it does not require us to define which explanatory variable is the exposure and which ones are the potential confounders, since all explanatory variables are treated in the same way. This is particularly important in studies designed to examine the effect of a wide range of exposures rather than just the effect of a specific one.

Similar regression models can be applied to data from studies of other designs. Let us consider again the hypothetical cohort study on Pap smear use and cervical cancer described in Example 14.3 (Section 14.2.3). In Table 14.8, we calculated the crude rate ratio to measure the effect of Pap smear testing on cervical cancer. We then went on to calculate the effect of Pap smear adjusting for educational level (Table 14.9) using the Mantel–Haenszel technique. We can also use the Mantel–Haenszel technique to adjust simultaneously for educational level, marital status and age at first intercourse. The results are shown in Table 14.16.

Using the Mantel–Haenszel technique to adjust simultaneously for educational level, marital status and age at first intercourse involved the formation of 18 (=2×3×3) strata. However, only seventeen cervical cancer cases occurred in women who reported having ever had a Pap smear. Consequently, there were empty cells in several strata.

Table 14.16.
Hypothetical cohort study on Pap smear testing and cervical cancer described in Example 14.3. Results obtained using the Mantel–Haenszel technique.

Variables adjusted for	Cervical cancer rate ratio for Pap smear use	95% confidence interval
None	0.32 (crude)	0.20–0.52
Educational level[a]	0.32	0.20–0.52
Educational level and marital status[b]	0.40	0.25–0.66
Educational level, marital status and age at first intercourse[c]	0.43	0.27–0.72

[a] Categorized as 'low educational level' and 'high educational level'.

[b] Categorized as marital status 1=married; 2=single; 3=divorced/widowed.

[c] Categorized as age at first intercourse 1=<18 years; 2=18–22 years; 3=22+ years.

We can use a special regression modelling technique, called *Poisson regression*, to analyse the data from this hypothetical cohort study on Pap smear and cervical cancer. The results are shown in Table 14.17.

As with logistic regression, we start by using a model which includes only one explanatory variable, Pap smear use (model 1 in Table 14.17). This model gives us the Poisson estimate of the cervical cancer rate ratio for Pap smear use. This value corresponds to the crude cervical cancer rate ratio obtained earlier. This model gives us another value called 'constant', which corresponds to the cervical cancer incidence rate in women who reported never having had a Pap smear (see Table 14.8). From these values, we can calculate the incidence rate in the exposed as $0.00074 \times 0.32 = 0.0002368 = 24$ per 100 000 person-years (the same as the value obtained in Table 14.8).

We then move on to add to our model another explanatory variable, for instance, educational level (model 2 in Table 14.17). This model gives us the Poisson estimate of the cervical cancer rate ratio for Pap smear use adjusted for educational level, which is 0.32 (95% CI = 0.20–0.52). This is the same value obtained when the Mantel–Haenszel technique was used to control for educational level (Table 14.16). In contrast with the Mantel–Haenszel technique, this model also gives us

Cervical cancer rate ratio for high versus low educational level adjusted for Pap smear use = 0.73 (95% CI = 0.65–0.82)

In the last model (model 4) shown in Table 14.17, we included Pap smear use, educational level, marital status and age at first intercourse as explanatory variables. The Poisson estimate of the rate ratio for Pap smear use adjusted for educational level, marital status and age at first intercourse is 0.46 (95% CI = 0.29–0.75), similar to that obtained with the Mantel–Haenszel method (RR_{MH} = 0.43; 95% CI = 0.27–0.72) (Table 14.16). But with the Poisson regression, we also obtained the following additional rate ratios:

Cervical cancer rate ratio for high versus low educational level adjusted for Pap smear use, marital status and age at first intercourse = 0.77 (95% CI = 0.68–0.87)

Variable	Baseline rate (per person year)	Cervical cancer rate ratio	95% confidence interval
Model 1			
constant	0.00074		0.0007–0.0008
Pap smear use[a]		<u>0.32</u>	0.20–0.52
Model 2			
constant	0.008		0.008–0.009
Pap smear use[a]		<u>0.32</u>	0.20–0.52
Educational level[b]		0.73	0.65–0.82
Model 3			
constant	0.005		0.004–0.005
Pap smear use[a]		<u>0.41</u>	0.25–0.66
Educational level[b]		0.74	0.66–0.84
Marital status2[c]		2.68	2.28–3.15
Marital status3		1.89	1.61–2.21
Model 4			
constant	0.008		0.006–0.009
Pap smear use[a]		<u>0.46</u>	0.29–0.75
Educational level[b]		0.77	0.68–0.87
Marital status2[c]		2.68	2.27–3.15
Marital status3		1.60	1.36–1.87
Age at first intercourse2[d]		0.52	0.46–0.59
Age at first intercourse3		0.13	0.09–0.19

[a] Categorized as 'never' (baseline) and 'ever'.
[b] Categorized as 'low educational level' (baseline) and 'high educational level'.
[c] Categorized as marital status 1=married (baseline), 2=single, 3=divorced/widowed.
[d] Categorized as age at first intercourse 1= >18 years (baseline), 2=18–22 years, 3=22+ years.

Table 14.17.
Hypothetical cohort study on Pap smear and cervical cancer described in Example 14.3. Results obtained from Poisson regression models with increasing numbers of explanatory variables. (The values underlined correspond to those obtained with the Mantel–Haenszel technique shown in Table 14.16.)

Cervical cancer rate ratio for single versus married women adjusted for Pap smear use, educational level and age at first intercourse = 2.68 (95% CI = 2.27–3.15)

Cervical cancer rate ratio for divorced/widowed versus married women adjusted for Pap smear use, educational level and age at first intercourse = 1.60 (95% CI = 1.36–1.87)

Cervical cancer rate ratio for age at first intercourse 18–22 versus < 18 years adjusted for Pap smear use, educational level and marital status = 0.52 (95% CI = 0.46–0.59).

Cervical cancer rate ratio for age at first intercourse 22+ versus < 18 years adjusted for Pap smear use, educational level and marital status = 0.13 (95% CI = 0.09–0.19)

Logistic regression is used for estimating odds ratios. It may therefore be used in a case–control study, a cross-sectional study, or if estimating 'risks' rather than 'rates', in a cohort study. *Poisson regression* models are used for estimating rate ratios using person-time data. Other commonly used regression models in epidemiology are:

Conditional logistic regression: logistic regression analysis is suitable for unmatched case–control studies or frequency-matched case–control studies. Individually matched case–control studies require a slightly different approach called conditional logistic regression analysis. This modelling technique is the only way we can adjust for confounders other than the matching factor(s) used in the design of these studies.

Cox's proportional hazards model: this type of regression model is used when the *time to an event* is of particular interest (as in survival analysis).

14.7 Conclusions

In summary, the Mantel–Haenszel method is a very useful technique to adjust for confounders, and this approach is often adequate for data with few confounders. However, in order to adjust simultaneously for several confounders, regression modelling methods may be necessary.

It is important, however, to stress that any analysis should start by using the Mantel–Haenszel method to obtain preliminary crude effect estimates and effect estimates adjusted for each confounder separately. The cross-tabulations used for stratification in this technique allow the investigator to observe most of the important relationships and interactions that are present and to detect errors and inconsistencies in the data that might not otherwise be evident.

Regression models can then be used in a second stage of the analysis to adjust simultaneously for several confounders. One of the main disadvantages of regression modelling is that we lose sight of the data, so that it is often regarded as a 'black box' approach. Statistical modelling should not be used by people who are not familiar with it and who do not understand the assumptions upon which it is based.

Box 14.1. Key issues

- Any analysis of data should be planned carefully. In general, it should involve the following steps:

    1. Produce simple tables to check the consistency of the data.

    2. Calculate crude measures of effect.

    3. Stratify by levels of the potential confounding factor.

    4. Compute stratum-specific effect estimates.

    5. Check uniformity of the stratum-specific estimates by visual inspection or by performing tests of statistical significance.

    6. If the effect is thought to be uniform across strata, calculate a pooled adjusted summary estimate of the effect using the Mantel–Hanszel method. Calculate confidence intervals for the adjusted estimate and the Mantel–Hanszel χ^2 test.

    7. If the effect is not thought to be uniform (i.e., if interaction is present), report stratum-specific estimates, confidence intervals and χ^2 for each estimate.

    8. Use regression modelling techniques to adjust simultaneously for several confounders.

- The simple classical methods based on stratification should always be used in the initial phase of an analysis. The cross-tabulations used in stratification keep the investigator in touch with the data.

- Regression models can be used in a second stage of the analysis to adjust simultaneously for several confounders. In contrast to the classical methods, regression modelling is, to a certain extent, a 'black box' approach and because of this, it may lead to serious errors. These methods are complex statistical procedures that should never be used by those who are unfamiliar with them.

Further reading

* In this chapter, we have presented formulae to calculate Mantel–Haenszel rate ratios, risk ratios and odds ratios. Formulae to calculate adjusted estimates of risk and rate differences can be found in Greenland & Robins (1985).

* Stratification and regression modelling techniques are covered in a much more comprehensive (although more statistically elaborate) way in Breslow & Day (1980, 1987) and Clayton & Hills (1993).

Appendix 14.1.
Confidence intervals and statistical tests for adjusted relative measures of effect

Note that there are several methods to calculate confidence intervals for adjusted relative measures of effect, which may yield slightly different values from those obtained here. These calculations can easily be performed by statistical computing packages such as EPI INFO, STATA or EGRET.

A14.1.1 Adjusted odds ratio
Confidence interval for Mantel–Haenszel odds ratio

The standard error (SE) of the logarithm of the Mantel–Haenszel odds ratio (OR_{MH}) can be estimated as

$$SE\ (\ln OR_{MH}) = \sqrt{\frac{\Sigma(b_i c_i/N_i)^2\ v_i}{(\Sigma b_i c_i/N_i)^2}}$$

in which $\sum b_i c_i/N_i$ corresponds to the denominator of the formula used to calculate the OR_{MH} and $v_i = 1/a_i + 1/b_i + 1/c_i + 1/d_i$

Thus, in the ovarian cancer study (Example 14.1; Table 14.2), we have

$$\Sigma b_i c_i/N_i = (32 \times 8)/77 + (4 \times 50)/81 = 3.32 + 2.47 = 5.79$$
$$v_1 = 1/9 + 1/32 + 1/8 + 1/28 = 0.30$$
$$v_2 = 1/15 + 1/4 + 1/50 + 1/12 = 0.42$$
$$\Sigma(b_i c_i/N_i)^2\ v_i = (3.32^2 \times 0.30) + (2.47^2 \times 0.42) = 3.31 + 2.56 = 5.87$$

Thus,

$$SE\ (\ln OR_{MH}) = \sqrt{5.87/(5.79)^2} = 0.42$$

An 'approximate' 95% confidence interval for the $\ln OR_{MH}$ can then be estimated as

$$95\%\ CI\ (\ln OR_{MH}) = (\ln 0.95) \pm 1.96 \times 0.42 = -0.05 \pm 1.96 \times 0.42 = -0.87\ \text{to}\ 0.77$$

An 'approximate' 95% confidence interval for the OR_{MH} can be obtained by taking anti-logarithms:

$$95\%\ CI\ (OR_{MH}) = e^{-0.87}\ \text{to}\ e^{0.77} = 0.42\ \text{to}\ 2.16$$

The Mantel–Haenszel χ^2 test

The Mantel–Haenszel χ^2 test can be used to determine whether OR_{MH} is significantly different from one. The test is just an extension of the Mantel–Haenszel χ^2 test for a single 2×2 table presented in Section A6.1.3. The null hypothesis is that there is no association between the exposure and the disease (that is, the odds ratio is equal to one) within any of the individual strata. In order to perform this test, we must first obtain the following, from each stratum i:

(i) The observed value of a_i:

$$O(a_i) = a_i$$

(ii) The expected value of a_i, assuming the null hypothesis of no association:

$$E(a_i) = n_{1i}m_{1i}/N_i$$

(iii) The variance of a_i, assuming the null hypothesis of no association:

$$V(a_i) = n_{1i}n_{0i}m_{1i}m_{0i}/(N_i^2(N_i - 1))$$

We then sum each of these quantities over all the strata. In Example 14.1 (Table 14.2), we obtain

$$\Sigma O(a_i) = 9 + 15 = 24$$

$$\Sigma E(a_i) = (41 \times 17)/77 + (19 \times 65)/81 \ 9.05 + 15.25 = 24.30$$

$$\Sigma V(a_i) = (41 \times 36 \times 17 \times 60)/(77^2 \times 76) + (19 \times 62 \times 65 \times 16)/(81^2 \times 80) = 3.34 + 2.33 = 5.67$$

We would expect the difference between our observed and expected values to be small if the null hypothesis were true. To test whether the differences obtained are greater than would be expected by chance, we calculate

$$\chi^2 = (\Sigma O(a_i) - \Sigma E(a_i))^2 / \Sigma V(a_i)$$

and obtain a P-value by referring our result to the χ^2 distribution with one degree of freedom (d.f.).

In our example, $\chi^2 = (24 - 24.30)^2/5.67 = 0.016$ on 1 d.f. This gives $P = 0.93$, from which we conclude that after adjusting for oral contraceptive use, there is no evidence of any association between smoking and ovarian cancer. So $OR_{MH} = 0.95$ is not statistically significantly different from 1.

A14.1.2 Adjusted risk ratio
Confidence interval for Mantel–Haenszel risk ratio

The standard error (SE) of the logarithm of Mantel–Haenszel risk ratio (R_{MH}) can be estimated by

$$SE\ (\ln R_{MH}) = \sqrt{\frac{\Sigma(n_{1i}m_{1i}m_{0i} - a_ib_iN_i)/N_i^2}{(\Sigma a_im_{0i}/N_i)(\Sigma b_im_{1i}/N_i)}}$$

where the expressions $\Sigma a_im_{0i}/N_i$ and $\Sigma b_im_{1i}/N_i$ correspond, respectively, to the numerator and denominator of the formula used to calculate R_{MH}.

In our occupational study (Example 14.2; Table 14.6)

$\Sigma a_im_{0i}/N_i = 264$

$\Sigma b_im_{1i}/N_i = 132$

$\Sigma(n_{1i}m_{1i}m_{0i} - a_ib_iN_i)/N_i^2 = (240{\times}4000{\times}16\ 000 - 80{\times}160{\times}20\ 000)/20\ 000^2 +$

$(600{\times}80\ 000{\times}80\ 000 - 400{\times}200{\times}160\ 000)/160\ 000^2$

$= 37.76 + 149.50 = 187.26$

Thus,

$$SE\ (\ln R_{MH}) = \sqrt{187.26/(264 \times 132)} = 0.073$$

95% confidence interval ($\ln R_{MH}$) = ($\ln 2.0$) $\pm$ 1.96 $\times$ 0.073 = 0.547 to 0.833

An 'approximate' 95% confidence interval for R_{MH} can be obtained by taking anti-logarithms:

95% confidence interval (R_{MH}) = $e^{0.547}$ to $e^{0.833}$ = 1.73 to 2.30

The Mantel–Haenszel χ^2 test

The Mantel–Haenszel χ^2 test to assess whether R_{MH} is statistically significantly different from unity is similar to that used above for odds ratio. The null hypothesis is that there is no association between the exposure and the disease within any of the individual strata, that is that the risk ratio is equal to one in each stratum.

In our occupational study (Example 14.2; Table 14.6)

$\Sigma O(a_i) = 80 + 400 = 480$

$\Sigma E(a_i) = \Sigma n_{1i}m_{1i}/N_i = 240{\times}4000/20\ 000 + 600{\times}80\ 000/160\ 000 = 48 + 300 = 348$

$\Sigma V(a_i) = \Sigma n_{1i}n_{0i}m_{1i}m_{0i}/(N_i^2(N_i-1)) = (240{\times}19\ 760{\times}4000{\times}16\ 000)/(20\ 000^2{\times}19\ 999)$

$+ (600{\times}159\ 400{\times}80\ 000{\times}80\ 000)/(160\ 000^2{\times}159\ 999)$

$= 37.94 + 149.44 = 187.38$

We can now calculate the χ^2 test:

$$\chi^2 = (\Sigma O(a_i) - \Sigma E(a_i))^2 \,/\, \Sigma V(a_i) = (480 - 348)^2/187.38 = 92.99$$

and obtain a *P*-value by referring our result to the χ^2 distribution with 1 d.f. In this example, $P < 0.0001$. Thus, it is very unlikely that these results are due to chance.

A14.1.3   Adjusted rate ratio
Confidence interval for Mantel–Haenszel rate ratio

As with any other estimate, it is useful to be able to construct a 95% confidence interval round a Mantel–Haenszel rate ratio (RR_{MH}). The standard error of the logarithm of a rate ratio can be estimated by

$$SE\,(\ln RR_{MH}) = \sqrt{\frac{\Sigma V(a_i)}{(\Sigma a_i y_{0i}/y_i)(\Sigma b_i y_{1i}/y_i)}}$$

We can obtain an 'approximate' 95% confidence interval around the logarithm of the RR_{MH} as

$$\ln RR_{MH} \pm 1.96 \times SE\,(\ln RR_{MH})$$

An 'approximate' 95% confidence interval for RR_{MH} can then be obtained by taking anti-logarithms.

Note that $\Sigma a_i y_{0i}/y_i$ and $\Sigma b_i y_{1i}/y_i$ are, respectively, the numerator and the denominator of the formula for the Mantel–Haenszel rate ratio, which were calculated for Example 14.3 in Section 14.2.3. Thus, we only need to calculate $\Sigma V(a_i)$:

$$\Sigma a_i y_{0i}/y_i = 16.24$$

$$\Sigma b_i y_{1i}/y_i = 50.23$$

$$V(a_i) = \Sigma n_i y_{1i} y_{0i}/y_i^2 = (710\times38\ 346\times828\ 149)/866\ 495^2 +$$
$$(431\times32\ 838\times690\ 552)/723\ 390^2 = 30.03 + 18.68 = 48.71$$

$$\ln RR_{MH} = \ln\,(0.32) = -1.14$$

$$SE\,(\ln RR_{MH}) = \sqrt{48.71/(16.24 \times 50.23)} = 0.244$$

$$\text{95\% confidence interval }(\ln RR_{MH}) = -1.14 \pm 1.96 \times 0.244 = -1.62 \text{ to} -0.66$$

$$\text{95\% confidence interval }(RR_{MH}) = e^{-1.62} \text{ to } e^{-0.66} = 0.20 \text{ to } 0.52$$

The Mantel–Haenszel χ^2 test

We may want to perform a significance test to test whether the true rate ratio is different from one. Our null hypothesis is that the true rate ratio in *all* strata is one. In order to calculate the test, we need first to compute the following for each stratum i:

(i)   Observed value of $a_i = O(a_i) = a_i$

(ii)   Expected value of $a_i = E(a_i) = n_i y_{1i}/y_i$

(iii)   Variance of $a_i = V(a_i) = n_i y_{1i} y_{0i}/y_i^2$

An overall test of significance (that the common rate ratio is unity) is given by

$$\chi^2 = (\Sigma O(a_i) - \Sigma E(a_i))^2 / \Sigma V(a_i)$$

where the summation is over all strata. The value calculated should be looked up in tables of the χ^2 distribution with one degree of freedom.

Thus, in Example 14.3,

$\Sigma O(a_i) = 13 + 4 = 17$

$\Sigma E(a_i) = (710 \times 38\ 346/866\ 495) + (431 \times 32\ 838/723\ 390)$
$= 31.42 + 19.57 = 50.99$

$\Sigma V(a_i) = 48.71$, which was obtained above for the calculation of the confidence interval.

$\chi^2 = (17 - 50.99)^2/48.71 = 23.72$

This χ^2 on 1 d.f. corresponds to $P < 0.001$.

Chapter 15
Size of a study

15.1 Introduction

It is important to ensure at the design stage that the proposed number of subjects to be recruited into any study will be appropriate to answer the main objective(s) of the study. A small study may fail to detect important effects on the outcomes of interest, or may estimate them too imprecisely, no matter how good its design may be in other respects. A study larger than necessary, while less common in practice, may waste valuable resources.

Example 15.1. *Suppose that a trial was set up to assess the value of a new treatment for breast cancer. A total of 200 women with newly diagnosed breast cancer were randomly allocated to receive either the new or the standard treatment. All patients were followed up for one year after their entry into the trial (or until death if it occurred earlier). The outcome of interest was the proportion of women still alive by the end of the trial. The results are shown in Table 15.1.*

		New treatment	Standard treatment	Total
	Yes	80 (a)	70 (b)	150 (n_1)
Alive one year after entry into the trial	No	20 (c)	30 (d)	50 (n_0)
	Total	100 (m_1)	100 (m_0)	200 (N)

$p_1 = 80/100 = 80\%$

$p_0 = 70/100 = 70\%$

Risk difference $= p_1 - p_0 = 10\%$

95% confidence interval $= -2\%$ to $+22\%$

$\chi^2 = 2.65; P > 0.10$

Table 15.1.
Number of patients with breast cancer still alive one year after entry into the trial by type of treatment administered: hypothetical data.

In Example 15.1, the χ^2 test of the difference between these two proportions gives a value of 2.65, which corresponds to $P > 0.10$. Thus the difference between the two proportions could easily have arisen by chance. However, we cannot conclude from this that there is no true difference between the treatments, since the 95% confidence interval for the difference between the proportions of patients still alive one year after entry into the trial is -2% to $+22\%$. Therefore the data from this trial are consistent with a proportion of surviving patients on the new treatment up to 22% higher or 2% lower than the proportion of those on the standard treatment.

Thus, although the trial has shown that the new treatment does not perform appreciably worse than the standard treatment, it is unclear whether the two treatments have similar effects or whether the new treatment increases survival substantially. This is because the sample size of this trial was far too small to provide an appropriate answer to the question being addressed.

In the rest of this chapter, we will show how sample size estimates can be obtained in the simplest situation where two groups are to be compared. The calculations are based on the statistical methods presented in Chapter 6 and its appendix and readers should be familiar with their content before proceeding.

There are two main approaches to sample size calculations. One is based on the concept of *power* of a study, i.e., its ability to detect a statistically significant result if the true magnitude of the effect is as anticipated. Thus, this approach to sample size calculations focuses on the *significance test* that will be performed at the end of the study. In Example 15.1, we may estimate the sample size necessary to ensure that the study will have a certain probability ('power') of yielding a *P*-value less than 0.05 if the true difference in survival between the two treatments is 10%. The second approach focuses on the *precision* of the estimate, i.e., on the level of sampling error we regard as acceptable. As we saw in Chapter 6, the confidence interval provides an indication of how precise our sample estimate is in relation to the true population value. Thus, this approach focuses on the *width of the confidence interval* that will be obtained when the results of the study are analysed. In the breast cancer trial, we may estimate the sample size necessary to ensure that the trial will be able to estimate the true difference in survival within ± 2.5% of its value (i.e., the confidence interval will extend 2.5% to either side of the sample estimate).

In this chapter, we start by considering sample size calculations based on power and then move to calculations based on precision. The chapter ends with a discussion of how to apply such calculations to more complex study designs and other practical issues that need to be taken into account in estimating sample sizes. It is, however, important to emphasize at this stage that any sample size calculations involve some guesswork, since we have to start by anticipating the results of the proposed study and, therefore, these calculations should be regarded as *providing only a rough estimate of the required study size*. Moreover, as we shall see later in this chapter, other aspects (e.g., costs, availability of eligible subjects, logistic problems), independent of statistical considerations, also have to be taken into account in any practical situation.

15.2 Power of a study

The power of a study is the probability of obtaining a 'statistically significant' result, that is, a *P*-value below a certain pre-established 'signifi-

cance' level (usually 0.05) if the true magnitude of the effect is as anticipated. However, as discussed in Section 6.3, there is a close link between
P-values and confidence intervals. Therefore, power can also be interpreted as the *probability of obtaining an estimate whose confidence interval does
not include the value stipulated by the null hypothesis*. The null hypothesis
states that the exposure has no effect on the outcome of interest corresponding to a value of zero, if the exposure effect is measured on an
absolute scale (e.g., risk or rate difference), or one, if measured on a ratio
scale (e.g., risk or rate ratio).

Figure 15.1(*a*) illustrates the relationship between
the null hypothesis value, the anticipated effect estimate and its confidence interval when the exposure
is associated with an increase in the occurrence of the
outcome of interest. For the study to have appropriate power to detect such an effect, the lower limit of
the confidence interval of the anticipated effect estimate has to be above the value stipulated by the null
hypothesis. Similarly, when the exposure is associated with a decrease in incidence (i.e., the exposure is
protective), the upper limit of the confidence interval
has to be below the null hypothesis value (Figure
15.1(*b*)). Thus, the power of the study to detect a 'statistically significant' effect, if the true effect is as
anticipated, is the probability that the lower limit of
the confidence interval falls above (or, if the exposure
is protective, the upper limit falls below) the null
hypothesis value.

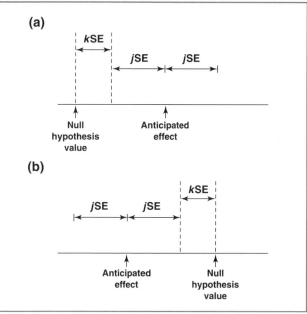

The position of the lower limit (or the upper limit,
if the exposure is protective) of the confidence interval of the anticipated
effect estimate is determined by the *width of the confidence interval (± jSE)*
(Figure 15.1), which in turn depends upon the *study size* (the bigger the
study, the smaller the standard error (SE) and, therefore, the narrower the
confidence interval) and upon the *significance (confidence) level chosen (j)*.
For a 95% confidence interval, *j* would be equal to 1.96 (Table 15.2); that
is, the confidence interval will extend 1.96SE to each side of the sample
estimate. For a 99% confidence interval, *j* will be 2.576 and, therefore, the
confidence interval will be wider. The wider the confidence interval, the
lower the power of a study of a given size.

Suppose that the study were repeated several times. The effect estimates
obtained each time and their confidence intervals would differ because of
sampling variation. If the effect estimates obtained each time were plotted, we would obtain a Normal sampling distribution with a standard error
of SE. Similarly, if the lower limits (or upper limits, if the exposure is protective) of each of the confidence intervals were plotted, we would obtain
a Normal distribution, with the same standard error SE, centred around
the anticipated value of the lower (or upper) limit. The power of a study is

Figure 15.1.
Diagram illustrating the relationship of
the null hypothesis value, the anticipated effect and its confidence interval
when the exposure is associated with
(*a*) an increase or (*b*) a decrease in
the occurrence of the outcome of interest (adapted from Clayton & Hills,
1993).

Significance level	*j*
0.10	1.645
0.05	1.960
0.01	2.576

Power	*k*
0.95	1.645
0.90	1.282
0.75	0.674
0.50	0.0
<0.50	<0

Table 15.2.
Values of *k* and *j* for different significance levels and powers.

the probability that the lower limit of the confidence interval would fall above the null hypothesis value (or the upper limit would fall below it, if the exposure is protective). This probability depends upon the *number of standard errors (k)* between the null hypothesis and the anticipated position of the lower limit (or upper limit, if the exposure is protective) of the confidence interval of the anticipated effect estimate (Figure 15.1). It can be shown mathematically that if *k* is equal to 1.645, the study will have 95% power (Table 15.2). In other words, if the study were to be conducted repeatedly, we would expect only 5 out of 100 resulting 95% confidence intervals to include the null hypothesis value, if the true magnitude of the effect is as anticipated. When the anticipated location of the lower (or upper) confidence limit is exactly at the null hypothesis, so that $k = 0$, the power is 0.50 and there is an even chance of obtaining a significant result. If $k < 0$, the power will be less than 50%. In general, a power of less than 80% is regarded as unacceptable.

Thus, to summarize, the power of a study depends upon:

1. The *magnitude of the anticipated effect* (i.e., the distance between the null hypothesis value and the anticipated effect). The greater the effect, the higher the power to detect it as 'statistically significant' for a study of a given size.

2. The *width of the confidence interval (jSE)*, which determines the position of the lower limit (or the upper limit, if the exposure is protective). The wider the confidence interval, the lower the power of a study of a given size. This in turn depends on:

    (*a*) The study size. The bigger the study, the smaller the standard error (SE) and, therefore, the narrower the confidence interval.

    (*b*) The significance (confidence) level chosen (*j*). For instance, a 95% confidence interval (*j* = 1.96) will be narrower than a 99% confidence interval (*j* = 2.576) for a sample of a given size.

It is useful to construct power curves to show how the power varies with the study size for different significance levels and different magnitudes of the anticipated effect. Figure 15.2 shows some examples of such curves for the breast cancer trial described in Example 15.1.

In most real situations, researchers have a very good idea of the number of eligible subjects they will be able to recruit into their study. This number is usually determined by availability of eligible subjects, logistics of recruitment, costs, etc. In these circumstances the relevant question is not '*How large should the study be?*' but '*Is the available number of subjects enough to provide a clear answer to the study objectives?*'. To answer this last question, we need to estimate the power of the study with the proposed number of subjects. If these calculations reveal that the power will be too low, it will be necessary to estimate by how much our sample size needs to be increased to ensure that the study will achieve the desired power. This is the approach suggested by Clayton & Hills (1993), which we will follow in the rest of this section.

15.2.1 Comparing two proportions (prevalences or risks)

To calculate the power of our breast cancer trial (Example 15.1) to detect a 10% difference in survival between the two treatments, we need to calculate first the SE of the difference between the two proportions of women still alive by the end of the first year. As we saw in Section A6.1.2, the SE of the difference between two proportions can be estimated, approximately, as

$$SE(p_1 - p_0) = \sqrt{\frac{p_1^2(1-p_1)}{a} + \frac{p_0^2(1-p_0)}{b}}$$

Thus, in our example,

$$SE = \sqrt{\frac{0.80^2(1-0.80)}{80} + \frac{0.70^2(1-0.70)}{70}} = 0.061$$

Figure 15.1(a) shows that the distance between the anticipated effect and the null hypothesis value (in our example, 0.10–0) is the sum of the two components, one deriving from the width of the confidence interval (jSE) and the other from the distance between the anticipated position of the lower limit of the confidence interval and the null hypothesis (kSE). Hence,

$$0.10 = j\,SE + k\,SE$$

If the significance level is set to 0.05 ($j = 1.96$) and SE = 0.061,

$$0.10 = 1.96 \times 0.061 + k \times 0.061$$

$$k = -0.32$$

This value of k corresponds to a power of less than 50% (Table 15.2). Thus, the probability of the trial being able to detect a statistically significant 10% difference in survival between the two treatments, even if such a difference truly exists, is below 50% because the confidence interval is too wide, due to the large SE. This is illustrated in Figure 15.3.

If we assume that the true difference in survival is 10% and we fix the significance level to 0.05 (j=1.96), we can calculate the value of the standard error that will be required to ensure that the power of the trial is 0.95 ($k = 1.645$):

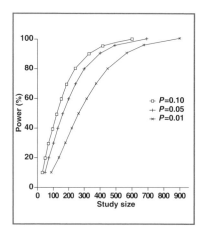

Figure 15.2.
Power for detecting a one-year survival difference of 10% when baseline survival is 70% (equivalent to 14% increase in survival) for various sample sizes and significance levels.

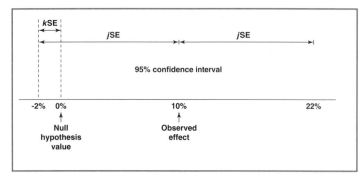

Figure 15.3.
Power calculation for the breast cancer clinical trial illustrated in Example 15.1: observed effect = 10% (= 80%–70%) difference in survival; sample size = 100 in each group; significance level = 0.05; power < 0.50.

$$1.96 \times SE + 1.645 \times SE = 0.10$$

$$\text{Required } SE = 0.10/(1.960 + 1.645) = 0.028$$

This value of the SE is much smaller than the value of 0.061 obtained with 100 subjects in each group. To reduce the SE to the required value, it is necessary to increase the size of the study. Clayton & Hills (1993) have provided the following formula to calculate a factor by which the study size must be increased in order to achieve the specified power:

$$(\text{Current value of SE/Required value of SE})^2$$

Thus, in our trial,

> Current value of SE = 0.061
> Required value of SE = 0.028
> Scale factor = 4.8

The initial sample size was 100 in each group. To ensure that the study will have 95% power to detect a 10% difference in survival at the 5% significance level, we need to multiply this original sample size by 4.8. Thus, we need to enrol *480 subjects in each treatment group*.

As we saw in Section A6.1.3, the significance test is the same regardless of the type of measure of effect (ratio or difference) used to compare the two groups. Power calculations are based on the significance test that will be performed at the end of the study and, as a logical consequence, *similar sample size estimates would be obtained if the calculations were based on the ratio of the two proportions (80%/70%) rather than on their difference (80%–70%)*. The approach would be similar to the one followed above, except that the calculations would be based on the SE of the ratio of the two proportions rather than on the SE of their difference. Since the confidence interval around a ratio of proportions is asymmetric, taking only values from zero to infinity (Section A6.1.2), we first convert the estimated survival risk ratio into its natural logarithm (denoted by ln):

$$\ln (0.80/0.70) = \ln (1.14) = 0.134$$

We can now calculate an 'approximate' standard error of the logarithm of the ratio of two proportions (R) by using the formula given in Section A6.1.2:

$$SE (\ln R) = \sqrt{(1/a + 1/b - 1/m_1 - 1/m_0)}$$

$$= \sqrt{(1/80 + 1/70 - 1/100 - 1/100)} = 0.082$$

The distance between the logarithm of the anticipated effect and the logarithm of the null hypothesis value of 1 is equal to

$$\ln (1.14) - \ln (1) = 0.134 - 0 = 0.134$$

Thus,

$$0.134 = j \times SE + k \times SE$$

The value of the required SE to ensure that the study will have 95% power ($k = 1.645$) to detect a risk ratio of 1.14 at the 5% significance level ($j = 1.96$) will be

$$0.134 = 1.96 \times SE + 1.645 \times SE$$

$$\text{Required SE} = 0.134/(1.960 + 1.645) = 0.037$$

Therefore,

$$\text{Scale factor} = (0.082/0.037)^2 = 4.8$$

This value is exactly the one we obtained before when the calculation was based on the difference between the two proportions rather than on their ratio. Thus, the sample size required to detect a 10% increase in survival from 70% to 80% is equivalent to the sample size required to detect a risk ratio of 80%/70% = 1.14.

15.2.2 Comparing two rates

Similar sample size calculations can be performed for intervention trials and cohort studies in which the rate ratio (or rate difference) is the appropriate measure of effect.

In Example 15.2, we can predict the values of a and b by using the total person-time of observation in the proposed cohort study (y) and the estimated lung cancer incidence rate in the unexposed (r_0). Since lung cancer is a rare condition, we can estimate the total person-time of observation as

$$y = 40\ 000 \times 5 \text{ years} = 200\ 000 \text{ pyrs}$$

assuming there were no losses to follow-up and no other competing causes of death.

If 40% of the cohort is exposed to the risk factor under study, 0.60 is unexposed. Thus,

$$y_1 = 200\ 000 \times 0.40 = 80\ 000 \text{ pyrs}$$
$$y_0 = 200\ 000 \times 0.60 = 120\ 000 \text{ pyrs}$$

Since the anticipated rate ratio (RR) is equal to 2.0, the expected numbers of lung cancer cases among exposed and unexposed workers are

$$a = 80\ 000 \text{ pyrs} \times (2 \times 50 \text{ per } 100\ 000 \text{ pyrs}) = 80$$
$$b = 120\ 000 \text{ pyrs} \times 50 \text{ per } 100\ 000 \text{ pyrs} = 60$$

Example 15.2. *Suppose we plan to conduct a cohort study to assess the effect of an occupational exposure on the incidence of lung cancer. We intend to recruit 40 000 middle-aged men into the study and follow them up for five years. 40% of the workers are known to be exposed to the hazard and we expect the lung cancer rate in those exposed to be twice that of workers unexposed (i.e., anticipated rate ratio = 2.0). It is estimated that the incidence rate of lung cancer in the unexposed group is 50 per 100 000 pyrs. The results to be obtained from this cohort study will be presented as in Table 15.3.*

Table 15.3.
Results from a hypothetical cohort study.

	Exposure		Total
	Yes	No	
No. of cases	a	b	n
Person-years at risk	y_1	y_0	y
Rate per 100 000 pyrs	r_1	r_0	r

We can now complete Table 15.3 with the results we expect to obtain from this cohort study if our assumptions are correct (Table 15.4).

Table 15.4.
Anticipated results from the proposed cohort study illustrated in Example 15.2.

	Exposure		Total
	Yes	No	
No. of cases	80 (a)	60 (b)	140 (n)
Person-years at risk	80 000 (y_1)	120 000 (y_0)	200 000 (y)
Rate per 100 000 pyrs	100 (r_1)	50 (r_0)	70 (r)

As shown in Section A6.1.2, an 'approximate' SE of the logarithm of a rate ratio can be calculated as

$$\text{SE (ln RR)} = \sqrt{(1/a + 1/b)}$$

Thus, in our example,

$$\text{SE (ln RR)} = \sqrt{(1/80 + 1/60)} = 0.171$$

The number of SEs between the logarithm of the anticipated rate ratio (ln (2.0) = 0.693) and the logarithm of the null hypothesis value (ln (1) = 0) is

$$0.693 - 0 = j \times 0.171 + k \times 0.171$$

$$j + k = 0.693/0.171 = 4.05$$

For a significance level of 0.05, j would be equal to 1.96 and, hence,

$$k = 4.05 - 1.96 = 2.09$$

This value of k corresponds to a power greater than 0.95 (Table 15.2). Thus, the probability that this cohort study will detect a true rate ratio of 2.0 (at the 0.05 significance level) is greater than 95%. Similar sample size estimates would be obtained if the calculations were based on the anticipated rate difference of 50 per 100 000 pyrs (100 per 100 000 pyrs − 50 per 100 000 pyrs).

If the power of the study with the proposed number of subjects were too low, we could have calculated by how much the sample size would have to be increased in order to achieve the required level by using the procedure described above when comparing two proportions.

15.2.3 Comparing two odds

A similar approach can be used in case–control studies. To estimate the power of the case–control study in Example 15.3, we need to guess the values of a, b, c and d. Since the controls are supposed to be representative of the population from which the cases will arise, we would expect 33.5% of them to be exposed and the rest to be unexposed to the factor under investigation. Thus

$$c = 200 \times 0.335 = 67$$
$$d = 200 - 67 = 133$$

Example 15.3. *Suppose we wish to conduct a study of 200 cases and 200 controls to detect an odds ratio of 0.5 for a particular exposure. The prevalence of this exposure in the population from which the cases arise is known to be 33.5%. The results to be obtained from this case–control study will be presented as in Table 15.5.*

	Exposure		Total
	Yes	**No**	
Cases	a	b	n_1
Controls	c	d	n_0
Total	m_1	m_0	N

Table 15.5.
Results from a hypothetical case-control study.

We can now calculate the odds of exposure among the controls as

$$c/d = 67/133 = 0.5$$

Since we anticipate an odds ratio equal to 0.5, we can calculate the odds of exposure among the cases as

$$a/b = 0.5 \times 0.5 = 0.25$$

Thus,

$$a = 0.25 \times b$$

Since $a + b = 200$, it follows that

$$b = 160$$
$$a = 200 - 160 = 40$$

We can now complete Table 15.5 with the values of a, b, c and d we expect to observe in the proposed case–control study (Table 15.6).

Table 15.6.
Anticipated results from the hypothetical case–control study described in Example 15.3.

	Exposure		Total
	Yes	No	
Cases	40 (a)	160 (b)	200 (n_1)
Controls	67 (c)	133 (d)	200 (n_0)
Total	**107 (m_1)**	**293 (m_0)**	**400 (N)**

With these data, we can calculate an 'approximate' SE of the logarithm of the anticipated odds ratio by using the formula given in Section A6.1.2:

$$SE = \sqrt{(1/a + 1/b + 1/c + 1/d)}$$

Thus, in our case–control study,

$$SE = \sqrt{(1/40 + 1/160 + 1/67 + 1/133)}$$
$$= 0.232$$

To calculate the power of the study for a significance level of 0.05 ($j = 1.960$), we need first to calculate ln (OR) = ln (0.5) = –0.693. This is a negative value, but since we are interested in the absolute distance between the anticipated value and the null hypothesis we can ignore the minus sign and proceed as usual:

$$0.693 = 1.96 \times SE + k \times SE$$
$$0.693 - 1.96 \times 0.232 = k \times 0.232$$

$$0.238 = k \times 0.232$$
$$k = 1.03$$

A k value of 1.03 corresponds to a power around 0.85 (Table 15.2). If we wish to increase the power to 0.95, the study size has to be increased:

$$0.693 = 1.96 \times SE + 1.645 \times SE$$

$$\text{Required } SE = 0.693/(1.96 + 1.645) = 0.192$$

$$\text{Factor} = (0.232/0.192)^2 = 1.46$$

Thus, the proposed sample size must be increased by a factor of 1.46, that is from 200 to 292, if we wish to increase the power of the study from around 0.85 to 0.95.

Example 15.4. *Consider again the breast cancer trial (Example 15.1). For the trial to have 95% power to detect a 10% difference in survival at the 5% significance level, the sample size has to be increased from 100 to 480 subjects in each of the two treatment groups (Section 15.2.1). With this new sample size, we anticipate the following results (Table 15.7 and Figure 15.4).*

		New treatment	Standard treatment	Total
Alive one year after entry into the trial	Yes	384 (*a*)	336 (*b*)	720 (n_1)
	No	96 (*c*)	144 (*d*)	240 (n_0)
	Total	**480 (m_1)**	**480 (m_0)**	**960 (*N*)**

$p_1 = 384/480 = 80\%$

$p_0 = 336/480 = 70\%$

Risk difference = $p_1 - p_0 = 10\%$

95% confidence interval = +4.6% to + 15.4%

$\chi^2 = 12.79$; $P < 0.001$

Table 15.7.
Anticipated results of a hypothetical trial to assess the value of a new treatment on the one-year survival from breast cancer. Anticipated effect = 10% (= 80%–70%) difference in survival; significance level = 0.05; power = 0.95; sample size = 480 women in each treatment group.

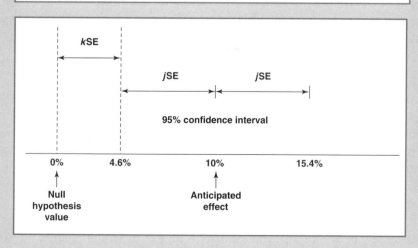

Figure 15.4.
Anticipated effect and its 95% confidence interval for the hypothetical breast cancer trial described in Example 15.4: anticipated effect = 10% (= 80%–70%) difference in survival; significance level = 0.05; power = 0.95; sample size = 480 women in each treatment group.

15.3 Sample size calculations based on precision

The approach to sample size calculations discussed in the previous section focused on the statistical significance test to be conducted at the end of the study. The main limitation of this approach is that it may produce very imprecise estimates of the effect on the outcome(s) of interest; thus, although the confidence interval will not include the null hypothesis value, it may still be too wide to be informative.

In Example 15.4, although the anticipated confidence interval does not include the null hypothesis value of no difference between the two treatments, its width is compatible with an improvement in one-year survival which ranges from 4.6% to 15.4% (Table 15.7; Figure 15.4). This is not a very precise estimate. Indeed, the range is wider than 10%, the difference we anticipate. We may consider more acceptable a width of ±2.5% either side of the sample estimate of 10%, so that the confidence interval of the difference in the proportion of women still alive by the end of the first year will range from 7.5% to 12.5%.

Sample size calculations based on power may be appropriate for new exposures, when it is not known whether there will be any impact at all on the outcomes of interest. If, however, other studies have already shown that the exposure is associated with either an increase or a decrease in incidence, there is not much point in testing the null hypothesis, and the objective should be to estimate the magnitude of the effect as precisely as possible. In these situations, it is more appropriate to choose a sample size that will yield a confidence interval of a predefined width.

> *Example 15.5. Suppose we wish to conduct a cross-sectional survey in a certain area to estimate the prevalence of current oral contraceptive use among women aged 20–44 years. We plan to take a random sample from the population of all women aged 20–44 years living in the study area. We would like to calculate the sample size required to ensure that the study will be able to estimate the true prevalence of current oral contraceptive users in the study area within 5% of its value (i.e. the confidence interval that we will obtain when the results of the study are analysed will extend 5% to either side of the sample estimate).*

15.3.1 Estimating a single crude proportion (prevalence or risk)

We can estimate the sample size necessary to ensure that the confidence interval for a single proportion (prevalence or risk) is of a predetermined width.

In Example 15.5, we plan to take a random sample of n women aged 20–44 years. If among them, a are current users, we estimate the prevalence of oral contraceptive use as

$$p = a/n$$

As we saw in Section 6.1, this estimate is subject to sampling error, but the 95% confidence interval will give a range of values within which the true population prevalence will lie with 95% confidence.

$$SE(p) = \sqrt{\frac{p^2(1-p)}{a}}$$

Suppose we wish our confidence interval around the sample estimate to be of a certain width ($\pm w$). The value of w depends upon the standard error SE and the significance level (j) chosen:

$$w = j \times SE$$

For a 95% confidence interval, $j = 1.96$, that is the interval extends 1.96 standard errors either side of the estimate ($w = 1.96 \times SE$).

Hence, we can estimate the prevalence of oral contraceptive use (p) with a pre-defined degree of precision by choosing an appropriate sample size (n). We must first guess the value of p. Suppose that statistics on oral contraceptive sales indicate that the prevalence of use is about 50% and we want to estimate it to within ±5%. Thus

$$p = 0.50$$
$$w = j \times SE = 0.05$$

Choosing a 95% confidence level,

$$1.96 \times SE = 0.05$$
$$SE(p) = 0.05/1.96 = 0.0255$$

Since $p = 0.5$, we can estimate a from the formula for the SE:

$$SE(p) = \sqrt{\frac{p^2(1-p)}{a}} = 0.0255$$

$$\sqrt{(0.5^2 \times 0.5)/a} = 0.0255$$
$$0.125/a = 0.0255^2$$
$$a = 192$$

Finally, we can calculate the sample size (n) required as

$$p = a/n$$
$$0.5 = 192/n$$
$$n = 384$$

Thus, we need to enrol 384 women into the study. When planning a study, it is a good idea to find out what sample size will be required for various levels of precision (Table 15.8 and Figure 15.5).

Table 15.8.
Sample sizes required to estimate a true prevalence of 0.50 with 95% confidence intervals of different widths (±*w*).

Width (±*w*)	Sample size (*n*)
0.01	9612
0.02	2403
0.03	1068
0.04	600
0.05	384
0.06	266
0.07	196
0.08	150
0.09	118
0.10	96
0.15	43

Figure 15.5.
Anticipated 95% confidence intervals for a true prevalence of 0.50 for various sample sizes.

Prevalence (*p*)	Sample size (*n*)
0.10	138
0.20	245
0.30	322
0.40	367
0.50	384
0.60	367
0.70	322
0.80	245
0.90	138

Table 15.9.
Sample size required to ensure that the 95% confidence interval for different levels of prevalence (*p*) will extend *w* = 0.05 to each side of the sample estimate.

Thus, to estimate a true prevalence of oral contraceptive use of 50% within ±1% (i.e., from 49% to 51%), we would need to recruit 9612 women.

It is also important to calculate the required sample size for different values of the anticipated prevalence *p*. As we can see in Table 15.9, the sample size required does not vary much for values of *p* between 0.3 and 0.7, being greatest when *p* = 0.50. Thus, to be on the safe side, we can set *p* = 0.50 and obtain the maximum sample size (*n*) required.

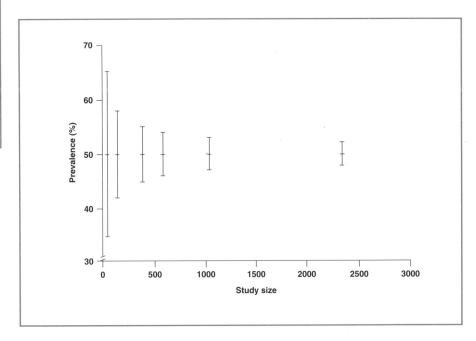

15.3.2 Estimating a single crude rate

A similar approach can be used to estimate the sample size necessary to ensure that the confidence interval for a single rate is of a predetermined width.

> **Example 15.6.** *Suppose we wish to determine the incidence rate of a particular condition in a certain population. Based on data from previously conducted studies, we expect the rate to be about 50 per 10 000 pyrs. We want to determine the size of the sample that will be required to estimate the incidence rate in that population within ±5 per 10 000 pyrs.*

In Example 15.6, we plan to take a random sample of individuals from the study population. Thus, for a 95% confidence level (*j* = 1.96)

$$w = 1.96 \times SE$$
$$5 \text{ per } 10\,000 \text{ pyrs} = 1.96 \times SE(r)$$
$$SE(r) = 2.55 \text{ per } 10\,000 \text{ pyrs}$$

An 'approximate' standard error of a rate can be calculated as indicated in Section A.6.1.1:

$$SE(r) = \frac{r}{\sqrt{a}}$$

where r is the estimated rate and a is the number of cases that occurred during the observation period. Thus, in our example,

$$\frac{50 \text{ per } 10\ 000 \text{ pyrs}}{\sqrt{a}} = 2.55 \text{ per } 10\ 000 \text{ pyrs}$$

$$a = 384$$

We can now calculate the person-time at risk (y) required to originate 384 cases:

$r = a/y$

50 per 10 000 pyrs = $384/y$

$y = 76\ 800$ pyrs

This level of total person-years at risk can be achieved by following 76 800 individuals for one year or 38 400 for two years, etc.

15.3.3 Estimating a difference or ratio of two proportions (risks or prevalences)

Let us consider again the breast cancer trial (Examples 15.1 and 15.4). Suppose we want to ensure that the width of the confidence interval for the difference in proportions will be equal to $\pm w = 2 \times 2.5\%$. Thus

$$w = 1.96 \times SE\ (p_1 - p_0) = 0.025$$

The required SE should be

$$0.025/1.96 = 0.0128$$

and

$$SE(p_1 - p_0) = \sqrt{\frac{p_1^{2}(1-p_1)}{a} + \frac{p_0^{2}(1-p_0)}{b}} = 0.0128$$

Since $a = 0.80m_1$, $b = 0.70m_0$ and $m_0 = m_1$, it follows that

$m_0 = m_1 = a/0.80$

$b = 0.70 \times (a/0.80) = 0.875\ a$

The above formula for the standard error can then be re-written as

$$SE = \sqrt{\frac{0.80^2(1-0.80)}{a} + \frac{0.70^2(1-0.70)}{0.875a}} = 0.0128$$

$(0.0128)^2 = 0.128/a + 0.147/0.875a$
$0.000164 = ((0.128 \times 0.875) + 0.147)/0.875a$
$0.875a = 0.259/0.000164 = 1579.3$
$a = 1805$
$m_1 = m_0 = 1805/0.80 = 2256$
$b = 2256 \times 0.70 = 1579$

Thus, to obtain a 95% confidence interval for the survival difference between the two treatments with a width of 2.5% either side of the anticipated effect of 10% (i.e., from 7.5% to 12.5%), we need to enrol 2256 subjects in each treatment group.

Similarly, we can calculate the sample size required to estimate a ratio of two proportions with a pre-defined level of precision. The approach would be similar to the one just illustrated, except that the calculations would be based on the formula for the SE of a ratio of proportions (see Section A6.1.2).

15.3.4 Estimating a rate difference or a rate ratio

A similar approach can be used in studies where the appropriate measure of effect is the rate ratio.

Example 15.7. The incidence of stomach cancer among men aged 50–59 years in a particular population is 65 per 100 000 person-years. Suppose that we are planning to conduct a trial in that population to assess whether a particular intervention reduces the rate of stomach cancer in men of that age-group. Eligible subjects will be randomized to receive either the intervention or the placebo in a ratio of 1:1. You expect the rate among those who receive the intervention to be 60% of the rate in those administered placebo (i.e., a 40% reduction in risk). We wish the confidence interval for the rate ratio estimate to have a width (on a logarithmic scale) of 1.30 either side of the sample estimate (i.e., from 0.46 (= 0.60/1.30) to 0.78 (= 0.60 × 1.30)). The results from this trial will be presented as in Table 15.3.

An 'approximate' 95% confidence interval of the logarithm of a rate ratio (r_1/r_0) can be estimated as

$$95\% \text{ confidence interval} = \ln RR \pm 1.96 \times SE (\ln RR)$$

In Example 15.7

$w = \ln(1.30) = 1.96 \times SE(\ln RR)$

$SE(\ln RR) = 0.262/1.96 = 0.134$

An 'approximate' standard error of the logarithm of an estimated rate ratio (RR) can then be obtained as follows:

$SE(\ln RR) = \sqrt{(1/a + 1/b)}$

In our example,

$0.134 = \sqrt{(1/a + 1/b)}$

Since the same number of subjects are to be allocated to each arm of the trial and we anticipate a rate ratio of 0.6, then

$a = 0.6 \times b$
$0.134 = \sqrt{(1/0.6b + 1/b)} = \sqrt{(1.6/0.6b)}$
$(0.134)^2 = 1.6/0.6b$
$0.6b = 1.6/0.018 = 88.89$
$b = 88.89/0.6 = 148$
$a = 0.6 \times 148 = 89$

The stomach cancer incidence rate for those given placebo is believed to be 65 per 100 000 pyrs. Thus, we need 227 692 pyrs (= 148/0.000065 pyrs) of follow-up in each arm of the trial in order to accumulate 148 stomach cancer cases among those receiving the intervention and 89 among those given placebo. This will ensure that the result of the trial will have the desired level of precision. This can be achieved by following 227 692 men for one year, 113 846 for two years and so on.

A similar approach can be used to calculate sample size estimates based on precision in situations where the appropriate measure of effect is the rate difference rather than the rate ratio, except that the calculations would be based on the formula of the SE of a difference in rates (see Section A6.1.2).

15.3.5 Estimating an odds ratio

Consider Example 15.8

Example 15.8. Suppose we wish to conduct a study to detect an odds ratio of 2.0 for an exposure present in 33.5% of the population from which the cases will arise. A similar number of cases and controls will be recruited into the study. We want to ensure that the 95% confidence interval for the odds ratio will have a width (on a logarithmic scale) of 1.25 either side of the sample estimate (i.e., from 1.6 (= 2.0/1.25) to 2.5 (= 2.0 × 1.25)). The results from this case–control study will be presented as in Table 15.5.

A 95% confidence interval of the logarithm of an odds ratio can be estimated as

$$\text{95\% confidence interval} = \ln\text{OR} \pm 1.96 \times \text{SE}(\ln\text{OR})$$

In our example,

$$w = \ln(1.25) = 1.96 \times \text{SE}(\ln\text{OR})$$
$$\text{SE}(\ln\text{OR}) = 0.223/1.96 = 0.114$$

An 'approximate' standard error of the logarithm of the estimated odds ratio can be obtained as

$$\text{SE}(\ln\text{OR}) = \sqrt{(1/a + 1/b + 1/c + 1/d)}$$

The odds of exposure among the cases is expected to be twice the odds of exposure among the controls:

$$a/b = 2 \times (c/d)$$

and the prevalence of exposure among the controls is expected to be 33.5%:

$$c = n_0 \times 0.335$$
$$d = n_0 \times 0.665$$

Hence,

$$a/b = 2 \times \frac{n_0 \times 0.335}{n_0 \times 0.665} = 1.008$$

$$a = 1.008 \times b$$
$$n_0 = n_1 = a + b = 1.008b + b = 2.008b$$

$$0.114 = \sqrt{\frac{1}{1.008b} + \frac{1}{b} + \frac{1}{2.008b \times 0.335} + \frac{1}{2.008b \times 0.665}}$$

$$0.114^2 = 1/b \times (1/1.008 + 1 + 1/0.673 + 1/1.335)$$
$$0.013 = 4.227/b$$
$$b = 325$$
$$a = 328$$
$$c = (325 + 328) \times 0.335 = 219$$
$$d = (325 + 328) \times 0.665 = 434$$
$$n_0 = a + b = 325 + 328 = 653$$
$$n_1 = c + d = 219 + 434 = 653$$

Thus, we need to recruit 653 cases and 653 controls into our case-control study.

15.4   Other considerations concerning study size

The methods described in this chapter should be regarded only as providing a rough estimate of the required study size, as they are based on guesses or approximate estimates of the parameters, on subjective decisions about the size of an effect that we would wish to detect, and on the use of approximate formulae. They only give an idea of the sort of size needed.

In practice there will be constraints on resources, which may limit the maximum possible sample size. Resources in terms of staff, vehicles, laboratory capacity, time and money are all likely to be limited, and it is usually necessary to achieve a balance between the results of the study size calculations and what can reasonably be managed given the resources. Trying to do a study that is beyond the capacity of the available resources is likely to be unfruitful, as data quality will suffer, and the study may collapse before completion, wasting the investment that had already been put into it. On the other hand, if the calculations show that a study of a manageable size will have a power and/or yield a precision that is unacceptably low, it may be worth considering involving other centres.

Study size calculation should always be carried out for several different scenarios, not just one (e.g., different levels of power/precision and of estimates of the effect measure), in order to give a clear picture of the scope of the study. A useful approach in deciding on the trade-off between cost and power is to construct power curves for one or two key outcome variables, to show how the power or precision varies with the study size for different values of the effect measure (as shown in Figure 15.2).

15.4.1 Studies designed to look at multiple exposure–outcome relationships

Many epidemiological studies are designed to look at several exposure-outcome relationships. We can use the methods described in this chapter to calculate the study size necessary to allow us to detect the most important exposure–outcome relationships. Ideally, we would then select the largest of these as our actual study size. We may find that the study size required to detect one or more of the exposure–outcome relationships in which we are interested is clearly beyond the available resources. For instance, we may be interested in examining the relationship between birthweight and the occurrence of benign breast diseases and breast cancer. The study size calculations may reveal that our sample will be sufficient to ensure that the study will have enough power or precision to examine the relationship between birthweight and benign breast diseases but will be far too small to examine the relationship between birthweight and breast cancer incidence. If we are unable to increase the sample size to the desired level, we will have to restrict the objectives of the study and consider benign breast disorders as the only outcome of interest.

15.4.2 Refusals and losses to follow-up

Refusals and/or losses to follow-up are likely to occur in epidemiological studies because subjects move away from the study area, die from some cause unrelated to the outcome of interest, refuse to continue with the study, etc. These losses reduce the size of the study available for analysis and, therefore, decrease the power or precision of the study. We can compensate for these losses by increasing the initial study size. For example, if study size calculations suggest that 320 subjects are required, and a 20% loss to follow-up is expected, the study size should be increased to about 400 (400 − 400 × 0.20 = 320). Note, however, that although this strategy will ensure that the study will have the required power or precision, it will not avoid the possibility of *selection bias*, as the individuals who refuse to participate or are lost to follow-up may differ in important respects from those who remain in the study.

15.4.3 Unequal sized groups

There are situations where we may wish to study groups of different sizes. For example, when the number of available cases and controls is large and the cost of obtaining information from both groups is comparable, the optimal control-to-case ratio is 1:1. However, if the available number of cases for the study is limited, or when the cost of obtaining information is greater for cases than controls, the number of controls per case can be increased to achieve the necessary power or precision. For example, a study with 100 cases and 100 controls has the same power as a study with 75 cases and 150 controls, or one with 63 cases and 252 controls, or one with 55 cases and 550 controls. It is usually not recommended to increase the control:case ratio beyond 4:1, because there is only a small increase in statistical power with each additional control beyond this point. This small increase in power is generally not worth the increase in logistics and costs of recruiting a much larger total number of subjects unless the data for the controls are available at very little extra cost.

15.4.4 Confounding and interaction

The sample size estimations presented here refer to *crude* measures. In most studies, however, it is essential to control for confounding variables by calculating *adjusted* measures. These adjustments usually lead to a loss of power or precision of the study. However, this loss is substantial only when a very strong confounding variable is present (Smith & Day, 1984).

In contrast, and as discussed in the previous chapter, studies designed with the aim of detecting interactions require much larger sample sizes than those designed to look for simple effects (Smith & Day, 1984). In practice, this restricts the number of studies that can be carried out explicitly to examine interactions.

15.4.5 Special study designs

The sample size calculations for case–control studies presented in this chapter referred to *unmatched* studies. Methods for calculation of adequate sample sizes for matched case–control studies are given in Breslow & Day (1980).

The methods presented in this chapter assume that *individuals* rather than *groups* are the units of study. The calculations would be different if, for instance, the unit of study were communities (see Smith & Morrow, 1996).

Box 15.1. Key issues

- Sample size calculations can be made to ensure that:

  1. the study has enough *power*, i.e., ability to detect a statistically significant result if the true magnitude of the effect is as anticipated. Thus, this approach focuses on the significance test that will be performed at the end of the study.

  2. the sample estimates are *precise*, i.e., the level of sampling error is low. This approach focuses on the width of the confidence interval.

- Sample size calculations based on power may be appropriate to identify new exposures when it is not known whether they will have any effect at all on the outcome(s) of interest. If, however, it is already known that the exposure is associated with the outcome, the objective of the study should be to quantify the magnitude of the effect as precisely as possible rather than just testing the null hypothesis of no effect. In these circumstances, sample size calculations should be based on precision.

- Sample size calculations should be taken as providing only a rough idea of the number of subjects that need to be recruited. Other considerations such as availability of subjects, resources, costs, etc. should be considered carefully.

Further reading

* The power calculations presented in Section 15.2 follow the approach suggested by Clayton & Hills (1993).

* Sample size calculations for more complex designs of cohort, case–control and intervention studies are given respectively in Breslow & Day (1987, 1980) and Smith & Morrow (1996).

Chapter 16
Cancer prevention

16.1 Introduction

The preceding chapters of this book have focused on principles and methods needed to study the determinants of disease and their effects. The ultimate goal of epidemiology, however, is to provide knowledge that will help in the formulation of public health policies aimed at preventing the development of disease in healthy persons.

Nearly all important issues in cancer prevention are linked to the natural history of the disease 'cancer', which can be summarized as shown in Figure 16.1. Here, point A indicates the biological onset of the disease and the start of the pre-clinical phase. This may be the point at which an irreversible set of events (e.g., gene mutation) takes place. As a result of progression of the disease, symptoms and/or signs appear that bring the patient to medical attention and diagnosis at point C. This is the end of the pre-clinical phase, which is the period from A to C, and the beginning of the clinical phase of the natural history. The disease may then progress to cure (D_1), to permanent illness and disability (D_2) or to death (D_3). The time from initial symptoms and/or signs to cure, permanent illness or death may reflect the effects of treatments given, as well as the underlying characteristics of the untreated disease.

Implicit in this scheme is the notion that a disease evolves over time and that, as this occurs, pathological changes may become irreversible. The aim of prevention is to stop this progression.

There are various levels of prevention:

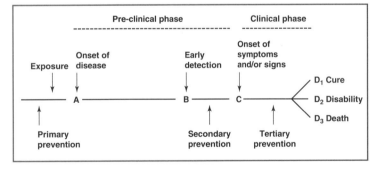

Figure 16.1.
Natural history of the disease 'cancer' and levels of prevention.

* *Primary prevention* is prevention of disease by reducing exposure of individuals to risk factors or by increasing their resistance to them, and thus avoiding the occurrence of event A.

* *Secondary prevention* (applied during the pre-clinical phase) is the early detection and treatment of disease. Screening activities are an important component of secondary prevention. In Figure 16.1, point B indicates the point in time at which the disease is first detectable by an appropriate screening test. For example, it might refer to the time at which a cancer mass reaches the min-

imum size that can be seen by X-ray examination. Thus, the distance from point B to C represents the 'detectable pre-clinical phase'. The location of point B varies markedly from one individual to another, and also depends on the screening technique used.

* *Tertiary prevention* (appropriate in the clinical phase) is the use of treatment and rehabilitation programmes to improve the outcome of illness among affected individuals.

In the rest of this chapter, we consider each of these levels of prevention in detail.

16.2 Primary prevention

The purpose of primary prevention is to limit the incidence of cancer by controlling exposure to risk factors or increasing individuals' resistance to them (e.g., by vaccination or chemoprevention). Clearly, the first step is to identify the relevant exposures and to assess their impact on the risk of the disease in the population.

16.2.1 How important is a particular exposure?

Relative and absolute measures of exposure effect

Much of epidemiology is concerned with identifying the risk factors for a disease, health problem or state of health. In assessing the strength of the association between a particular exposure and a particular outcome, we calculate measures known as *relative measures of effect*. As shown in Section 5.2.1, there are three types of relative measure (risk ratio, rate ratio and odds ratio) which are often collectively called relative risk.

Relative measures of effect provide answers to the question: *How many times more likely are people exposed to a putative risk factor to develop the outcome of interest relative to those unexposed, assuming that the only difference between the two groups is the exposure under study?* The magnitude of the relative risk is an important consideration (but not the only one—see Chapter 13) in establishing whether a particular exposure is a cause of the outcome of interest.

Once we have established that an exposure is *causally* associated with the outcome of interest, it is important to express the absolute magnitude of its impact on the occurrence of the disease in the exposed group (see Section 5.2.2). If we have information on the usual risk (or rate) of a particular disease in the absence of the exposure, as well as in its presence, we can determine the *excess risk* (also known as *attributable risk*) associated with the exposure.

Excess risk = risk (or rate) in the exposed – risk (or rate) in the unexposed

It is useful to express the excess risk in relation to the total risk (or rate) of the disease among those exposed to the factor under study. This measure is called *excess fraction* (also known as *excess risk percentage* or *attributable risk percentage*). It describes the proportion of disease in the *exposed group* which is attributable to the exposure.

Excess fraction (%) = 100 × (excess risk / risk (or rate) in the exposed)

Alternatively, it can be calculated by using the following formula:

Excess fraction (%) = 100 × (relative risk – 1) / relative risk

Example 16.1. *Suppose that a cohort study was conducted in the town of Minas Gerais (Brazil) to assess the relationship between cigarette smoking and lung cancer in men. We assume, for simplicity, that smokers and non-smokers were similar with respect to other risk factors for lung cancer such as age and occupational exposures. The results are shown in Table 16.1.*

	Smokers	Non-smokers	All
Number of cases	120	10	130
Person-years	54 545	50 000	104 545
Rate per 100 000 pyrs	220	20	124

Table 16.1.
Lung cancer incidence in smokers and non-smokers: hypothetical data.

In this study, the rate ratio is

220 per 100 000 pyrs / 20 per 100 000 pyrs = 11

and the excess risk associated with smoking (assuming causality) is

Excess risk = 220 per 100 000 pyrs – 20 per 100 000 pyrs = 200 per 10 000 pyrs

To assess what proportion 200 per 100 000 pyrs is of the rate among smokers (220 per 100 000 pyrs), we can calculate the excess fraction:

Excess fraction (%) = 100 × (200 per 100 000 pyrs / 220 per 100 000 pyrs) = 91%

This is the proportion of lung cancer cases in smokers attributable to smoking.

Excess fraction provides an answer to the question: *What is the proportion of new cases of disease in the exposed that can be attributed to exposure?* Another way of using this concept is to think of it as the decrease in the incidence of a disease that would have been seen if the exposed had never been exposed. Thus, in Example 16.1, a maximum of 91% of lung cancer cases in smokers could theoretically have been prevented if they had never smoked.

If the exposure is *protective,* analogous measures can be calculated. They are usually called *risk reduction* (also known as *prevented risk*) and *prevented fraction* (also known as *prevented risk percentage*).

Risk reduction = risk (or rate) in the unexposed – risk (or rate) in the exposed

Prevented fraction (%) = 100 × (risk reduction / risk (or rate) in the unexposed)

Example 16.2. A large randomized trial was carried out to assess the value of a smoking cessation programme (the intervention) in reducing the occurrence of lung cancer among smokers. By the end of the trial, the incidence of lung cancer was 155 per 100 000 pyrs among those who received the intervention and 240 per 100 000 pyrs among the controls. Thus, the maximum benefit achieved by the intervention was

Risk reduction = 240 per 100 000 pyrs – 155 per 100 000 pyrs = 85 per 10 000 pyrs

Thus, 85 new cases of lung cancer per 100 000 pyrs were prevented by the smoking cessation programme.

Prevented fraction (%) = 100 × (85 per 100 000 pyrs/ 240 per 100 000 pyrs) = 35%

Thus 35% of the expected lung cancer cases among smokers were prevented by the smoking cessation programme.

Prevented fraction tends to be appreciably smaller than excess fraction (Example 16.2). This is because it is generally impossible to eliminate the exposure completely and, even if possible, the incidence of the disease in those who stop being exposed may never fall to the level in those who have never been exposed.

Calculation of excess risk (or risk reduction) requires information on the incidence of disease in the exposed and unexposed groups. This information is directly available in cohort and intervention studies. For case–control studies, however, it is not possible to calculate the excess risk using the formula given above, because incidence of disease among the exposed and unexposed groups is not known. We can still calculate excess fraction using the formula based on relative risk, which in these studies is estimated by the odds ratio. Alternative formulae can, however, be used in population-based case–control studies to calculate excess risk. These are presented in Appendix 16.1.

Measures of population impact

The measures of effect discussed so far compared the incidence of the disease in the *exposed* group with the incidence in the unexposed group. To assess the extra disease incidence in the *study population* as a whole that can be attributed to the exposure, we can calculate a measure called the *population excess risk* (also known as *population attributable risk*). This is defined as

Population excess risk = risk (or rate) in the population – risk (or rate) in the unexposed

or, similarly, as

Population excess risk = excess risk × proportion of the population exposed to the risk factor

---

Example 16.3. *Returning to the hypothetical study described in Example 16.1, the proportion of smokers in the whole cohort was 52%. If this 52% of the study population that smoked had never smoked, their incidence of lung cancer would have been reduced from 220 to 20 cases per 100 000 pyrs.*

Population excess risk = (220 per 100 000 pyrs – 20 per 100 000 pyrs) × 0.52 = 104 per 100 000 pyrs

Similarly, the population excess risk can be calculated by subtracting the rate in the unexposed group from the rate in the total study population. The rate in the total study population was 124 per 100 000 pyrs (Table 16.1). Thus,

Population excess risk = 124 per 100 000 pyrs – 20 per 100 000 pyrs = 104 per 100 000 pyrs

Thus, 104 cases of lung cancer per 100 000 pyrs could have been prevented in the whole study population if none of the smokers had ever smoked.

Analogously to the excess risk among exposed individuals, the *population excess risk* is a measure of the risk of disease in the *study population* which is attributable to an exposure (Example 16.3). We can express the population excess risk in relation to the total risk of the disease in the whole population. This measure is the *population excess fraction* (also known as *population attributable fraction*).

$$\text{Population excess fraction (\%)} = 100 \times \frac{\text{population excess risk}}{\text{rate (or risk) in the total population}}$$

Alternatively, it can be calculated by using the following formula:

$$\text{Population excess fraction (\%)} = 100 \times \frac{p_e \, (\text{relative risk} - 1)}{p_e \, (\text{relative risk} - 1) + 1}$$

where p_e represents the prevalence of exposure in the population under study.

> **Example 16.4.** *In Example 16.3, the population excess fraction would be*
>
> *Population excess fraction (%) = 104 per 100 000 pyrs/124 per 100 000 pyrs = 84%.*
>
> *This means that (assuming causality) approximately 84% of the lung cancer incidence in the study population is attributable to smoking. Thus, 84% of the lung cancer cases in this population would have been prevented if the smokers had never smoked.*

Population excess fraction is an important measure. It provides an answer to the question: *What proportion (fraction) of the new cases of disease observed in the study population is attributable to exposure to a risk factor?* It therefore indicates what proportion of the disease experience in the population could be prevented if exposure to the risk factor had never occurred (Example 16.4).

Note that the excess fraction among the exposed is always greater than the population excess fraction, since the study population includes already some unexposed people who, obviously, cannot benefit from elimination of the exposure.

Sometimes it is useful to calculate the population excess fraction for a much larger population than the study population. For instance, public health planners are particularly interested in using data from epidemiological studies conducted in subgroups of the population to estimate the proportion of cases in a region or in a country that are attributable to a particular exposure (Example 16.5). In this case, it is necessary to obtain data on the prevalence of exposure in these populations from other sources.

Table 16.2 shows how the population excess fraction varies in relation to the level of prevalence of the exposure in the population under study (p_e) and the magnitude of the relative risk. It is clear that the proportion of cases in a particular population that can be attributed to a particular exposure depends both on the magnitude of the relative risk and on the prevalence of the exposure in the population. For instance, tobacco smoking, with a relative risk of about 5, and occupational exposure to aromatic amines, with a relative risk of about 500, are implicated as causes of bladder cancer. Despite the fact that the relative risk is much smaller for smoking than for aromatic amines, the population excess fraction is sub-

Example 16.5. Returning to the previous example, a recent household survey conducted in the region of Minas Gerais revealed that the prevalence of smoking among men was 35%. Thus, the proportion of lung cancer cases occurring among men in the whole region that can be attributed to smoking can be calculated as

$$Population\ excess\ fraction\ (\%) = 100 \times \frac{0.35 \times (11-1)}{0.35 \times (11-1)+1} = 78\%$$

Thus, in this hypothetical example, 78% of the lung cancers in the whole male population of Minas Gerais could be attributed to smoking. Note that this is lower than the value for the study population itself, the explanation being that the prevalence of smoking was lower in the whole male population of Minas Gerais (35%) than in the study population (52%).

stantially higher for smoking because this exposure is far commoner than exposure to aromatic amines. It has been estimated that the population excess fraction for smoking in England is 46% in men (Morrison *et al.*, 1984), whereas the population excess fraction for all occupational exposures (including exposure to aromatic amines) is only between 4 and 19% (Vineis & Simonato, 1986). Thus, a much larger number of bladder cancer cases would be prevented by eliminating smoking than by eliminating occupational exposures.

Prevalence of exposure (p_e) (%)	Relative risk		
	2	5	10
10	0.09	0.29	0.47
25	0.20	0.50	0.69
50	0.33	0.67	0.82
75	0.43	0.75	0.87
95	0.49	0.79	0.90

Table 16.2.
Population excess fractions for different levels of prevalence of the exposure and various magnitudes of the relative risk.

These measures of population impact suffer from a number of limitations. Firstly, it has to be assumed that the risk factor is causally associated with the disease of interest. The criteria that may be used to assess whether an observed association is likely to be causal were discussed in Chapter 13. Secondly, it has to be assumed that there is no confounding or bias in the measures of incidence among exposed and unexposed groups. So far in our discussion we have, for simplicity, assumed that the exposed and unexposed groups were similar except for the exposure under study. This is rarely the case except in large randomized intervention trials. In our previous examples, for instance, we should have taken into account differences in the age distribution between smokers and non-smokers. This can be done by using techniques similar to those described in Chapter 14 to calculate *adjusted measures*. We can then use these adjusted measures to calculate absolute measures of effect and measures of population impact using the same formulae as before. Thirdly, we must remember that estimates of relative risk are generally derived from case–control, cohort or intervention studies. These studies are often conducted in special subgroups of the population such as migrants, manual workers, etc. However, levels of exposure and intrinsic susceptibility in these subgroups may be quite different from those in the general population. It is therefore important that the extrapolation of data from these studies to other populations is undertaken with caution. For instance, many cohort studies are based purposely on groups with exposure to much higher levels than the general population (e.g., occupational cohorts) and the relative risks obtained from them should not be used as such to provide estimates of population excess fractions for other populations with much lower levels of exposure. This may be overcome if levels of exposure are properly measured (rather than just 'exposed' versus 'unexposed') and estimates of population excess fractions take them into account.

We can calculate the proportion of a particular cancer in a certain population that is caused by diet, by alcohol, by smoking, etc. These percentages may add up to more than 100%. This is because each individual calculation of population excess fraction does not take into account the fact that these risk factors interact with each other. For instance, in calculating the proportion of laryngeal cancer due to smoking, we ignore the fact that some of the cancers that occurred among smokers only occurred because they were also exposed to alcohol.

16.2.2 Role and evaluation of primary preventive measures

Once the risk factors have been identified and their impact in the population estimated, it is important to consider methods to either eliminate or reduce the exposure to them. Primary prevention involves two strategies that are often complementary. It can focus on the whole population with the aim of reducing average risk (the *population strategy*) or on people at high risk (the *high-risk individual strategy*). Although the high-risk individual strategy, which aims to protect susceptible individuals, is most efficient for the people at greatest risk of a specific cancer, these people may contribute little to the overall burden of the disease in the population. For example, organ transplant patients are particularly susceptible to non-melanoma skin cancer (Bouwes Bavinck *et al.*, 1991). The tumour tends to develop in highly sun-exposed areas of the body. Primary prevention campaigns for organ-transplanted patients involving reduction of sun exposure and sunscreen use are likely to be of great benefit to these patients, but will have little impact on the overall burden of disease in the population, because organ transplant patients represent a very small proportion of the population. In this situation, the population strategy or a combination of both strategies should be applied.

The major advantage of the population strategy is that it is likely to produce greater benefits at the population level and does not require identification of high-risk individuals. Its main disadvantage is that it requires the participation of large groups of people to the benefit of relatively few. For example, adoption by a population of measures to reduce sun exposure may reduce the risk of skin cancer at a population level, but will be of little apparent benefit to most individuals, since the disease is rare even among those exposed. This phenomenon is called the *prevention paradox* (Rose, 1985).

Various approaches have been used to reduce or eliminate exposure to a particular risk factor, some examples of which are given in Box 16.1.

Box 16.1. Examples of approaches used to reduce or eliminate exposure to a hazard risk factor

• Health education on an individual or community basis (e.g., media campaigns promoting use of sunscreens).

• Regulation of carcinogens in occupational settings and in the environment (e.g., improvement of radiation protection).

• Price regulation (e.g., imposing taxes on cigarette and alcohol purchases).

• Advertising restrictions (e.g., banning of tobacco advertising or forcing the printing of health warnings on cigarette packages).

• Time and place restrictions on consumption (e.g., banning smoking in public places).

If specific preventive measures to reduce the incidence of a particular cancer have been adopted, it is essential to establish whether the effort has had any positive effect. Evaluation of primary preventive efforts at the population level is performed mainly in terms of monitoring changes in cancer incidence in relation to changes in exposure to risk factors. Thus, time trends in cancer incidence may be compared with temporal changes in exposure to a particular risk factor to show whether the desired effect is being achieved. This is illustrated in Figure 16.2, which shows trends in *per caput* consumption of cigarettes in the USA in relation to the timing of implementation of tobacco-control initiatives and important historical events, and trends in lung cancer mortality.

The following issues should be taken into account when interpreting incidence trends in relation to changes in exposure to risk factors. First, if the downward trend started long before the introduction of the preventive measure, it is difficult to attribute a recent decrease in incidence to the preventive measure under investigation. Second, given the long induction period of cancer, it may take many years or even decades before any effect of a preventive measure becomes apparent in incidence or mortality trends

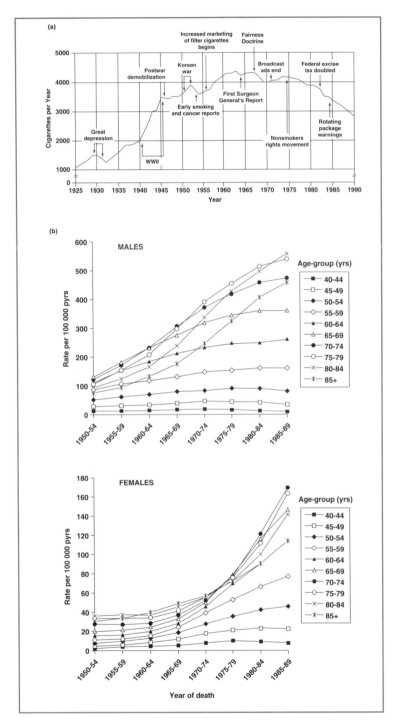

Figure 16.2.

(a) *Per caput* consumption of cigarettes among persons aged 18 years and over, United States of America, 1925–90 (reproduced from US Department of Health and Human Services, 1991) and (b) age-specific mortality trends from lung cancer, United States of America, 1950–89 (reproduced from Gilliland & Samet, 1994).

(except if the risk factor acts at late stages of carcinogenesis), as illustrated in Figure 16.2. Third, if the measures undertaken are directed to only a small fraction of the population (e.g., a region), the evaluation should be limited to the same sub-population, otherwise the effect may be missed. Fourth, when implementation has been confined to one area, comparisons of the changes in the intervention area versus 'control' areas may be possible.

Individual-based studies of subjects who have adopted potentially healthier habits or lifestyles are relatively few and were in the past confined mainly to the investigation of the risk of cancer in ex-smokers. Such studies show a marked decline in risk, which is related to the time since cessation of smoking, and they constitute the most powerful evidence for the effectiveness of stopping smoking in preventing cancer (Rose & Colwell, 1992; Gupta *et al.*, 1990). More recently, the potential of other changes in lifestyle (e.g., changes in diet) in cancer primary prevention have also been (or are currently being) assessed in large intervention trials (e.g. Alpha-Tocopherol, Beta Carotene Cancer Prevention Study Group, 1994; Hennekens *et al.*, 1996; Omenn *et al.*, 1996; Chlebowski & Grosvenor, 1994).

Individual-based studies have also helped to assess the effectiveness of preventive measures in the workplace. For instance, women first employed before 1925 in the watch dial-painting industry in the USA had greatly increased risks of mortality from bone cancer and from leukaemia and other haematological diseases, but risks declined for those employed in subsequent years (Table 16.3). The reduction in risk coincided with changes in work regulations in the industry, which included the prohibition of tipping or pointing of brushes between the lips in 1925–26 (Figure 16.3). These measures greatly reduced the exposure of the workers to radium.

Year of first employment	Bone cancer		Leukaemia and blood diseases	
	SMR (O/E)[b]	Observed no. of cases (O)	SMR (O/E)[b]	Observed no. of cases (O)
1915–19	233**	7	7.4*	2
1920–24	154**	20	3.3*	4
1925–29	10	1	1.0	1

[a] Data from Polednak *et al.* (1978)
[b] Expected numbers derived from cause-specific mortality rates for US white females
* $P < 0.05$; ** $P < 0.001$.

Table 16.3.
Mortality of women employed in US watch dial-painting industry and followed to end of 1975, by year of first employment.[a]

Other approaches to primary prevention are being evaluated, such as the use of mass vaccination campaigns (e.g., hepatitis B vaccine against liver cancer (Gambia Hepatitis Study Group, 1987)) and of chemoprevention (e.g., tamoxifen in prevention of breast cancer in high-risk women (Powles *et al.*, 1994)).

16.3 Secondary prevention

Secondary prevention refers to detection of cancer at an early stage, when treatment is more effective than at the time of usual diagnosis and treatment. With such measures it is possible to prevent the progression of the disease and its complications (including death).

16.3.1 Screening

Screening represents an important component of secondary prevention. It involves application of a relatively simple and inexpensive test to asymptomatic subjects in order to classify them as being likely or unlikely to have the disease which is the object of the screen. The positive cases can then be subjected to conventional diagnostic procedures and, if necessary, given appropriate treatment. Screening activities are based on the assumption that early detection and treatment will retard or stop the progression of established cases of disease, while later treatment is likely to be less effective. The ultimate objective of screening for a particular cancer is to reduce mortality from that disease among the subjects screened.

The concept of screening is not as straightforward as it may at first appear, however. Early treatment does not always improve prognosis and, even if it does, the true benefits of any type of screening have to be assessed in relation to its risks and costs and in relation to the benefits that may be derived from other public health activities. The final value of any screening programme can be established only by rigorous evaluation.

Any cancer screening activity requires (1) a suitable disease; (2) a suitable test and (3) a suitable screening programme.

Suitable disease

To be suitable for control by a programme of early detection and treatment, a disease must pass through a pre-clinical phase during which it is detectable (see Figure 16.1), and early treatment must offer some advantage over later treatment. Obviously, there is no point in screening for a

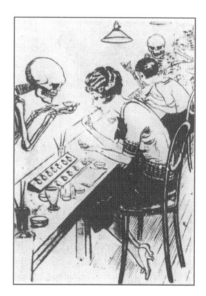

Figure 16.3.
New York newspaper cartoon alluding to the radium poisoning of watch dial painters

disease that cannot be detected before symptoms bring it to medical attention and, if early treatment is not especially helpful, there is no point in early detection.

Detectable pre-clinical phase

The pre-clinical phase of a cancer starts with the biological onset of the disease (point A in Figure 16.1). The disease then progresses and reaches a point at which it can be detected by the screening test (point B in Figure 16.1). From this point onwards, the pre-clinical phase of the disease is said to be 'detectable'. The starting point of this detectable pre-clinical phase depends partly on the characteristics of the individual and partly on the characteristics of the test being used. A test which can detect a very 'early' stage of the cancer is associated with a longer detectable pre-clinical phase than a test which can detect only more advanced lesions.

The proportion of a population that has detectable pre-clinical disease (its prevalence) is an important determinant of the utility of screening in controlling the disease. If the prevalence is very low, too few cases will be detected to justify the costs of the screening programme. At the time of initial screening, the prevalence of the pre-clinical phase is determined by its incidence and its average duration (recall the discussion on prevalence in Section 4.2). In subsequent screening examinations, however, the prevalence of the pre-clinical phase is determined mainly by its incidence, the duration being relatively unimportant if the interval between examinations is short. Therefore, the number of cases detected by the programme is greatest at the first screening examination, while the shorter the interval between examinations, the lower the number of cases detected per examination (and the higher the cost per case detected).

Early treatment

For screening to be of benefit, treatment given during the detectable pre-clinical phase must result in a lower mortality than therapy given after symptoms develop. For example, cancer of the uterine cervix develops slowly, taking perhaps more than a decade for the cancer cells, which are initially confined to the outer layer of the cervix, to progress to a phase of invasiveness. During this pre-invasive stage, the cancer is usually asymptomatic but can be detected by screening using the Papanicolaou (or Pap) smear test. The prognosis of the disease is much better if treatment begins during this stage than if the cancer has become invasive.

On the other hand, if early treatment makes no difference because the prognosis is equally good (or equally bad) whether treatment is begun before or after symptoms develop, the application of a screening test will be neither necessary nor effective and it may even be harmful (see below).

Relative burden of disease

Prevalence, incidence or mortality rates can be used to assess whether a cancer has sufficient public health importance to warrant instituting a screening programme. Even if a disease is very rare but it is very serious and easily preventable, it may be worth screening for it. The final judgement will depend on the benefits, costs and cost/benefit ratio in relation to other competing health care needs.

Suitable test

For a screening programme to be successful, it must be directed at a suitable disease with a suitable test. In order to assess the suitability of a screening test, it is necessary to consider its validity and acceptability.

Validity

The preliminary assessment of a screening test should involve studies of its reliability, which is evaluated as intra- and inter-observer variation (see Section 2.6). Although even perfect reliability does not ensure validity, an

---

Box 16.2. Sensitivity, specificity and predictive value of a screening test

		Gold standard	
		Positive	**Negative**
Screening test	Positive	*a*	*b*
	Negative	*c*	*d*

True positives = *a*   False positives = *b*
True negatives = *d*   False negatives = *c*

- The *sensitivity* of the screening test is the proportion of individuals classified as positives by the gold standard who are correctly identified by the screening test:

    Sensitivity = $a/(a + c)$

- The *specificity* of the screening test is the proportion of those classified as negatives by the gold standard who are correctly identified by the screening test:

    Specificity = $d/(b + d)$

- The *predictive value of a positive screening test result* represents the probability that someone with a positive screening test result really has the disease:

    Predictive value of a positive screening test = $a/(a + b)$

- The *predictive value of a negative screening test result* represents the probability that someone with a negative screening test result does not really have the disease:

    Predictive value of a negative screening test = $d/(c + d)$

---

unreliable test will not be sufficiently valid to be of use. On the other hand, a test that is highly valid must be highly reliable.

The validity of the screening test can be expressed by its sensitivity and specificity. These measure the ability of the test to identify correctly diseased and non-diseased people (see Box 16.2 and Section 2.6 for a review of the concepts). In the ideal situation, tests would be 100% sensitive and 100% specific. In this perfect situation, the distribution of the screening test results among individuals with the disease is completely separated from the distribution in healthy individuals. In Figure 16.4(a), everyone affected by the disease will have a test result which is above a chosen cut-off value located between these two distributions. Unfortunately, reality is more complex. In general, the distributions of the screening test results in the disease-free and diseased subjects overlap (Figure 16.4(b)). In these situations, the location of the cut-off value to classify screening test results as positive or negative is arbitrary. In Figure 16.4(b), some disease-affected subjects, having values below the chosen cut-off value, will be missed by the screening test, whereas some disease-free people will be wrongly classified as positive. Thus, there is generally a trade-off between the sensitivity and specificity of a given screening test; its ability to detect as many true cases as possible (high sensitivity) can only be increased at the expense of an increase in the number of individuals without the disease who will erroneously be classified as positive by the screening test (low specificity) and vice versa (see Section 2.6.1 for a numerical example of this).

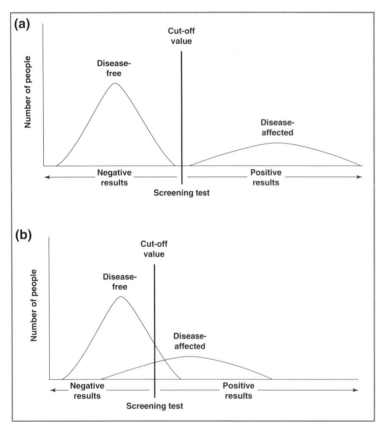

Figure 16.4.
Distribution of results from a screening test in disease-free and disease-affected individuals: (a) ideal distribution without overlap; (b) overlap of the distributions with the inevitable trade-off of sensitivity and specificity. In this example, where the screening test tends to give higher values for people with the disease than for those without it, moving the cut-off value to the left (i.e., lowering its value) increases sensitivity but decreases specificity; moving it to the right (i.e., increasing its value) increases specificity but decreases sensitivity.

Sensitivity is an indicator of the yield of cases (i.e., the number of truly diseased cases identified by the programme), whereas specificity is an indicator of the number of false-positive test results. Although one would like to detect all the subjects with the disease in a screening programme by using a test with a maximum sensitivity, such a policy might lead to an unacceptably low specificity, entailing high costs because of the need for further investigation of large numbers of false positives and a risk of poor motivation of subjects to participate in subsequent screening examinations. Hence, the choice of the cut-off point depends on the relative costs of false positives and false negatives.

In practice, however, it is difficult to estimate the sensitivity of the test, since it is not possible to apply a 'gold standard test' to the screened population to find out the total number of diseased subjects ($a + c$ in Box 16.2). The screening test gives us only the value of a, that is, the number of persons who had a positive screening test and were confirmed to have the condition after further diagnostic evaluation. The usual approach to estimating sensitivity is to follow up subjects (usually for one year) having negative screening results, in order to observe how many cancers eventually develop among them. These '*interval*' cases are regarded as false negatives (c). The sensitivity of the screening test can then be calculated as usual. However, the value of this approach is limited since it is difficult to achieve complete follow-up and because some of the 'interval' cancers may have been true negatives at the time of the screening examination (i.e., very fast-growing tumours).

It is easier to estimate specificity if the screening is aimed at a rare condition such as cancer. Practically all those screened (N) are disease-free and thus N can be used to estimate the total number of people not affected by the condition ($b + d$ in Box 16.2). Since all screen-positive subjects are further investigated, the number of false positives (b in Box 16.2) is also known and, therefore, the number of true negatives (d in Box 16.2) can be calculated as $N - b$. Specificity can then be estimated as $(N - b)/N$.

Acceptability and costs

In addition to having adequate validity, a screening test should be low in cost, convenient, simple and as painless as possible, and should not cause any complications. Many screening tests meet these criteria—the Pap smear test for cervical precancerous lesions is a good example. In contrast, although sigmoidoscopic screening might lead to a reduction in mortality from colon cancer, it is questionable whether such a test would be acceptable because of the expense, the discomfort and the risk of bowel perforation.

Suitable screening programme

The organized application of early diagnosis and treatment activities in large groups is often designated as *mass screening* or *population screening*, and the set of procedures involved described as a *screening programme*.

A screening programme must encompass a diagnostic and a therapeutic component, because early detection that is not followed by treatment is useless for disease control. The diagnostic component includes the screening policy and the procedures for diagnostic evaluation of people with positive screening test results. The screening policy should specify precisely who is to be screened, at what age, at what frequency, with what test, etc., and it should be dynamic rather than fixed. The therapeutic component is the process by which confirmed cases are treated. It should also be dynamic and be regulated by strict universal procedures which offer the best current treatment to all identified cases.

A screening programme is a complex undertaking involving the application of a particular test to a particular population in a particular setting. Circumstances vary in different countries, and it should not be assumed that a format suitable for one country will apply to another without rigorous prior testing and evaluation. Box 16.3 lists the essential features of an organized screening programme.

Box 16.3. Essential features of an organized screening programme

• There is a clear definition of the target population.

• The individuals to be screened are identifiable (e.g., list with names and addresses of all eligible individuals in the target population).

• Measures are available to ensure high coverage and attendance (e.g., personal letter of invitation).

• There are adequate field facilities for collecting the screening material and adequate laboratory facilities to examine it.

• There is an organized quality-control programme to assess the screen material and its interpretation.

• Adequate facilities exist for diagnosis and appropriate treatment of confirmed neoplastic lesions and for the follow-up of treated individuals.

• There is a carefully designed referral system for management of any abnormality found, and for providing information about normal screening tests.

• Evaluation and monitoring of the total programme is organized so that it is possible to calculate incidence and mortality rates separately for those participating and those not participating in the programme, at the level of the total target population. Quality control of these epidemiological data should be established.

(modified from Hakama *et al.*, 1986)

16.3.2 Evaluation of screening programmes

Even after a disease is determined to be appropriate for screening and a valid test becomes available, it will remain unclear whether a widespread screening programme for that disease should be implemented in a particular population. It is therefore necessary to evaluate a potential screening programme to assess whether it is worth introducing it as a public health measure to control a particular cancer. This involves consideration of two issues: first, whether the organization of the proposed programme is *feasible* and *cost-effective* (low cost per case detected), and second, whether it will be *effective in reducing the burden of the disease*. Both must be considered carefully. The implementation of a screening programme, no matter how cost-effective, will not be warranted if it does not accomplish its goal of reducing morbidity and mortality in the target population.

Process measures

The feasibility, acceptability and costs of a programme may be evaluated by *process measures*, which are related to the administrative and organizational aspects of the programme such as identification of the target population, number of persons examined, proportion of the target population examined, facilities for diagnosis and treatment in the health services, functioning of the referral system and its compliance, total costs, cost per case detected, etc. The major advantage of these process measures is that they are readily obtained and are helpful in monitoring the activity of the programme. Their main limitation is that they do not provide any indication of whether those screened have lower mortality from the cancer being targetted by the programme than those who were not screened.

A particularly useful process measure is the predictive value of a positive test. The predictive positive value (PPV) represents the proportion of persons found to have the disease in question after further diagnostic evaluation out of all those who were positive for the screening test ($a/(a+b)$ in Box 16.2). A high PPV suggests that a reasonably high proportion of the costs of a programme are in fact being spent for the detection of disease during its pre-clinical phase. A low PPV suggests that a high proportion of the costs are being wasted on the detection and diagnostic evaluation of false positives (people whose screening result is positive but did not appear to have the disease on subsequent diagnostic investigation). It is important to emphasize, however, that the PPV is a proportional measure; a high PPV might be obtained even if the frequency of case detection is unacceptably low. For instance, the PPV may be 80% indicating that 80% of those who screened positive were truly diseased. However, if only 10 subjects screen positive, the number of cases detected by the programme will be only 8! The main advantage of this measure is that it is available soon after the screening programme is initiated and, in contrast to sensitivity, no follow-up is necessary for it to be estimated.

The PPV of a screening test depends upon both the number of true positives a and the number of false positives b (see Box 16.2). Thus, it can be increased by either increasing the number of true positives or decreasing the number of false positives. The number of true positives may be increased by increasing the prevalence of detectable pre-clinical disease, for instance, by screening less frequently so as to maintain the prevalence of pre-clinical disease in the target population at a higher level. The number of false positives may be reduced by increasing the specificity of the test, that is, by changing the criterion of positivity or by repeating the screening test after a positive test. A low PPV is more likely to be the result of poor specificity than of poor sensitivity. It is the specificity of a test that determines the number of false positives in people without the disease, who are the vast majority of people tested in virtually any programme. The sensitivity is less important for a rare disease because it operates on fewer people. By contrast, a small loss of specificity can lead to a large increase in the number of false positives, and a large loss of PPV.

Effectiveness in reducing mortality

The second, and definitive, aspect of evaluating a screening programme is whether it is effective in reducing morbidity and mortality from the disease being screened. Even if a screening programme will accurately and inexpensively identify large numbers of individuals with pre-clinical disease, it will have little public health value if early diagnosis and treatment do not have an impact on the ultimate outcome of those cases.

Obtaining an accurate estimate of a reduction in mortality requires a long-term follow-up of large populations. Consequently, *intermediate outcome measures* such as stage at diagnosis and survival (case-fatality) have been used which may be available in the early years of a screening programme. For example, in a successful screening programme, the stage distribution of the cancers detected should be shifted towards the less advanced stages and the risk of dying from cancer (case-fatality) should be lower for cases detected through screening than for symptom-diagnosed cases.

There are, however, critical shortcomings associated with the use of these intermediate endpoints. Absence of a change in the parameters may mean that the screening is not successful, but they do not provide an adequate measure of evaluation because they suffer from a number of biases, namely, length bias, lead-time bias and overdiagnosis bias.

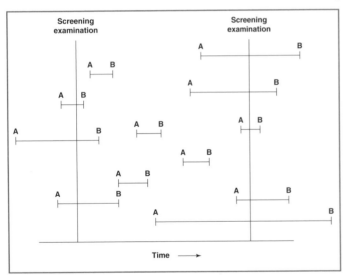

Figure 16.5.
Diagram illustrating length bias (see text). Each line represents a case from the point where it becomes detectable by the screening test (A) to the point where clinical symptoms or signs occur

(a) *Length bias.* Length bias refers to the phenomenon occurring when cases detected by a screening programme are not a random sample from the general distribution of all cases of pre-clinical disease in the screened population. This is likely to happen when screening tests are applied at moderately long intervals (say once every 2–5 years), so that cases with a long pre-clinical phase are more likely to be detected than those with faster-growing tumours (Figure 16.5). Hence, the cases detected by screening may be those with lesions having a more favourable prognosis, while cases with similar onset date but more rapid disease progression are detected by clinical symptoms. The resulting length bias could lead to an erroneous conclusion that screening was beneficial when, in fact, observed differences in survival (case-fatality) were a result merely of the detection of less rapidly fatal cases through screening.

(*b*) *Lead-time bias.* If an individual participates in a screening programme and has disease detected earlier than it would have been in the absence of screening, the amount of time by which diagnosis is advanced as a result of screening is the *lead time.* Since screening is applied to asymptomatic individuals, by definition every case detected by screening will have had its diagnosis advanced by some amount of time. Whether the lead time is a matter of days, months, or years, however, will vary according to the disease, the individual, and the screening procedure. Cases progressing rapidly from pre-clinical to clinical disease will gain less lead time from screening than those that develop slowly, with a long pre-clinical phase. The amount of lead time will also depend on how soon the screening is performed after the pre-clinical phase becomes detectable. Because of the lead-time phenomenon, the point of diagnosis is advanced in time and survival as measured from diagnosis is automatically lengthened for cases detected by screening, even if total length of life is not increased. This is referred as lead-time bias.

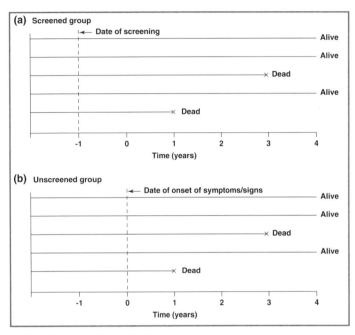

Figure 16.6.
Diagram illustrating lead-time bias. The lines represent the survival experience of each cancer case in the screened and unscreened groups (see text).

Suppose that 100 individuals were screened for a particular cancer for which there is no effective treatment. On average, the test succeeds in identifying the cancer one year before it becomes clinically evident. A similar unscreened group of 100 patients was also assembled. These two groups were followed up for five years and five persons were detected as having this cancer in each of them.

Let us examine the survival experience of the five cases in each of the groups. The course of their illness is shown in Figure 16.6. The 1.5-year survival for the screened group is 100% (all of them were still alive 1.5 year after being screened), whereas the 1.5-year survival for the unscreened group was only 80% (one case died one year after the onset of symptoms), even though the two groups have the same duration of survival (given our initial assumption of no effective treatment).

The problem with this analysis is that the starting point for monitoring survival is different between the screened and unscreened cases, always to the apparent detriment of the cases detected without screening. The appropriate approach is to compare the mortality experience of the 100 screened people with the mortality experience of the 100 unscreened people *from the time of screening*. In the above example, the mortality rate in the screened group is two deaths in 496 person-years (98 persons × 5 years, plus 1 person × 4 years, plus 1 person × 2 years). The rate is the same in the unscreened group, since the number of person-years, counted from the time the screening would have taken place had it been done, is identical to that for the screened group.

There are two ways in which the effect of lead time on the evaluation of the efficacy of a screening programme can be taken into account. The first is to compare not the length of survival from diagnosis to death, but rather the mortality rates in the screened and unscreened groups (as done in the above example). Alternatively, if the lead time for a given disease can be estimated, it can be taken into account, allowing comparison of the survival experience of screen- and symptom-detected cases. For example, the average lead time for breast cancer has been estimated as approximately one year (Shapiro *et al.*, 1974). Thus, to evaluate the efficacy of a breast cancer screening programme, the two-, three-, four-, five- and six-year survival risks of the screened cases should be compared, respectively, with the one-, two-, three-, four- and five-year survival risks of the unscreened cases. However, determinations of lead time are difficult to carry out and cannot be generalized, since they depend on the ability of the screening procedure to detect pre-clinical conditions.

(c) Overdiagnosis. It is possible that many of the lesions detected by the screening programme would never have led to invasive cancer and death. These lesions are known as 'pseudo-cancer'. Thus, the true benefit of identifying pre-clinical lesions through screening may be much smaller than is perceived.

In short, although intermediate outcome measures, such as stage distribution and case fatality (survival), may appear to be suitable as surrogate endpoints in a screening programme, they are subject to lead time bias, length bias and overdiagnosis bias. Thus, the ultimate outcome measure which should be evaluated in screening programmes aimed at detecting early cancer (e.g., breast and colon cancer screening) is reduction in mortality. When screening is aimed at detecting both pre-cancerous conditions and early cancers (e.g., cervical cancer screening), reduction in the incidence of invasive cancer and reduction in mortality are suitable outcome measures. This implies that any screening programme should be planned in such a way that its evaluation in terms of change in mortality (and incidence) in the total target population is possible.

An illustration of how intermediate outcomes may be misleading is given in Example 16.6. In this example, intermediate outcomes seemed to indicate that the use of chest X-ray and cytology was effective in lung cancer screening. However, no reduction in mortality was observed. Similar results have consistently been found in all randomized trials that have addressed this issue.

Example 16.6. A total of 6364 cigarette-smoking males aged 40–64 years were randomized into an intervention group which received six-monthly screening by chest X-ray and sputum cytology during three years, and a control group which received a single examination at the end of the third year. Lung cancer cases detected by screening were identified at an earlier stage, were more often resectable, and had a significantly better survival than symptom-detected cases. There was, however, no significant difference in mortality between the intervention and control groups (Kubik et al., 1990).

Studies to evaluate the effectiveness of a screening programme
Intervention studies

The randomized trial is the best study design for evaluating the effectiveness of a screening programme, because it provides the opportunity for a rigorous experimental evaluation. When the sample size is sufficiently large, control of confounding is virtually assured by the process of randomization. Patient self-selection or volunteer bias, which is problematic for the comparison of screened and unscreened groups in observational studies, cannot influence the validity of the results of randomized trials, since the screening programme is allocated at random by the investigators after individuals have agreed to participate in the trial.

There are various problems with randomized trials, however. First, there can be contamination of the control group (awareness of the screening programme may lead subjects in the control group to seek screening). Second, a large number of subjects may be required in screening trials for diseases with low incidence rate, such as most cancers, and/or if the trial is designed to show small benefits (as in Example 16.7). Third, it may be unacceptable to randomize some subjects to be non-screened if a screening programme has already been introduced despite the lack of experimental evidence (e.g., screening for cervical cancer).

Example 16.7. A randomized controlled trial was set up in Sweden in 1977 to assess the efficacy of mass screening with single-view mammography in reducing mortality from breast cancer. A total of 162 981 women aged 40 years or more and living in the counties of Kopparberg and Östergötland were randomized to either be or not be offered screening every 2 or 3 years, depending on age. The results to the end of 1984 showed that among women aged 40–74 years at the time of entry, there was a 31% reduction in mortality from breast cancer in the group invited for screening (Tabár et al., 1985).

Observational studies

While randomized trials can provide the best and most valid evidence concerning the efficacy of a screening programme, as with the evaluation of etiological hypotheses, most evidence on the effects of screening programmes will come from the non-experimental study designs because of issues of costs, ethics and feasibility. Especially in the numerous situations where randomized trials are not possible, such as with well established procedures like the Pap smear, observational approaches can provide useful and necessary information. Interpretation of the results from these studies is less straightforward, however.

Ecological studies have been used to examine trends in disease rates in relation to screening frequencies within a population, or to compare the relationship between the frequencies of screening and disease rates for different populations (as in Example 16.8). Such studies can be useful in suggesting that a relationship exists between screening and a decline in morbidity or mortality, but the inherent limitations of ecological studies must be borne in mind. First, since the information from such studies concerns populations rather than individuals, it is not possible to establish that those experiencing the decreased mortality are in fact the same persons who were screened (the *ecological fallacy*; see Section 11.2.2). Moreover, such studies cannot allow for control of potential confounding factors. Finally, the measure of screening frequency employed is usually an average value for the population, so that it is not possible to determine an optimal screening strategy for an individual. Thus, ecological studies may suggest the

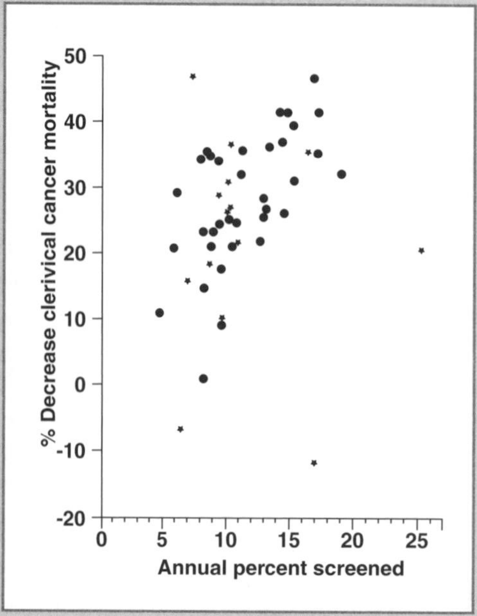

Figure 16.7.
Change in cervical cancer mortality between 1950–54 and 1965–69 in relation to estimated average annual percentage of women aged 19 years and over screened during 1953–68, by state of the USA. The stars indicate the less populous states (i.e., accumulated female population aged 19 years or over of less than five million during the study period) (reproduced, by permission of Wiley-Liss Inc., a subsidiary of John Wiley & Sons, Inc., from Cramer, 1974).

Example 16.8. To assess whether declines in cervical cancer mortality in the USA were related to screening, the change in cervical cancer mortality between 1950–54 and 1965–69 in the various states was examined in relation to the proportion of women screened in each one. The results are shown in Figure 16.7. There was a positive correlation between the magnitude of the decrease in mortality rates and the screening effort in each state. The positive relationship becomes more evident if the less populous states are excluded from the analysis (correlation coefficient (r) = 0.60; P<0.0005 (Cramer, 1974). These results were consistent with a beneficial effect of cervical cytological screening. However this relationship may be confounded by other factors such as socioeconomic changes.

possibility of a benefit of a screening programme, but they cannot test that hypothesis.

Cohort studies require long-term follow-up of screened and unscreened subjects. However, in interpreting the results of such studies, the potential effects of self-selection of participants must be taken into account (Example 16.9).

Example 16.9. *To examine the protective effect of Pap-smear screening for cervical cancer, a cohort study was conducted in two counties in Sweden (Uppsala and Gävleborg) where organized cytological screening was introduced in 1967 and 1972, respectively. A total of 386 990 women resident at any time during 1968 to 1992 in these two counties were identified through the Population Register and enrolled into the study. Each woman's screening history was ascertained from computerized registers of Pap smears taken in the area and record-linkages allowed complete follow-up with regard to cancer incidence, out-migration and survival through to 1992. A total of 938 newly diagnosed cases of squamous cell cervical cancer occurred during the follow-up of this cohort. Women who were ever screened were found to have about half the risk of those never screened (rate ratio = 0.55; 95% confidence interval 0.51–0.61) (Sparén, 1996).*

In cohort studies such as that described in Example 16.9, the people undergoing screening are not chosen randomly and individuals who choose to be screened may differ both from those who refuse screening and from the population at large (selection bias). These volunteers may have very different prognoses compared with their unscreened counterparts. In general, volunteers tend to have better health and lower mortality rates than the general population and are more likely to adhere to prescribed medical regimens. On the other hand, those who volunteer for a screening programme may represent the 'worried well', that is, asymptomatic individuals who are at higher risk of developing the disease because of medical or family history, or any number of lifestyle characteristics. Such individuals may have an increased risk of mortality regardless of the efficacy of the screening programme. The direction of the potential selection bias may be difficult to predict and the magnitude of such effects even more difficult to quantify.

Case–control studies of screening involve comparison of the screening histories of subjects who do, or do not, exhibit the outcome which screening aims to prevent (death from cancer or incidence of invasive disease). Although case–control studies are increasingly used to evaluate screening programmes, they cannot replace experimental studies because they are liable to confounding and bias (for instance, cases may differ from controls in their ability to recall past screening). However, once a form of screening is widespread, case–control studies may make use of existing records so that recall bias should not arise. The first study of this kind compared the history of Pap smear screening in 212 hospital cases of invasive cervical cancer with age-matched neighbourhood controls (Clarke & Anderson, 1979). Fewer cases than controls had received a Pap smear during the five years before the year of diagnosis. The risk of invasive cervical cancer among women who had not had a Pap smear was about three times that of women who were screened, after controlling for socioeconomic status. The authors attempted to examine the impact of potential recall bias by comparing the data obtained through a sample of personal interviews with data from physicians' records. There was no evidence that the information obtained during the interviews was affected by recall bias.

> *Example 16.10. In Cali (Colombia), screening for cervical cancer has been offered to all sexually active women and routinely performed in pre-natal clinics since the late 1960s. To evaluate the role of Pap smear in preventing invasive carcinoma of the cervix in this population, a case–control study was carried out. A total of 204 cases with newly diagnosed invasive cervical cancer during the years 1977–81 were identified through the Cali population-based cancer registry and successfully interviewed. For each case, a neighbourhood control matched to year of birth of the case ± 2 years was selected. Cases and controls were interviewed about history of Pap smears performed for screening purposes during the period 12–72 months before the date on which the case was diagnosed. Examinations performed within 12 months of diagnosis were ignored because they were likely to be symptom- or disease-related. For each control, the inquiry covered the same calendar time interval as that of the matching case, as determined by her date of diagnosis. The risk of developing invasive carcinoma was 10 times greater in unscreened than in screened women (Aristizabal et al., 1984).*

The use of case–control studies to evaluate screening programmes raises some special methodological issues. Tests done for diagnostic rather than screening purposes should not be considered and, for the controls, the screening history should be restricted up to the time of diagnosis of the case (as in Example 16.10) to ensure that cases and controls are fully comparable with respect to period of exposure to screening.

Case–control studies can be set up as an integral part of established screening programmes, in order to assess the screening policy (e.g., the age at which screening should be initiated or stopped, or the optimal frequency of screening).

16.3.3 Targeting high-risk groups

One way of reducing the costs of a screening programme is to target the screening towards groups of individuals at higher than average risk of developing the disease of interest. Most cancer screening programmes are limited to certain age-groups. For instance, it is not worth screening women under age 40 for breast cancer, because very few cases occur at these ages.

Screening programmes can also be targeted exclusively to high-risk groups defined on the basis of factors such as family history, medical history or occupation. For instance, targeting breast cancer screening programmes exclusively to women with a positive family history would increase the proportion of cases detected among screened women, but the large majority of cases in the population would be missed since they occur among people without a family history of this disease. Thus, restricting a screening programme to selected high-risk groups is useful only if a substantial fraction of all the cases in a population occur in these high-risk groups.

16.4 Tertiary prevention

Tertiary prevention consists of alleviation of disability resulting from disease in order to improve the outcome of illness among affected individuals. It includes not only the treatment itself, but also all rehabilitation attempts to restore an affected individual to a useful, satisfying, and, where possible, self-sufficient role in society.

Randomized clinical trials are the only acceptable method to evaluate cancer treatments (see Chapter 7). However, data from population-based cancer registries may provide a more representative picture for evaluating comprehensive cancer care in a particular population, since they will include all cancer cases in the population regardless of the treatment they might or might not have received. These issues are further discussed in Section 17.6.2.

Box 16.4. Key issues

- Epidemiology is a key discipline of public health which provides the scientific background for formulation of policies aimed at preventing the development of disease in healthy persons.

- There are three levels of cancer prevention:

    (a) *Primary prevention* aimed at preventing the onset of the disease either by reducing exposure to risk factors or by increasing the individuals' resistance to them. Measures of population impact are very useful in helping to identify exposures that are potentially responsible for large numbers of cases of a particular cancer in the population.

    (b) *Secondary prevention* aimed at reducing mortality from a particular cancer through early detection and treatment. Screening programmes are an important part of secondary prevention.

    (c) *Tertiary prevention* aimed at improving the prognosis and quality of life of affected individuals by offering them the best available treatment and rehabilitation programme.

Further reading

* A comprehensive discussion of cancer screening programmes is given in Cole & Morrison (1978).

Box 16.4. (Cont.)

- *Screening* involves the use of a simple and inexpensive test to detect early stages of cancer at which treatment is more effective than at the time of usual diagnosis. Mass screening programmes should only be directed towards the control of cancers for which there is an effective treatment that will reduce mortality, if applied at early stages. There should also be valid, inexpensive and acceptable tests for the detection of the cancer at early stages.

- The performance of a screening test in terms of its acceptability, feasibility and costs can be monitored by *process measures* related to the administrative and organizational aspects of the programme (e.g., proportion of the target population examined, functioning of the referral system, cost per case detected, etc.). Predictive value of a positive test is a particularly useful measure because it provides an indication of whether most of the effort of the programme is being used to identify cases at an early stage or whether they are mainly wasted on the evaluation of false positives. Although process measures are useful for monitoring the activity of the programme they do *not* indicate whether those screened will have lower mortality than those not screened.

- The ultimate outcome measure to be used in evaluating the *effectiveness* of a screening programme aimed at detecting early cancer (e.g. mammography) is reduction in mortality. When the programme is aimed at detecting both pre-cancerous conditions and early cancer (e.g., Pap-smear screening), reduction in the incidence of invasive cancer and reduction in mortality are suitable outcome measures. *Intermediate outcome measures* such as stage distribution and case-fatality (survival) have also been used, but although they give an indication of whether the programme is likely to be effective, they are subject to length bias, lead time bias and overdiagnosis bias.

- The effectiveness of a screening programme should ideally be assessed by conducting a randomized intervention trial. In practice, most of the evidence on the effects of screening programmes comes from observational studies.

Appendix 16.1

Calculation of absolute measures of exposure effect and measures of population impact in case–control studies

In *population-based case–control studies* in which the incidence rate in the total population of interest is known and the distribution of exposure among the controls is assumed to be representative of the whole population, these parameters can be used to estimate incidence rates in the exposed and unexposed groups.

A population contains a mix of exposed and unexposed people. Thus, the overall incidence rate (r) of the disease in a population is equal to the weighted average of the incidence rates in its exposed (r_1) and unexposed (r_0) groups, the weights being the proportions of individuals in each group. Suppose that a proportion p_e of the population is exposed to the factor under study. Thus, the proportion of unexposed people in that population is equal to $(1 - p_e)$. Hence, the rate in the population will be

$$r = r_1 p_e + r_0 (1 - p_e)$$

Since the relative risk (estimated by the odds ratio (OR) in case–control studies) is the ratio of the incidence rates among the exposed and unexposed, the incidence rate among the exposed (r_1) members of a population is equal to the relative risk times the rate in the unexposed ($OR \times r_0$). Hence,

$$r = (r_0 \times OR \times p_e) + r_0 (1 - p_e)$$

$$= r_0 ((OR \times p_e) + (1 - p_e))$$

$$r_0 = \frac{r}{(OR \times p_e) + (1 - p_e)}$$

Once the incidence rate among the unexposed is determined, it can be multiplied by the odds ratio to provide an estimate of the incidence among the exposed. Given these two incidence rates (r_1 and r_0), the *excess risk* and the *excess fraction* can then be calculated as usual.

Example A16.1. In a hypothetical population-based case–control study conducted in London, cases with lung cancer were nine times more likely to have smoked cigarettes regularly in the past five years than men without lung cancer. The population lung cancer incidence rate in London was 40 per 100 000 pyrs and the proportion of smokers among the controls 60%. Thus,

$$r_0 = \frac{40 \text{ per } 100\,000 \text{ pyrs}}{(9 \times 0.6) + (1 - 0.6)} = 6.9 \text{ per } 100\,000 \text{ pyrs}$$

$r_1 = 9 \times 6.9 \text{ per } 100\,000 \text{ pyrs} = 62.1 \text{ per } 100\,000 \text{ pyrs}$

Excess risk = 62.1 per 100 000 pyrs – 6.9 per 100 000 pyrs = 55.2 per 100 000 pyrs

Excess fraction (%) = 100 × (55.2 per 100 000 pyrs / 62.1 per 100 000 pyrs) = 89%

Note that the excess fraction could also have been calculated by using the formula given in Section 16.2.1:

$$\text{Excess fraction (\%)} = 100 \times \frac{(OR - 1)}{OR}$$

$$\text{Excess fraction (\%)} = 100 \times \frac{(9 - 1)}{9} = 89\%$$

The *population excess risk* and the *population excess fraction* can then be determined as

Population excess risk = excess risk × proportion of the population exposed to the factor (p_e)

$$\text{Population excess fraction (\%)} = 100 \times \frac{\text{population excess risk}}{\text{rate in the total population } (r)}$$

The *population excess fraction* can also be calculated by using the formula given in Section 16.2.1:

$$\text{Population excess fraction (\%)} = 100 \times \frac{p_e (OR - 1)}{p_e (OR - 1) + 1}$$

Example A16.2. *In the above example, the population excess risk and the population excess fraction can be calculated as follows:*

Population excess risk = 55.2 per 100 000 pyrs × 0.6 = 33.1 per 100 000 pyrs

$$\text{Population excess fraction (\%)} = 100 \times \frac{0.6\,(9-1)}{0.6\,(9-1)+1} = 83\%$$

Thus, 83% of the lung cancer cases in the whole population of London could be attributed to smoking.

In *hospital-based case–control studies*, it is not possible to calculate the excess risk or the population excess risk, since incidence rates in the exposed and unexposed cannot be estimated. However, the following formulae can be used to calculate *excess fraction* and *population excess fraction*:

$$\text{Excess fraction (\%)} = 100 \times \frac{(\text{OR}-1)}{\text{OR}}$$

$$\text{Population excess fraction (\%)} = 100 \times \frac{p_e\,(\text{OR}-1)}{p_e\,(\text{OR}-1)+1}$$

Chapter 17
The role of cancer registries

17.1 Aims of cancer registries

The cancer registry is an organization for the systematic collection, storage, analysis, interpretation and reporting of data on subjects with cancer. There are two main types of cancer registry: hospital-based and population-based cancer registries.

Hospital-based cancer registries are concerned with the recording of information on the cancer patients seen in a particular hospital. The main purpose of such registries is to contribute to patient care by providing readily accessible information on the subjects with cancer, the treatment they received and its result. The data are used mainly for administrative purposes and for reviewing clinical performance. Although these data may be used, to a certain extent, for epidemiological purposes (see Section 17.7), these registries cannot provide measures of the occurrence of cancer in a defined population because it is not possible to define their catchment populations, that is the populations from which all the cases arise.

Population-based cancer registries seek to collect data on all new cases of cancer occurring in a well defined population. Usually, the population is that which is resident in a particular geographical region. As a result, and in contrast to hospital-based registries, the main objective of this type of cancer registry is to produce statistics on the occurrence of cancer in a defined population and to provide a framework for assessing and controlling the impact of cancer in the community. Thus, the emphasis is on epidemiology and public health.

The uses of population-based cancer registration data may be summarized as follows:

(1) They describe the extent and nature of the cancer burden in the community and assist in the establishment of public health priorities.

(2) They may be used as a source of material for etiological studies.

(3) They help in monitoring and assessing the effectiveness of cancer control activities.

Some of these functions can be fulfilled using mortality data derived from vital statistics systems. Cancer registration data, however, provide more comprehensive, more valid and more detailed information on patient characteristics than can be obtained from death certificates. Moreover, reliable cause-specific mortality data are available in most developed countries but in only a few developing countries. Thus, cancer registries may be the only way of obtaining information on the burden and patterns of cancer in developing countries, as well as providing a focus for research into etiology and prevention.

The discussion in the rest of this chapter will focus on population-based cancer registries unless otherwise specified.

17.2 A brief history of cancer registration

The first serious efforts to estimate the number of new and existing cancer cases in a given population were made at the turn of the century in various European countries. In Germany, an attempt was made in 1900 to register all cancer patients who were under medical treatment. Questionnaires were sent to every physician in the country to record the prevalence of cancer on 15 October 1900 (Anon., 1901). The same approach was adopted between 1902 and 1908 in Denmark, Hungary, Iceland, the Netherlands, Portugal, Spain and Sweden. These efforts were not very successful, however, mainly due to poor collaboration by the physicians. Similar surveys were conducted in the United States of America.

The first population-based cancer registry was set up in Hamburg (Germany) in 1926. Three nurses visited hospitals and medical practitioners in the city at regular intervals. They recorded the names of new cancer patients and transferred data to a central index in the health department. This index was compared once a week with official death certificates. Other population-based cancer registries were set up in subsequent decades, so that by 1955, almost twenty had been established in various countries (Table 17.1).

At present, more than 200 population-based cancer registries exist in various parts of the world. They cover about 5% of the world's population, but the proportion is much greater in developed countries than in developing ones. Moreover, in developing countries, registries are more likely to cover urban areas, where access to diagnostic and treatment services is better.

Nationwide cancer registration operates in some countries such as England & Wales, Scotland, the Nordic countries, Canada, Australia, New Zealand, Israel, Cuba, Puerto Rico and The Gambia. The Danish Cancer Registry, founded in 1942, is the oldest functioning registry covering a national population. In most countries, however, population-based cancer registries cover only a proportion of the population (e.g., Colombia, India, Italy, United States). Some specialized registries that cover only the registration of specific age-groups (e.g., childhood cancers in Oxford, UK) or particular cancer sites (e.g., gastro-intestinal cancers in Dijon, France) have also been established. In addition, hospital-based cancer registries have been set up in a large number of hospitals worldwide.

The International Association of Cancer Registries (IACR) was formed in 1966. The main objective of this association is to develop and standardize the collection methods across registries to make their data as comparable as possible.

A more detailed account of the history of cancer registration is given in Wagner (1991).

Country (region)	Year of establishment	Notification
Germany (Hamburg)	1929	Voluntary
USA (New York State)	1940	Compulsory
USA (Connecticut)	1941 (registered cases retrospectively back to 1935)	Compulsory (since 1971)
Denmark	1942	Compulsory (since 1987)
Canada (Saskatchewan)	1944	Compulsory
England and Wales (SW Region)	1945	Voluntary
England and Wales (Liverpool)	1948	Voluntary
New Zealand	1948	Compulsory
Canada (Manitoba)	1950	Voluntary
Slovenia	1950	Compulsory
Canada (Alberta)	1951	Compulsory
USA (El Paso)	1951	Voluntary
Hungary (Szabolcs, Miskolc, Vas)	1952	Compulsory
Norway	1952	Compulsory
Former USSR	1953	Compulsory
Former German Democratic Republic	1953	Compulsory
Finland	1953	Compulsory (since 1961)
Iceland	1954	Voluntary

[a] Reproduced with permission from Wagner (1991).

Table 17.1.
Population-based cancer registries established before 1955.[a]

17.3 Cancer registration methodology

The aim of a population-based cancer registry is to collect information on every case of cancer identified within a specified population over a given period of time. To ensure this, it is necessary to guarantee that the following basic requirements are fulfilled before setting up a population-based cancer registry:

(a) Clear definition of the catchment population. The registry should be able to distinguish between residents of the area and those who have come from outside and it should be able to register cases in residents treated outside the area.

(b) Availability of reliable population denominators from the census or other statistical offices.

(c) Generally available medical care and ready access to medical facilities, so that the great majority of cancer cases will come into contact with the health care system at some point in their illness and, therefore, will be correctly diagnosed.

(d) Easy access to case-finding sources such as hospitals, pathology departments, death certificates and other sources of clinical data within the catchment area and in the surrounding areas.

17.3.1 Data collection

The way in which a registry operates depends, inevitably, on local conditions and on the material resources available. Usually, the main sources of information of a population-based registry include: (1) information from treatment facilities, such as cancer centres and major hospitals (and sometimes, if appropriate, private clinics, hospices, homes for the elderly and general practitioners); (2) information from diagnostic services, especially pathology departments, but also haematological, biochemical and immunological laboratories, X-ray and ultrasound departments, and other imaging clinics; (3) death certificates from the death registration system (if they are available).

The information is collected from these sources by either active collection or passive reporting. *Active collection* involves registry personnel actually visiting the different sources and abstracting the data on special forms. This is the usual method in registries in developing countries. *Passive reporting* involves health-care workers completing the notification forms developed and distributed by the registry, or sending copies of discharge abstracts to the registry. A mixture of both procedures, with an emphasis on the latter, is followed in most registries in developed countries. In certain countries, notification of cancer cases is compulsory, although this does not necessarily ensure completeness.

The data items to be collected by a registry are dictated by the purpose for which the registry has been established, by the method of data collection used and by the resources available to the registry. However, the emphasis should be on the *quality of the data collected rather than on the quantity*. It is advisable that registries in developing countries should start by attempting to collect only information on the basic items listed in Table 17.2.

A unique *registration number* (cancer registry number) is assigned by the registry to each patient. If a patient has more than one primary tumour, the same number is given to each tumour. Multiple primaries are then distinguished on the basis of their incidence date and their topography and morphology.

Other *identification items* such as name, sex and date of birth (or, approximate age, if the date of birth is not known) are important to avoid multiple registrations of the same patient or tumour, to obtain follow-up data and to conduct any type of record linkage. Patient's usual address is essential for establishing the residence status, to exclude all non-residential patients, to conduct analysis by area of residence and for follow-up of the patients. Data on ethnicity is important in populations containing distinct ethnic groups.

The *incidence date* is primarily the date of first consultation or admission to a hospital or clinic for cancer, as this is a definite, consistent and reliable point in time which can be verified from records. This date is chosen as the anniversary date for incidence calculations and as the starting date for survival analyses (see Section 17.6.2). If this information is not available, the incidence date should be taken as the date of first diagnosis by a physician or the date of the first pathological report. A special problem arises when

Item	Comments
The patient	
Personal identification	
Registration number	Assigned by the registry
Name	According to local usage
Sex	
Date of birth or age	Estimate if not known
Demographic	
Address	Usual residence
Ethnic group	If relevant
The tumour	
Incidence date	
Most valid basis of diagnosis	Non-microscopic or microscopic
Topography (site)	Coded using ICD-O[b]
Morphology (histology)	Coded using ICD-O
Behaviour	Coded using ICD-O
Source of information	Type of source: physician, laboratory, hospital, death certificate or other
	Actual source: name of physician, laboratory, hospital, etc.
	Dates (e.g. dates of relevant appointments, hospital admissions, diagnostic procedures)

[a] Modified from MacLennan (1991).
[b] *International Classification of Diseases for Oncology* (Percy *et al.*, 1990).

Table 17.2.
Basic data items to be collected by population-based cancer registries.[a]

cancer is first ascertained from a death certificate and attempts to follow back are unsuccessful. The date of death of such 'death certificate only' (DCO) cases should be taken as their incidence date.

Information on the *most valid basis of diagnosis* is of great interest in assessing the quality of the registration data. The minimum requirement of a cancer registry is to discriminate between tumours that were microscopically verified and those which were not. If possible, further information should be obtained to distinguish neoplasms that were diagnosed on the basis of a clinical history only, clinical history plus other investigations (e.g., X-ray), exploratory surgery, autopsy, cytology, etc. For future checking purposes, it is important that the registry collects data on the source(s) of case-finding (e.g., name of physician, hospital, laboratory), dates of relevant medical events (e.g., hospital admission, biopsy) and any other details that will help to trace the patient's medical records (e.g., hospital number, biopsy number, laboratory reference number).

Inclusion of data items other than those listed in Table 17.2 increases the complexity and cost of the registration process and, hence, should be done only if justified by local needs and if the necessary resources are available. A list of optional items is given in Table 17.3; the most relevant ones are clinical extent of disease before treatment (stage at presentation) and follow-up data.

The data from the various case-finding sources are usually abstracted by using a standard registration form developed according to the needs of the

Table 17.3.
Optional items of information which may be collected by population-based cancer registries.[a]

The patient

Identification

    Personal identification number (e.g., national identity number or social security number)

Demographic and cultural items

    Place of birth

    Marital status

    Age at incidence date

    Nationality

    Religion

    Occupation and industry

    Year of immigration

    Country of birth of father and/or mother

The tumour and its investigations

    Certainty of diagnosis

    Method of first detection

    Clinical extent of disease before treatment

    Surgical-cum-pathological extent of disease before treatment

    TNM system

    Site(s) of distant metastases

    Multiple primaries

    Laterality

Treatment

    Initial treatment

Follow-up

    Date of last contact

    Status at last contact (alive, dead, emigrated, unknown)

    Date of death

    Cause of death

    Place of death

---

[a] Modified from MacLennan (1991).

registry. Two main considerations should be kept in mind when developing a registration form:

(1) The information on cancer cases should be collected and classified so that it accords with the data available from the census or other statistical offices. This is fundamental to ensure comparability between the numerators (i.e., numbers of cancer registrations) and the relevant denominators (i.e., population figures) in the calculation of incidence rates.

(2) Although data should be collected (and reported) according to local needs and interests, an effort should be made to ensure that comparisons with data from other national and international cancer registries will be possible.

17.3.2 Classification and coding of neoplasms

As mentioned in Appendix 2.2, it is recommended that cancer registries use the *International Classification of Diseases for Oncology* (ICD-O) (Percy *et al.*, 1990) to code the topography (site of primary tumour) and morphology (histological type) of the tumours. The fifth digit in the ICD-O morphology codes describes the behaviour of the tumour—benign, borderline, *in situ*, malignant. The topography of a tumour is the most important data item recorded and provides the main basis of tabulation of registry data.

17.3.3 Data quality

Two main issues should be considered when evaluating the quality of the data in a cancer registry: its *completeness* and its *validity*. A population based-registry should, by definition, register every single case that occurs in its catchment population. However, case ascertainment is rarely complete. Various methods, such as comparisons with death certificates and hospital records, have been used to determine the degree of completeness of registration. It is also important to ascertain the extent to which the registry eliminates registrations of cases from outside the catchment population and avoids multiple registrations of the same person or of the same tumour.

The validity of the data can be assessed in various ways. The proportion of cases with microscopic verification of diagnosis is a very useful index, as is the proportion registered during life (not simply from a death certificate). Cancer registries should develop their own internal quality control checks so that attention is drawn to missing information and inconsistent data. Many registries frequently re-abstract and re-code a sample of cases to assess the quality of their data. A full discussion of quality control methods is given by Parkin *et al.* (1994).

17.3.4 Reporting of results

The collection of information on cancer cases and the production of cancer statistics are only justified if use is made of the data collected. A population-based cancer registry should make its data and findings available in the form of reports and articles in scientific journals. The reports should include background information on the registry, registration procedures, catchment population, degree of data completeness and validity, methods of analysis and findings. Basic statistics should be produced and presented for diagnostic entities mainly according to topography of the tumour. The data should be presented in tabular and graphical form. Examples are given in Figure 17.1 and Table 17.4

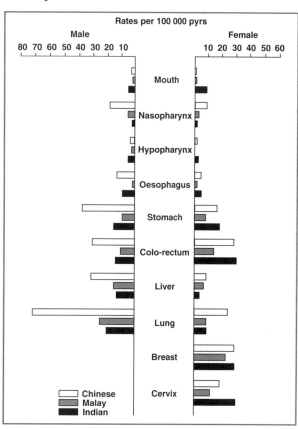

Figure 17.1.
Age-standardized incidence rates (to the world population) for selected cancer sites by sex and ethnic group, Singapore, 1978–82 (reproduced with permission from Lee *et al.*, 1988).

Site (ICD–9)	Number of cases by age group									Total	%	Incidence rate	
	Unknown	0–	15–	25–	35–	45–	55–	65–	75+			Crude	ASR[b]
All sites	10	69	89	255	241	266	362	264	74	1630	100.0	101.1	238.5
All sites but skin	8	69	88	253	236	264	359	259	72	1608		99.8	234.6
Oral cavity (140–145)	1	–	1	1	2	5	2	3	1	16	1.0	1.0	2.5
Nasopharynx (147)	–	–	1	5	1	1	1	4	–	13	0.8	0.8	2.0
Other pharynx (148–149)	–	–	1	–	–	–	2	1	–	4	0.2	0.2	0.6
Oesophagus (150)	–	–	–	1	16	25	63	35	13	153	9.4	9.5	30.4
Stomach (151)	–	–	–	2	10	15	14	20	6	67	4.1	4.2	13.5
Colon (153)	–	–	5	2	6	6	9	9	2	39	2.4	2.4	6.6
Rectum (154)	–	–	2	3	6	8	4	4	1	28	1.7	1.7	3.8
Liver (155)	–	2	10	22	37	41	46	46	9	213	13.1	13.2	34.6
Pancreas (157)	–	–	–	1	2	7	13	7	1	31	1.9	1.9	5.9
Larynx (161)	1	–	–	–	–	4	12	4	2	23	1.4	1.4	4.5
Bronchus, lung (162)	–	–	–	1	6	30	50	32	6	125	7.7	7.8	24.6
Pleura (163)	–	–	–	–	–	–	1	–	–	1	0.1	0.1	0.1
Connective tissue (171)	–	4	4	4	2	2	1	–	–	17	1.0	1.1	1.1
Melanoma of skin (172)	–	–	2	2	2	2	4	1	1	14	0.9	0.9	1.8
Other skin (173)	2	–	1	2	5	2	3	5	2	22	1.3	1.4	4.0
Breast (175)	–	–	–	–	1	3	1	–	–	5	0.3	0.3	0.6
Prostate (185)	3	–	–	–	2	11	37	41	18	112	6.9	6.9	29.2
Penis (187)	–	–	–	–	1	4	3	2	3	13	0.8	0.8	2.8
Bladder (188)	–	1	–	3	5	19	18	16	6	68	4.2	4.2	13.2
Kidney (189)	–	10	1	–	1	2	1	2	–	17	1.0	1.1	1.7
Eye (190)	–	5	1	1	–	1	1	1	–	10	0.6	0.6	0.9
Brain, nervous system (191–192)	–	7	6	4	5	2	4	1	–	29	1.8	1.8	2.4
Thyroid (193)	–	–	1	1	1	1	4	1	–	9	0.6	0.6	1.2
Hodgkin's disease (201)	–	2	1	4	2	2	2	–	–	13	0.8	0.8	1.0
Non-Hodgkin lymphoma (200, 202)	–	12	4	13	11	10	6	2	–	58	3.6	3.6	4.7
Multiple myeloma (203)	–	–	–	1	5	4	8	1	1	20	1.2	1.2	2.7
Lymphoid leukaemia (204)	–	8	3	1	1	1	2	4	–	20	1.2	1.2	2.5
Myeloid leukaemia (205)	–	8	6	6	5	6	2	1	–	34	2.1	2.1	2.7
Other leukaemia (207–208)	–	–	–	–	–	–	1	1	–	2	0.1	0.1	0.6
Kaposi's sarcoma	2	7	28	171	97	44	27	4	–	380	23.3	23.6	24.6
Other and uncertain	1	3	11	4	9	8	20	16	2	74	4.5		

[a] Reproduced, by permission of Wiley-Liss Inc., a subsidiary of John Wiley & Sons Inc., from Bassett *et al.* (1995).
[b] ASR = Incidence rate age-standardized to the world population.

Table 17.4.
Example of the type of table used by cancer registries to report their data. Number of cancer registrations among African men resident in Harare, 1990–92. Harare Cancer Registry, Zimbabwe, 1990–92.[a]

17.4 Cancer registration in developing countries

It might seem that cancer registration should not be regarded as a priority for the health services of a developing country, given all the competing demands upon the limited resources allocated to health. However, cancer is already a significant health problem in many developing countries. More than half of the new cancer cases in the world occur in developing countries (Parkin *et al.*, 1993). The rapid increase in life expectancy (largely because of a reduction in mortality from infectious disease) together with the adoption of western lifestyles suggest that the burden of cancer in these countries is likely to increase in the near future.

Most often cancer registries provide the only opportunity of properly assessing the extent and nature of the cancer burden in developing countries, since very few of them have reliable cause-specific mortality data. Ideally, the objective should be to establish a population-based cancer registry which will be able to estimate the incidence of different tumours in a well defined community. However, because of the relative ease with which they can be established, cancer registries in developing countries often start on the basis of cases attending certain hospitals or departments of histopathology.

Population-based cancer registries in developing countries usually face enormous logistic problems due to lack of appropriately trained personnel and adequate resources. In addition, their success may be jeopardized by external factors beyond their control.

Lack of basic health services

The functioning of a cancer registry relies heavily on the availability of proper health services for diagnosis and treatment of cancer cases. In many developing countries, however, health facilities are scanty and tend to be concentrated in urban areas. For individuals seeking medical attention, the quality of diagnostic information may be poor and based on clinical examination only.

Lack of proper denominators

Population-based registries require information on the size and the nature of the population served, information which requires the availability of census data. Censuses are particularly difficult to conduct in developing countries, and so they tend to be conducted infrequently, and their results may become available late and with inadequate detail.

The population of many developing countries is particularly mobile because of the increasing tendency to migrate temporarily from rural areas to urban areas and because social and political circumstances may force whole communities to move from one area to another. Inter-censal estimates or post-censal projections of the population size and structure are, therefore, likely to be inaccurate.

These population changes present a special challenge to cancer registries which must make special efforts to distinguish residents from non-residents in their catchment area using, as far as possible, the same definitions as in the census.

Identity of individuals

The ability to distinguish individuals from events (e.g., hospital admissions) is a key feature of a cancer registry. Thus, the registry should have sufficient information on each individual to avoid multiple registrations of the same subject. The most universal and generally used identifier is the name. The utility of using names will vary depending on local custom. For instance, surname (or family name) may not be used—persons may be known only by their first name. Individuals may change their name when they get married or for other social reasons. Variations in spelling of names is a frequent problem, particularly if a large percentage of the population is illiterate. This is aggravated if there is a need to transliterate names to the Roman alphabet, in order to use computerized database systems.

Lack of follow-up

Active follow-up usually means that the registry attempts to contact physicians or patients on a regular basis to see if the patient is still alive. Because this is expensive, many registries rely on passive follow-up, matching with death certificates and assuming patients are alive otherwise. Mixed systems use death certificates plus updating the 'date last known alive' from hospital admissions, consultations, and other sources of data.

Active follow-up of the patients is usually very difficult in developing countries. Few registries have the necessary facilities for regular follow-up of patients. There are also problems with unreliable postal services, unstable addresses and mobility of the population. Passive follow-up is possible only in the few countries where a reliable death registration system exists.

17.5 The role of cancer registry data in epidemiology

Population-based cancer registries are important resources for cancer epidemiologists since they hold information on the distribution of cancer in well defined populations. This information may be analysed without the need for any additional data collection. Cancer site-specific *incidence rates* can be calculated and compared according to many different variables such as age, sex, country of birth, place of residence at the time of diagnosis, etc. Time-trend studies are also possible when data have been accumulated over long periods of time. The methods used in such analyses were discussed in Chapters 4 and 11. Systematic compilations of data from population-based cancer registries from all over the world are published in *Cancer Incidence in Five Continents* (Doll *et al.*, 1966; Waterhouse *et al.*, 1970, 1976, 1982; Muir *et al.*, 1987; Parkin *et al.*, 1992, 1997). These data are of great value for international comparisons.

In addition to incidence figures, population-based cancer registries that conduct adequate follow-up of their patients are able to estimate the *prevalence* of cancer. Prevalence figures give an indication of the burden of the disease in the community. Cancer registries generally assume that once diagnosed with cancer, an individual remains a prevalent case until death. Thus, prevalence may be estimated from data on incidence and survival. When a registry has been in operation for many years, so that all patients diagnosed with cancer before the establishment of the registry have died, the prevalent cases may simply be enumerated from the registry file, provided, of course, that the registry receives information on deaths and emigrations for all registered cases.

The cancer registry provides an economical and efficient method of ascertaining cancer occurrence in *intervention trials* (Example 17.1) and *cohort studies*, as long as the cancer patients are properly identified in their files so that case matching can be performed.

Population-based registries can also provide a source of cases for *case–control studies*. However, in general, cancer registries are not regarded as well suited for the conduct of these studies because of delays in registration. The main value of the registry is rather to evaluate the completeness and representativeness of the case series.

The registry may, however, carry out its own case–control studies using its database, comparing one type of cancer with a selection of the other cancers ('controls') (see Section 11.1.6). The variables usually available for these analysis are limited to those routinely collected by the registry. Registries may supplement these variables with additional information (e.g., smoking, diet,

Example 17.1. The Gambia Hepatitis Intervention Study is a large-scale vaccination trial in The Gambia, initiated in July 1986, in which about 60 000 infants received a course of hepatitis B vaccine and a similar number did not. New cases of liver cancer will be ascertained through the nation-wide cancer registration scheme (Gambia Hepatitis Study Group, 1987).

Example 17.2. The importance of some selected risk factors in the etiology of oesophageal cancer in Bulawayo, Zimbabwe, was assessed using data collected by the local cancer registry during the years 1963–77, when an attempt was made to interview all cancer patients using a standard questionnaire. Risk factors for oesophageal cancer were estimated by case–control analysis in which other non-tobacco- and non-alcohol-related cancers were taken as the 'control' group. Table 17.5 shows the analysis for men. There was a strong association with tobacco use, with an apparent dose–response effect. In contrast, alcohol intake appeared to have little effect on the risk of oesophageal cancer in this population (Vizcaino et al., 1995).

	Cases	Controls[b]	Odds ratio (95% confidence intervals)[c]
Tobacco use			
Non-smoker[d]	120	947	1.0
Ex-smoker	21	38	3.4** (1.9–6.2)
< 15 g daily	279	542	3.5** (2.7–4.5)
≥ 15 g daily	71	91	5.7** (3.8–8.4)
Not specified	56	116	2.8** (1.8–4.2)
Test for trend			$P < 0.001$
Alcohol intake			
None[d]	144	654	1.0
Occasionally	44	206	0.6* (0.4–0.9)
Weekly	121	387	0.8 (0.6–1.1)
Daily	212	539	0.9 (0.7–1.2)
Not specified	41	68	1.8* (1.1–3.0)

Table 17.5.
Risk factors for oesophageal cancer in men, south-western Zimbabwe, 1963–77.[a]

[a] Data from Vizcaino et al. (1995)
[b] Formed by all other non-tobacco- and non-alcohol-related cancers (i.e., after exclusion of cancers of the oral cavity and pharynx, liver, larynx, lung and bladder).
[c] Adjusted for age, province, occupation and for the other variable in the table.
[d] Baseline category
* $P < 0.05$; ** $P < 0.001$.

occupation, treatment, etc.) by interviewing samples of patients (Example 17.2), by extracting such information from medical records, or by record linkage with other relevant records.

Cancer registries have been particularly useful in the conduct of case–control studies to investigate the carcinogenic effects of cancer treatments (Example 17.3).

> **Example 17.3.** *A collaborative group of population-based cancer registries and major oncological centres carried out a case–control study to identify reasons for the observed increases in lung cancer risk following Hodgkin's disease. A total of 98 cases of lung cancer were identified in patients who had survived for at least one year following a diagnosis of Hodgkin's disease. For each case, three controls were selected from patients with Hodgkin's disease who did not develop subsequent lung cancer, matched to the case on registry or hospital, sex, year of birth and year of diagnosis of Hodgkin's disease. For both cases and controls, detailed information was abstracted from medical records concerning stage and treatment of Hodgkin's disease. Patients treated with chemotherapy alone had about twice the risk of developing lung cancer compared with those treated by radiotherapy alone or both modalities. There was also an increasing risk of lung cancer with increasing estimated radiation dose to the lung among patients treated with radiotherapy alone (Kaldor et al., 1992).*

17.6 The role of cancer registries in cancer control

The cancer registry is an essential part of any rational programme of cancer control. Its data can be used in a wide variety of areas of cancer control ranging from etiological research, through primary and secondary prevention to health-care planning and patient care. Although most cancer registries are not obliged to do more than provide the basis for such uses of the data, they possess the potential for developing and supporting important research programmes making use of the information they collect.

17.6.1 Planning of cancer control programmes

Accurate information on cancer occurrence is important in fixing priorities and targeting cancer control activities. Population-based cancer registries are in a unique position to provide this information.

The annual numbers of incident cases provide an indication of the resources needed for primary treatment, and the number of prevalent cases describe how many people are in need of regular long-term follow-up (although for certain cancers, no regular surveillance is required beyond the first 5–10 years after diagnosis). Table 17.6 shows the numbers of incident (new) and prevalent (new and old) cancer cases in South-east England in 1992. The ranking of the cancer sites is quite different for incidence and prevalence. This is due to differences in survival. Cancers with a good survival have high prevalence even if their incidence is low, whereas those with

Site	ICD-10	No. of incident cases, 1992[b]	No. of prevalent cases at 31 December 1992[b]	Five-year relative survival (%)[c]
Lung	C33–34	6434 (1)	8201 (4)	9
Prostate	C61	4096 (2)	13 564 (3)	49
Colorectal	C18–21	3492 (3)	14 470 (2)	43
Bladder	C67	2183 (4)	16 538 (1)	70
Stomach	C16	1516 (5)	2407 (7)	13
Non-Hodgkin lymphoma	C82–85	1009 (6)	4582 (5)	51
Oesophagus	C15	858 (7)	805 (10)	8
Pancreas	C25	833 (8)	586 (11)	6
Kidney	C64	644 (9)	2296 (8)	40
Brain	C71	523 (10)	1558 (9)	22
Melanoma of skin	C43	367 (11)	2855 (6)	71
All malignant neoplasms (excluding non-melanoma skin cancer)		**28 732**	**109 637**	**36**

[a] Data from Thames Cancer Registry (1995).
[b] Ranking of sites by decreasing frequency is given in parentheses.
[c] Patients aged 15 years and over, diagnosed during the years 1986–89.

Table 17.6.

Number (and ranking) of male incident and prevalent cancer cases, and five-year relative survival ratios for selected sites. South-east England, 1992.[a]

poor survival have lower prevalence even if their incidence is higher.

Up-to-date cancer statistics provide information on the present burden of cancer to the health care system in a population. To develop long-term programmes for cancer control, it is necessary to predict what the needs will be in the future. In other words, it is necessary to have reliable estimates of the numbers of incident and prevalent cases that will occur in coming years. Cancer registries are an important source of data upon which to base such predictions. The simplest predictions of cancer incidence rates are based on continuing the present age-specific time trends into the future. The forecast can be imp-roved if birth cohort effects can also be taken into account by using age–period–cohort statistical models (see Section 4.3.2). An example is given in Figure 17.2.

An even more sophisticated approach to predic-

Figure 17.2.

Annual age-adjusted incidence rates of cancers at selected primary sites in Finland: actual rates from 1953 to 1979 and predictions up to the year 2000 based on a statistical model which includes age, period and cohort effects (reproduced with permission from Läärä, 1982).

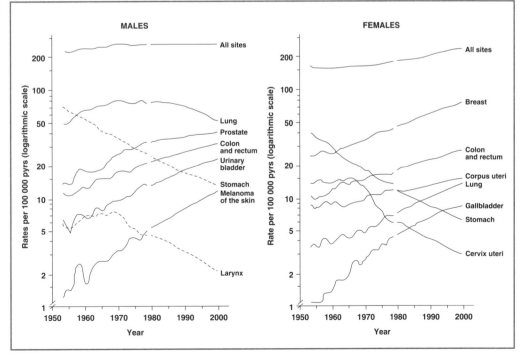

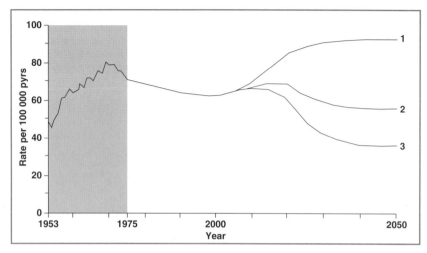

Figure 17.3.
Age-adjusted incidence rates (to the world population) of lung cancer in males in Finland in 1953–75, and forecasts for the rates in 1976–2050 derived from a simulation model based on the following assumptions: in each consecutive five-year period in 1976–2050, 10% of smokers will stop smoking, and one of the following three alternatives (three curves) holds true: (1) 60% of non-smokers aged 10–14 years, 30% of those aged 15–19 and 10% of those aged 20–24 will start smoking; (2) the percentages are 30, 15 and 5, respectively; and (3) the percentages are 15, 7.5 and 2.5, respectively (reproduced, by permission of Oxford University Press, from Hakulinen & Pukkala (1981)).

tion of future cancer incidence rates can be used if information on temporal changes on the prevalence of major risk factors is known and likely future changes can be predicted. This approach has been used to predict lung cancer incidence in relation to prevalence of smoking (as in Figure 17.3) and breast cancer in relation to changes in fertility.

Any predictions should be interpreted with caution, however, since they are based upon a considerable number of assumptions. To assess their robustness, it is advisable to provide forecasts under different possible scenarios, as in the example given in Figure 17.3.

17.6.2 Evaluation of cancer control programmes
Primary prevention

Cancer registries can play an important role in monitoring and evaluating the effectiveness of primary prevention measures. As mentioned in Section 16.2.2, trends in cancer incidence can be related to changes over time in exposure to risk factors. Occasionally, when implementation has been confined to one area, comparisons of the changes in the intervention area versus 'control' areas may be possible. It should be kept in mind when interpreting such relationships that it takes considerable time (generally decades) for the effect of a change in exposure to be reflected in cancer incidence data.

Screening and early detection

Cancer registries can play an important role in the evaluation and monitoring of screening programmes aimed at detecting pre-invasive conditions. Cancer registration data have been used in routine-data-based studies to examine trends in disease rates in relation to screening frequencies within a population and to compare disease rates between different populations with the coverage offered by their screening programmes (see Section 16.3.1). For instance, such studies have supported the hypothesis that regular use of the Pap smear test is effective in reducing the incidence of invasive cervical cancer.

Cancer registries can also contribute to the ascertainment of cancer occurrence in intervention trials and cohort studies designed to assess the value of screening programmes, and as an unbiased source of cases for case–control studies. The main issues to be considered in the design and interpretation of these studies were presented in Section 16.3.1.

When screening programmes are aimed at detecting early invasive cancers (e.g., breast cancer), reduction in mortality rather than incidence should be the ultimate measure of their effectiveness. However, once a screening programme is known to be effective, cancer registries may help to monitor its performance by providing data on so-called 'intermediate outcome measures'. Absence of a change in such intermediate end-points indicates that the screening has not been effective. Suitable monitoring statistics from cancer registries are:

(a) the incidence of interval cancers (i.e., cancers detected between screening tests) as compared to the incidence in the screened population before screening was introduced;

(b) the stage distribution of screen-detected cancers compared to the distribution of non-screen-detected cancers. A lack of shift in stage distribution towards early stages indicates that the programme is not effective.

(c) if screening is effective, screen-detected cancers should show better survival than non-screened cases.

It should, however, be stressed that *intermediate end-points are subject to several forms of bias* and therefore they may suggest that the programme is effective even though mortality data do not. These issues were discussed in Section 16.3.1.

Tertiary prevention

Survival statistics can be produced by population-based cancer registries that follow up their cases, either actively or passively. Although survival analysis of data from population-based registries cannot evaluate specific treatments (this can be done only in clinical randomized trials), it provides a useful evaluation of cancer care in the area covered by the registry, since all cancer cases will be included regardless of the type of treatment they may have received.

The methods used in survival analyses are those discussed in Chapter 12. The first requirement for the application of these methods is a *clear and well defined case definition*. This should clearly specify the site of the cancer and/or histology, age and sex of the patient and, if available, the extent of disease (stage) at the time of diagnosis. The nature of the cases to be included should also be defined. For example, a decision must be taken on whether to include cases for which the most valid basis of diagnosis is solely clinical. A decision should also be taken regarding cases registered on the basis of a death certificate only (DCO), for whom no information is available on the date of diagnosis of the cancer. The most usual practice is to omit these cases from the analysis, but if they represent a large proportion of registrations, it may be better to present two survival analyses, one including DCO cases and another excluding them. In both cases, the proportion of DCO registrations should be stated in survival reports.

The second requirement is a *clear and well defined starting point*. For population-based cancer registries, the starting date (from which the survival is calculated) is the *incidence date* (see Section 17.3.1).

The third requirement is a *clear and well defined outcome*. Death is generally the outcome of interest, but some registries collect enough data to allow them to conduct analyses using recurrence of tumour, or first recurrence of a particular complication, as the outcome of interest. It is also necessary to formulate clear criteria for deciding who should be considered 'lost to follow-up'. For instance, certain registries would assume that cases for which it was not possible to obtain follow-up data for more than 15 months should be taken as 'lost to follow-up'.

There are several problems in the interpretation of time trends in survival. Firstly, improvements in survival may be due, at least in part, to better ascertainment and recording of incident cases. Secondly, if there has been a trend towards earlier diagnosis (e.g., through introduction of a screening programme), survival may improve but the gain may be due entirely to increased lead time, with no change in mortality rate (see Section 16.3.1).

Despite these caveats, time trends in survival are useful to assess the extent to which advances in treatment have had an effect in the population. For instance, the dramatic improvements in survival observed in clinical trials in the treatment of childhood cancers conducted in the 1960s do seem to have been transposed into the community in many developed countries, as the population-based survival from many of these cancers shows significant increases over time (Table 17.7).

Comparisons of cancer survival estimates derived from population-based cancer registries are increasingly used to compare the effectiveness of cancer treatment across populations. However, survival reflects not only treatment but also prognostic factors such as stage at diagnosis, histological type and other characteristics of the disease. When data on such factors are not available, or when their definition is not properly standardized across registries, the reasons for any variations observed cannot be properly identified.

Table 17.7.
Time trends in five-year survival risk for certain childhood cancers (0–14 years) in Great Britain.[a]

Cancer	Five-year survival risk (%)	
	1962–64[b]	1971–74
Lymphoid leukaemia	14	39
Hodgkin's disease	39	79
Non-Hodgkin lymphomas	20	25
Wilms' tumour	26	57
Malignant bone tumours	22	29

[a] Data from Draper *et al.* (1982).
[b] 1968–70 data for lymphoid leukaemia.

In Example 17.4, survival in Khon Kaen was equal to, or better than, that in the USA for stomach, liver and lung cancers. Thus, improvements in treatment may be of reduced benefit in the control of these cancers in Thailand compared with the potential benefits of primary and secondary prevention (e.g., control of hepatitis B infection and liver fluke infestation for liver cancer; anti-smoking campaigns for lung cancer). In contrast, survival was lower for Khon Kaen residents than USA white residents for those cancers whose prognosis is associated with early diagnosis (breast, cervix and large bowel), indicating that interventions to promote early detection may provide potential benefits. Survival from leukaemia and lymphoma was also lower for residents in Khon Kaen, probably because of poor access to complex therapeutic regimens.

Example 17.4. The Khon Kaen Cancer Registry in the north-east of Thailand is one of the few population-based cancer registries in developing countries that collects follow-up data. These data are obtained from clinical records, death certificates and return-paid postcards sent annually to each patient thought to be alive. A total of 10 333 residents of Khon Kaen province registered with cancer during the years 1985–92 were followed up to the end of 1993. Table 17.8 shows five-year relative survival ratios for selected cancer sites. These survival ratios were compared with age-standardized survival data from two developed countries—the USA and Scotland (Sriamporn et al., 1995).

Site	ICD-9	Khon Kaen, 1985-92	US whites, 1983-88[b]	US blacks, 1983-88[b]	Scotland, 1983-87[b]
Stomach	151	23.4	17.2	19.0	12.8
Large bowel	153–154	41.9	58.9	50.0	42.3
Liver	155	9.2	5.9	3.5	4.2
Lung	162	15.4	14.7	10.3	7.7
Breast (females)	174	48.1	78.4	61.5	66.8
Cervix uteri	180	60.1	69.2	56.8	61.0
Non-Hodgkin lymphoma	200, 202	32.5	56.6	49.7	53.2
Leukaemia	204–208	19.4	45.7	31.7	41.6

[a] Data from Sriamporn *et al.* (1995).
[b] Standardized to the site-specific age distribution of Thai subjects.

Table 17.8.
Five-year relative survival ratios in Khon Kaen province (Thailand), USA and Scotland for selected cancer sites.[a]

17.7 Hospital-based cancer registries

Hospital-based cancer registries are more numerous and widespread than population-based cancer registries. The primary purpose of these registries is to contribute to patient care by providing readily accessible information on the patients with cancer, the treatment they received and its results. The data may also be used for clinical research and, to a certain extent, for epidemiological purposes.

One of the main advantages of hospital registries is that they have ready and instant access to medical records, the primary source of cases. The data items collected by a hospital registry tend to be more extensive than those collected by a population registry. There are, however, several limitations to the data from hospital registries:

(1) They are institution-based and not population-based. This means that no attempt is made to register all cancer cases occurring in any defined population; thus incidence rates cannot be determined. Patients who are hospitalized in more than one hospital are counted more than once in an area's hospital tumour registries. Information may not be shared among hospitals caring for the patient at different times. Changes over time in numbers of any type of cancer or patient characteristics may only reflect shifts by patients (or doctors) from one institution to another. The cancer cases in any one hospital (or group of hospitals) may not be representative of all cancer cases that are occurring in the area. For instance, certain institutions are referral centres for specific types of cancer or for particularly difficult or extensive tumours.

(2) Ascertainment of death is likely to be more incomplete in hospital-based registries than population-based registries because of limited access to, and use of, other sources such as death certificates, and limited sharing of information among hospitals.

(3) In contrast to most population-based cancer registries, hospital registries make little attempt to standardize methods of data collection between them. It is therefore difficult to compare their findings.

Hospital cancer registries produce reports on the numbers of cancers seen in the hospital per year by site, age and sex. These results may be presented as *proportional incidence ratios* (i.e., the frequency of cancers of a particular site in relation to the total number of cancer cases—see Sections 4.3.5 and 11.1.6 for a discussion of this type of measure). They may also provide information on methods of diagnosis, stage distribution, treatment methods, response to treatment, and survival at an institutional level. The hospital registry data may also be used to forecast future demands for services, equipment and manpower in a given hospital.

Although these registries cannot provide incidence rates in the general population, they may be used for epidemiological purposes. For instance, case–control studies may be set up to investigate the etiology of a particular cancer by comparing the characteristics of cases with those of a control group; this control group may be formed by patients with other types of cancer or by other hospital patients. The analysis will be similar to that shown in Example 17.2

Box 17.1. Key issues

- There are two main types of cancer registry:

  (a) Hospital-based cancer registries record information on all cancer patients observed in a particular hospital. Their main aim is to monitor and plan patient care at an institutional level. However, their data are of limited value for epidemiology, because it is not possible to define the population from which their cases arise.

  (b) Population-based cancer registries seek to collect data on all new cases of cancer which occur in a well defined population. As a result, and in contrast to hospital-based cancer registries, they can provide data on the occurrence of cancer in a particular population and, therefore, they are of particular value for epidemiology and public health.

- Population-based cancer registries play an important role in epidemiology by quantifying the incidence and prevalence of the disease in the community and as a source of ascertainment of cancer cases in intervention, cohort and case–control studies. Their data are also important in planning and evaluating cancer control programmes by helping to establish priorities and forecast future needs; by monitoring cancer occurrence in relation to the prevalence of important risk factors; by helping to assess and monitor the effectiveness of screening programmes; and by evaluating cancer care through survival statistics.

- The data items to be collected by a population-based cancer registry are determined by their aims, the data collection methods to be used, and the resources available. The emphasis should be on the quality of the data rather than their quantity. The completeness and validity of the data should be monitored regularly.

- Population-based cancer registries are particularly useful in developing countries where reliable cause-specific mortality data are rarely available.

Further reading

* Jensen *et al.* (1991) describe in great detail the planning of cancer registries in both developed and developing countries and the uses of registration data in epidemiology and public health planning.

* Parkin *et al.* (1994) provide practical recommendations on how population-based cancer registries can assess and monitor the quality of their data.

Chapter 18

Designing, planning and conducting epidemiological research

18.1 Introduction

In previous chapters of this book, we covered the basic methodological principles of study design, analysis and interpretation. In this chapter, we concentrate on practical aspects of how to design, plan and conduct an epidemiological study. Only general issues are covered. Each research project and each study setting presents unique problems which cannot be dealt with here.

The first step in the design of any epidemiological study is to have an 'idea' for a study. This is a creative process for which no guidelines or advice can be given. The idea for a study usually comes from one's own work and experience and from the realization that there is a need to obtain a clear answer to a particular research question. Once the idea for the study has been identified, the next step is a critical review of the existing literature to find out what exactly is known about the subject and to make sure that the question has not already been answered. Where appropriate, registers of clinical trials and/or directories of on-going research (such as that of the International Agency for Research on Cancer) should be consulted. It may also be helpful to contact experts in the subject. In addition to revealing what is already known about the question, this will help the investigator to become familiar with problems that other researchers have faced, when using various study methods.

Once all the relevant information on the topic has been gathered, the next step is to state the study hypotheses in a clear and practical way. There is a tendency to formulate hypotheses that are broad and vague. Instead, they should be stated in terms of clear, simple, answerable questions. All main and secondary hypotheses should be formulated at the beginning of a study to ensure that all the necessary data are collected. They should include a concise description of the exposure(s) or intervention(s) to be studied, the outcome(s) of interest, and the magnitude of the anticipated effect(s) in the population in which the study will be conducted.

18.2 Preparing a protocol and obtaining funding

If we are convinced that the study is worth doing and that it is feasible, the next step is to obtain the necessary funding. If the total cost of the project is small, it may be possible to conduct it with available local resources, but many epidemiological studies are expensive enterprises which require substantial external financial support.

18.2.1 Funding bodies

Funding bodies which may be potentially interested in the proposed research should be identified. Some funding bodies do not fund cancer research. Others have their own research agenda and will fund only projects that address the particular questions in which they are interested. In some countries, directories of funding bodies with their areas of interest and funding budget are published regularly.

It is important to obtain grant application forms from all potential funding bodies and read the documentation carefully, checking the areas they are particularly interested in funding, and the deadlines for submission of applications. Sometimes, their material include lists of proposals they have funded in the past. These lists give an idea of the areas they are likely to fund in the future and the amount of money usually allocated to individual projects. It may be beneficial to contact funding bodies at this stage to check whether the proposal is of potential interest to them; if the proposed study is outside their areas of interest, there is no point in making the effort of preparing and submitting an application.

Writing a protocol

The protocol of the study should be written according to the specifications of the funding body. Although the layout of the application forms varies from one funding body to another, they are generally divided into the following sections:

Study hypotheses

The main and secondary study hypotheses should be written in a clear and concise way, indicating the exposure(s) and outcome(s) of interest and the magnitude of the anticipated effect(s).

Background and justification

This section should include a brief review of the state of knowledge about the topic. It should 'justify' the need for the proposed study by clearly indicating its originality and the potential significance of its findings. The proposed research may be a logical extension of previous work conducted by the researchers or of an initial pilot study. The results of such studies should be presented here.

Study population and methods of recruitment

The geographical location and the demographic characteristics of the study population should be described. Any particular reasons for the choice of the study population should also be given. For instance, a particular study population may have been chosen because of its exceptionally high exposure to a particular risk factor or for logistic reasons such as ease of follow-up. Details should be given on how the study subjects will be recruited.

Study design

It must be made explicit whether this will be an intervention, cohort, case–control, cross-sectional or routine-data-based study. The choice of design needs to be justified (see Chapters 5 and 7–11).

Sample size

It is necessary to show that the proposed number of subjects in the study will provide adequate power or precision to detect or estimate a particular effect. Sample size estimates should be presented under different assumptions. A single estimate is rarely convincing (see Chapter 15).

Methods of data collection

The methods of data collection (e.g., interview, laboratory measurements, extraction of data from clinical records, etc.) should be described in sufficient detail to show that the plan has been adequately prepared and is feasible. Possible practical constraints and strategies to overcome them should be presented here.

Statistical analysis

A concise description of the statistical methods planned for use in the analysis of data should be given (see Chapters 6 and 14).

Ethics

The protocol of any study involving human subjects should provide answers to the following questions: What will the subjects be told? What will their collaboration entail? Will invasive procedures be used? Are there any risks for participants? How will consent be obtained (e.g., at an individual or community level; written or verbal)? What steps will be taken to ensure confidentiality of the data? It will be worth consulting at this stage the ethical guidelines proposed by the Council for International Organizations of Medical Sciences (CIOMS) and the World Health Organization (WHO) (1993). Most funding bodies will fund only projects that have been approved by the relevant ethical committees and some will wish to see samples of the information sheet and consent form to be given to the study subjects.

Timetable

A realistic timetable for carrying out the various activities of the study should be provided. This should incorporate milestones to be achieved at regular time intervals (e.g., every six months), which will help in monitoring the progress of the study.

References

References to key publications should be included in the grant proposal.

Budget

The budget is generally divided into staff costs, equipment (e.g., computers, freezers, centrifuges) and running expenses (e.g., office expenses, computer and laboratory consumables, travel costs). Each item must be justified and of reasonable cost. This will often involve discussions with the personnel office about staff costs and consulting price lists to get the best prices for supplies and equipment. In certain countries, allowances should be made for inflation and currency fluctuations when calculating the final budget.

It is also important to check whether the institution where the study is going to be based will charge 'overheads'. These correspond to the costs to the institution of administering the grant, organizing the payment of salaries, ordering supplies, providing office space, heat, electricity, air-conditioning etc. Some funding bodies refuse payment of overheads (e.g., the World Health Organization), whereas others will pay only up to a certain proportion of the total cost (e.g., the European Commission pays only 20% of the total cost). If the funding body does not pay overheads, it may be possible to include as running costs in the budget some expenses that might otherwise be covered by the overheads, such as telephone, fax and mailing costs.

Dissemination of results

Some funding bodies require applicants to state how they intend to inform study participants about the findings of the study and how they will be disseminated to relevant health authorities and the scientific community. This topic is further discussed in Section 18.4.

Box 18.1 presents a checklist on how to prepare grant applications. Before sending the grant application to the funding body, it is useful to send a draft to people who have experience of writing and reviewing applications, for comment. Although no one can foresee all the problems that may occur, many potential difficulties will be quickly spotted by experienced researchers. In particular, it is advisable to involve a statistician in the development of the study protocol.

The investigator should also inform all people whose approval or cooperation is either required or desirable. Proposed research in clinical or academic institutions should be presented to appropriate departmental heads and/or hospital administrators. Often there will be a committee specially designated to review and approve study protocols. Studies conducted in the community should be presented to local health officials. In addition to gaining the required approval, the investigator may receive valuable practical suggestions and other assistance from these individuals, such as introductions to physicians who may permit the study of their own patients. The investigator may also learn of other similar or related research that is under way. Cooperation with other investigators may help avoid duplication of effort and lead to sharing of resources and, possibly, even of data.

Box 18.1. Checklist on how to prepare grant applications

• Identify funding bodies potentially interested in the proposed research. Obtain grant application forms from them.

• Read their guidelines carefully. Check deadline for submission of applications.

• Check whether they require submission of any special documents (e.g., statement of willingness to participate in the study from all collaborators, confirmation of ethical approval) which may take some time to obtain.

• Make a list of the staff and equipment required. Consult personnel office to obtain estimates of staff salaries. Obtain list of prices for equipment. Make an estimate of running expenses (e.g., office expenses, computer consumables, travelling expenses). Check whether your organization charges overheads.

• Write the study protocol according to the instructions of the funding body, respecting the various section headings. Do not exceed the space and/or maximum number of words specified for each of the sections.

• Be concise and clear. Check spelling errors carefully. If you are writing the application in a language other than your mother tongue, it will be useful to show it to someone who is proficient in that language.

• Show the draft of the protocol to experts in the topic. Review the draft in the light of their comments.

• Make sure you send the original application and the requested number of copies to the funding body in time to reach its office before the closing date for submission of applications.

Review of grant proposals

Most funding bodies send the applications to experts in the particular subject. These experts are asked to evaluate the proposals by answering the following questions: Does the proposal address an important question? Is the study design appropriate? Are the applicants qualified to conduct research? Is the budget reasonable? Each referee will send a report with his/her comments to the funding body.

Most funding bodies have their own research review panel who will consider the applications and the referee's reports. The panel will rank the applications and award those on the top of the ranking scale. Occasionally, applicants may be invited to submit a revised application which takes into account the referees' comments. The revised application should address all the referee's comments and be submitted together with a covering letter detailing the revisions.

18.3 Conducting the study

Once funding for the study is secured, the researchers need to start planning the conduct of the study carefully and in detail.

18.3.1 Logistic organization

It is important to plan all the activities of the study at a very early stage. Three general principles should govern the logistic organization of a study. First, realistic milestones should be set up at the start of the study. Second, all study procedures and decisions should be properly documented. Third, expenses should be monitored closely.

A *timetable* of all the activities to be conducted should be established. An example is given in Box 18.2. The timetable should indicate targets to be achieved at regular time intervals. It must be realistic. For instance, it should take into account possible delays in delivering vital equipment, climatic factors which may affect the fieldwork, and staff holidays and sickness.

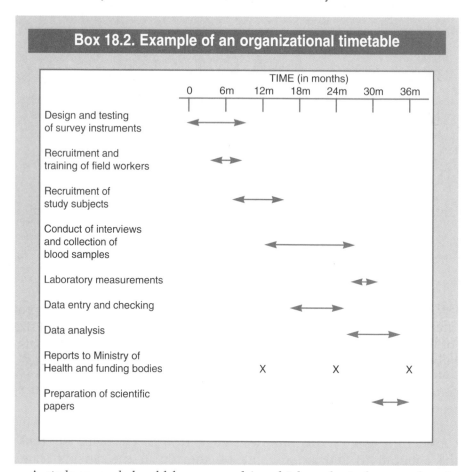

Box 18.2. Example of an organizational timetable

A *study manual* should be prepared in which each study procedure is documented in detail (e.g., step-by-step instructions for the administration and completion of questionnaires or for the collection of biological samples). The manual should be updated if any changes are made during the study. Copies of the relevant parts of the manual should be given to all research team members. In addition to the study manual, it is also important to keep a *study diary* in which all problems encountered are noted and the solutions adopted are recorded. This will be useful in maintaining consistency of decisions throughout the study.

A detailed *record of expenditure* should be kept to monitor expenses throughout the study and to facilitate submission of expenditure statements to the funding body. It is important to keep copies of salary payment sheets, invoices, receipts, order forms, etc. Grant accounts can be easily monitored by using a computer spreadsheet.

18.3.2 Recruitment, training and management of personnel

Epidemiological studies often require the recruitment of personnel (e.g., statisticians, interviewers, data-entry clerks, computer programmers, etc.). A job description should be written for each post indicating the responsibilities involved, and the minimum qualifications and experience required.

It is important to establish a clear line of management so that each staff member knows what his/her responsibilities are and to whom he/she should report. Proper training of personnel is fundamental to the success of the study and adequate time and resources should be allocated to this. Performance of each staff member should be monitored regularly and constructive feedback given. Successful work must be seen as a team effort.

18.3.3 Equipment

The equipment required will depend on the design of the study and the setting where it will be carried out. Routine-data-based studies may require only access to good computing facilities. In contrast, a large intervention trial conducted in a remote area may require everything from computer equipment to staff accommodation and transport facilities.

Computing equipment

The choice of computer equipment ('hardware') and computer programs ('software') (see Box 18.3) will be determined by the design and size of the study as well as by the availability of technical expertise for data-processing and statistical analysis and of local servicing facilities. However, the rate of development of computer equipment and software is such that any advice or guidelines soon become out-of-date. Thus, it is essential that professional advice, from a computing specialist, should be sought at the planning stage of the study so that advantage is taken of the most recent developments.

Hardware

Computers differ in their type of microprocessor, the size of their random access memory (RAM) and their storage capacity. The most commonly used microcomputers are based on the 486 and Pentium microprocessors. The RAM governs the size of program and the amount of data that the machine can actively work with at any time. The bigger the RAM the better. Most machines have at least 4 Mb of RAM, but if Windows is to be used, at least 16 Mb is desirable. The data storage capacity is determined by the capacity of the hard disk. In general, the hard disk capacity should be at least 500 megabytes (Mb), especially if Windows-based software is to be used, as these programmes tend to use a considerable amount of space on the hard disk.

Once the appropriate type of machine for the study has been selected, it is necessary to obtain price lists from different manufacturers. Machines with similar specifications are produced by many different manufacturers and the prices tend to differ widely. However, value for money is not the same as cheapness. Equipment reliability, warranty and free maintenance from the dealer are all important factors which need to be considered. The availability of good local servicing and repair facilities is another important consideration, particularly for studies in developing countries.

Microcomputers with similar features are available in two basic models: desktop/tower and laptop (portable) computers. Laptop computers have the advantage of being portable, but they are more expensive than desktop machines of equivalent computing capacity. However, since they work from rechargeable batteries, they avoid the need for an uninterruptible power supply (see below).

It is absolutely vital to take adequate precautions against the possibility of losing data that have been entered onto the computer. All the information on the computer should be regularly copied onto some other storage device to guard against the possibility of hard disk or computer failure. Floppy disks are adequate to store relatively small data-sets, but removable hard-disk units may be needed for very large data-sets. Alternatively, a 'tape-streamer' may be used to back-up the data onto a small magnetic tape. It is essential to make back-up copies of the data regularly, on both a daily and weekly basis, and to create multiple copies as a back-up to the back-up (see Section 18.3.6).

Unreliable power supplies can lead to loss of data and serious damage to the computing equipment. It is advisable to avoid sharing the mains circuit with equipment such as electric motors and air-conditioning systems that makes heavy but intermittent demands on the power supply. Power stabilizers (or mains filters) are small devices, sometimes incorporated into the plugs, which are designed to deal with rapid voltage fluctuations. However, they offer no protection against loss of data if there is a power failure. Uninterruptible power supplies (UPS) are devices that, in the event of a power failure, provide power (from batteries) for short periods, until the batteries run down. This gives enough time to save the work and switch off the computer without loss of information. Some UPSs shut down the computer automatically should the loss of the main power supply be prolonged.

Printers vary in price enormously. In general, the better the print quality, the higher the price. Dot-matrix printers are relatively cheap and the quality of their output is usually good enough for most requirements. An ink-jet or a laser printer may be required if there is a need to produce higher-quality documents such as grant proposals, questionnaires and study reports.

Box 18.3. Computing requirements

- Hardware (machines)
    Minimum requirements
    - computer
    - printer

    Optional requirements
    - back-up facilities (e.g., tape-streamer) or removable hard drive
    - uninterruptible power supply (UPS)

- Software (computer programs)
    Minimum requirements
    - operating system
    - database package
    - statistical package
    - word-processing package
    - virus-checking software

    Optional
    - data transfer software

Computing equipment can be used in most normal ambient conditions. It is advisable, however, to try to ensure that they are kept in a dust-free environment with temperatures below 25°C (to avoid overheating) and humidity of less than 80%. Thus, special equipment to ensure that ambient conditions are appropriate (e.g., air-conditioning systems) may be required, particularly in hot and humid locations.

Software

In order for a computer to work, it requires a set of instructions which control its operations. This set of instructions is called an operating system. In the past, most IBM-type microcomputers used the DOS operating system, but today the Windows operating system is almost universal. Windows allows several programs to be run simultaneously (which is not possible with DOS unless a special software package has been installed) and, therefore, it is easier to move data, text and figures between different programs.

Apart from the operating system, most epidemiological studies require a database package to enter and check the data, a statistical package to perform the statistical analyses, and a word-processing package for use in preparing the data-collection forms, progress reports and papers with the final results for publication. Many suitable computer packages are available. The best policy is to use well known packages that have been thoroughly tested by others; newly developed packages often contain 'bugs' (i.e., errors) that can cause major problems. Epi Info (version 6) is a very useful package for word-processing, questionnaire design, data entry and validation, and simple tabulations and statistical analysis. It has been developed by the Centers for Disease Control in the USA and the Global Programme on AIDS at the World Health Organization in Geneva. This software package was specifically developed for epidemiological studies, it is easy to use and it is distributed free of charge (apart from postage)[a].

Computers may become infected by a 'virus', which is a piece of software, written by unscrupulous people, designed to damage the computer or the data it holds. Precautions should be taken to prevent this happening and to detect any possible contamination immediately. Virus-checking software packages have been developed to routinely check for the introduction of viruses and to clean them from the computer. Floppy disks should be scanned for viruses before data are transferred into the computer. It is important to ensure that the program is updated every time new viruses appear.

If there is frequently a need to transfer data between computers (for instance, from a portable computer to a desktop computer), this can be done efficiently via a cable link which connects the serial or parallel ports of the two machines. Special software will be needed for such data transfer. Data can be transferred much more quickly this way than by using floppy disks. If constant access to the data is required from more than one computer, a network of computers can be created. However, this is more complex to set up and specialist help should be obtained.

Other equipment

It may be necessary to obtain office equipment such as desks, filing cabinets, a photocopying machine, a fax machine, etc. Studies involving collection of biological specimens may require laboratory equipment such as freezers, centrifuges, etc. (see Section 18.3.5). Field studies in remote areas may require staff accommodation and transport facilities.

18.3.4. Recruiting study subjects

The recruitment of study subjects may involve obtaining lists of potentially eligible subjects. Such lists may be obtained from local authorities (e.g., lists of all subjects resident in a particular area), from doctors or hospitals (e.g., lists of patients with a particular condition) or from cancer registries. If a list of all the residents of a particular geographical area is required as a sampling frame and no enumeration lists are available or those available are grossly inaccurate or out-of-date, it will be necessary to conduct a census of the defined study population before recruiting the study subjects.

---

[a] Details can be obtained from USD Incorporated (2075A West Park Place, Stone Mountain, GA 30087, USA; telephone +1 404 469 4098).

The recruitment of subjects usually involves writing letters and/or meeting the study subjects, their doctors, local health representatives, leaders of the communities, etc. to explain the objectives of the study and to obtain their support and consent.

Once recruited into the study, each subject should be given a *unique study identification number*. This number should remain constant throughout the study. It will help to keep confidentiality and blindness and will be used to link individual information obtained from different sources (e.g., questionnaires, clinical records and laboratory forms).

18.3.5 Collection of biological samples and laboratory measurements

Many cancer-related epidemiological studies involve collection of biological specimens such as blood, serum, plasma, urine, cell and tissue samples from study participants.

Collection and processing of biological specimens

Biological specimens may be specifically collected for the purpose of the epidemiological study or may derive from samples collected for clinical purposes. Clinical activities can be an easy source of biological materials, but the specimens are sometimes inadequate for an epidemiological investigation, particularly if collected by a number of different people using different methods of collection and processing. The amount of specimen available may be insufficient in volume or quality, specimens may have remained too long in less than optimal conditions of preservation or they may be contaminated with extraneous materials (see Box 18.4).

Blood can be collected by venepuncture or by finger (or heel) pricks. Finger (or heel) pricks tend to be more acceptable to study participants. The volume of blood obtained with this method, although smaller than that obtained by venepuncture, is usually sufficient for most laboratory assays. It is, therefore, important to check with laboratory staff the minimum amount of blood that needs to be collected to perform all the necessary laboratory assays. The timing of the blood collection may also be important (e.g., time since exposure, time of the day, time within the menstrual cycle, etc.). Some laboratory assays require fasting samples. Other factors such as a subject's posture and the use of a tourniquet can affect the concentration of certain blood components.

After collection, blood can be separated into several components including serum, plasma, red cells and white cells. Separation must be done shortly after the blood has been collected (ideally, within two hours). During this period, the specimens can be left at room temperature, but preferably at 4°C. Serum and plasma samples should be frozen as soon as possible after separation, and stored at –20°C. This is adequate for most assays, at least for several weeks. Some assays require immediate storage at –70°C or below (e.g., vitamin C measurements).

Some urinary assays require collection of 24-hour urine samples, whereas others can be performed in a single sample collected 'on the spot'. The collection of 24-hour urine samples is logistically more complex and less readily accepted by study subjects. Particular care is necessary in instructing study subjects in the collection of 24-hour urine, and in checking that instructions have been followed. It is usually necessary to leave the container with the individual overnight and to arrange for it to be collected the following day. Creatinine levels should be measured to take into account and correct determinations for possible losses of urine. A good check for the completeness of urine collection is the administration of 250 mg of *para*-aminobenzoic acid, which is completely recoverable in the urine over the 24 hours following its administration.

Before storing samples for long periods of time, it may be necessary to add appropriate fixatives and stabilizers. This should be checked with the laboratory staff. Biological samples are easily damaged by repeated freezing and thawing. Thus, samples should be divided into small portions before freezing. Ideally, the size of the aliquots should be such that each one contains just sufficient material to perform the assays required at a particular time.

All biological specimens should be properly labelled. To ensure confidentiality, the label should contain the unique study identification number of the subject but not any other personal details (e.g., name). The identification number will make it possible to link back the results from the laboratory assays to the records of the individual from whom the sample was taken. In some circumstances, it will be appropriate to include on the label the date of collection and the type of specimen, if not evident. It is important, however, to ensure that laboratory staff are kept 'blind' to the exposure (or outcome) status of the subjects from whom the samples were taken. Pre-printed, adhesive labels with each identification number duplicated several times are available commercially. Alternatively, they can easily be produced by a microcomputer. Waterproof marker pens should be used, except if samples are going to be frozen in salt–alcohol mixtures, in which case plain pencils should be used instead. The labelling must be done on the body of the container and never on the cap only. Numbers and letters must be written in a clear and standardized form (see Box 18.5). It is important to pre-test the labels to check how they stick and how pen/pencil writing is preserved during transport and storage.

Samples may be stored temporarily in a laboratory located where the fieldwork is being carried out before being sent to the laboratory where the assays will be conducted and/or to their permanent storage place. If a large number of samples is collected and stored, it is important to store them in a way that allows rapid retrieval of any particular sample. For instance, samples may be stored in batches according to the date they were collected or frozen. This information may be computerized so that any particular specimen can be easily and rapidly located.

Quality control of laboratory procedures

Laboratories should keep a record of the reagents, test kits, laboratory equipment, the batches of supplies and reagents used at different times, and the number of times each aliquot has been thawed and re-frozen.

> ### Box 18.4. Collection, processing, transport and storage of biological samples
>
> - Step-by-step instructions should be given in the study manual on how to collect, process, transport and store biological specimens.
>
> - All the methods for collection, processing, storage and transport of specimens should be pilot-tested before being implemented.
>
> - All biological samples should be considered potentially infectious. All personnel involved in their collection, processing, analysis or storage should take measures to protect themselves against the possibility of becoming infected (e.g., by wearing disposable gloves).
>
> - The quality of laboratory measurements should be closely monitored. This consists of:
>
>   *Internal quality control*
>   – Use in-built standard controls.
>   – Perform duplicate measurements.
>   – Send a random sample of specimens twice, laboratory staff being unaware that they are duplicates.
>
>   *External quality control*
>   – Send random duplicate samples to a reference laboratory.

Records should also be kept of reasons for considering a specimen as 'unacceptable' (e.g., insufficient material, inadequate processing, storage or transport) and of unusual events which may affect the results of a test (e.g., power failures, errors in test procedures).

Many laboratory tests have 'in-built controls' using standardized reagents of known concentration or quantity. In addition, many assays are performed in duplicate as a normal routine laboratory procedure. Although in-built controls and duplicate measurements are important to assess the quality of laboratory measurements, they are not sufficient (see Box 18.4). A random sample of specimens should be sent to the laboratory and tested twice, laboratory staff being unaware that they are duplicate samples. The reliability between the first and the second measurements gives an indication of the internal quality of the laboratory procedures (see Section 2.6.2). Ideally, reliability should be checked within batches, between batches and from one time period to another (e.g., week-to-week). It is important to measure intra-observer (by having duplicate samples processed by the same observer at different times), inter-observer (by having the same samples processed independently by two different staff members) and inter-product reliability (by analysing the same samples with different batches of reagents). High reliability does not ensure high validity of the measurements, however. Thus, it is desirable to send a random sample of duplicate specimens to an external reference laboratory, whose measurements will be taken as a 'gold standard' (see Section 2.6.1).

Laboratory results should be recorded in laboratory notebooks or, preferably, on specially prepared forms to facilitate computer entry. It is important to ensure that the forms are designed in a way that allows the recording of particular problems or features which may be of relevance to the interpretation of the measurements. For example, it should include items on the identity of the technicians involved with each test (to check for inter-observer variation), the batch of reagents used (to check for inter-product variability) and any technical problems that may arise (e.g., lost and broken samples, samples with insufficient material, errors in test procedures, etc.).

18.3.6 Data processing and editing

All the various steps of data processing and editing should be planned early at the design stage of the study. This should be done in consultation with a statistician and a computer programmer.

Design of data-collection forms

All forms to be used for recording data in a study should be carefully designed and pre-tested to ensure that the relevant data are collected and can be easily extracted for data processing. This general principle applies to all data-collection forms: questionnaires, laboratory forms, data extraction forms from hospital notes, etc. These issues were discussed in Chapter 2 and Appendix 2.1.

Data collection and recording

Adequate training is the single most important aspect of data quality control. It should focus on accuracy and completeness, with an emphasis on how and why the work of the entire project is dependent upon the quality of the data recorded. Field workers should be instructed how to write numbers and letters so that the coding and data entry clerks have no difficulty in reading the forms. Some letters and numbers are frequently confused and special instructions should be given regarding these. Examples are given in Box 18.5.

The leaving of blanks should be avoided since these can be interpreted in different ways. A blank may mean that the question was not appropriate, the answer was not known or, simply, that the question was mistakenly skipped by the interviewer. In addition, some computer programs interpret blanks as zeros, which may be a valid code. It is preferable to design the forms so that all options are covered (for example, the answers to a specific question may be: 'yes', 'no', 'not known' and 'not appropriate').

Information should be recorded in pencil or using a ball-point pen. Errors should be corrected by writing the correct response above or below

Box 18.5. Handwritten numbers and letters which are commonly confused and possible solutions to avoid confusion

Characters confused	Solution
1 and 7	This confusion arises if ones are written with an initial upward stroke (for example 1). If this is the situation, always write sevens with a horizontal line through them (as do the French), that is 7. A simpler solution may be to insist that ones are written with a single stroke (for example $/$).
O (oh) and 0 (zero)	Note 1. Write 0 (zero) with a line through them, that is $\emptyset$
4 and 9	Write 4 as 4
4 and 7	These digits may be confused if sevens are written with a horizontal line through them! Instruct field workers to ensure that the top of the seven is written horizontally
6 and 9 (upside down)	Relevant when coding laboratory samples (for example, is it 6l or l9?) Draw a horizontal line under all numbers, for example <u>19</u>
2 and Z	Note 1. Always write Z with a horizontal line through it, that is Z
5 and S	Note 1. Always write 5 using two pen strokes
O (oh) and Q	Note 1
I and 1	Note 1. Always write I with 'hat and shoes', not as a single stroke, that is I not $|$.
U and V	Avoid both letters as codes as far as possible (but they will be needed for names)

Note 1. Avoid using the alphabetical character in data fields that may contain alphabetical or numerical information.

[a] Reproduced with permission from Smith & Morrow, 1996)

the original response but never writing over the top of the incorrect response. Field workers and supervisors may use pens of different colours so that it is clear where corrections were made.

The data-collection activities should be supervised and the quality of the data monitored on a regular basis. Every data-collection activity should be designed in such a way that it can be checked. Checks should be designed with the objective of detecting errors rather than proving the high quality of the data.

Forms should be checked for their data completeness and consistency (Box 18.6). Interviewers' performance should be monitored regularly and constructive feedback given. If feasible, a random sample of subjects should be re-interviewed by the interviewer, co-worker and/or supervisor to assess the reliability of the measurements.

Interim tabulations and scatter plots of the most important variables should be produced regularly. These may help to detect problems. For instance, systematic patterns in the data (e.g., one interviewer with a much higher refusal level than the others) will indicate the need to check on particular aspects of data collection.

Box 18.6. Ensuring good data quality

• Ensure adequate training and supervision of field workers.

• Check samples of data-collection forms to assess their completeness and accuracy.

• Assess interviewer's performance by watching/listening to interview.

• Re-interview a random sample of subjects. The second interview may be conducted by the supervisor, by another interviewer, or by the same interviewer. Assess reliability of the data obtained in the two interviews.

• Tabulate the most important variables by interviewer to assess inter-interviewer variability.

Coding

Coding is the term used to describe the conversion of data from a data-collection form into a format that is suitable for analysis on a computer, by assigning a numerical code to every possible answer on the data-collection form. For instance, sex may be coded 1 for males and 2 for females; only the number 1 or 2 will be entered onto the computer file. Numerical data (e.g., number of children) do not require coding since the exact number can be entered.

Many data collection forms are 'pre-coded', that is, they are designed so that every possible answer is assigned a code in the form (see Appendix 2.1). The field worker selects one (or more) of these 'pre-coded' options. Such pre-coded forms have the advantages of being almost ready for computer entry by the data clerk and of minimizing transcription errors. However, later coding is still required for 'open' questions and for answers which do not fit into the pre-coded categories. These answers may be given additional codes if necessary.

An alternative approach is to code the data only after the form has been completed. The data-collection forms are designed so that there is a specific column for coding on the right- hand side of the page. The field workers (or the study subjects if the questionnaire is self-administered) are asked to ignore this column and fill in the answers in the spaces provided on the left-hand side. The answers are coded later by the field workers or by specially trained coding clerks and the codes are inserted in the right-hand column. The time between data recording and coding should be kept as short as possible so that inconsistencies in the data are revealed and the field worker can be asked to re-contact the subject to correct them.

Some aspects deserve special attention when developing coding instructions. Firstly, numerical variables such as number of children, weight or height should not be coded into pre-determined categories. Their actual values should be recorded so as to preserve the full detail of the data in analyses. Data may then be grouped in different ways, if appropriate. Secondly, specific codes should be given if a particular question is not applicable to a respondent (e.g., number of pregnancies for a man) or the answer is not known or the response was mistakenly left blank by the field worker (for example, 1 = yes; 2 = no; 7 = not recorded; 8 = not relevant; 9 = not known). Similarly, specific result codes should be developed in laboratory forms to allow for the coding of technical problems such as broken samples, insufficient material, error in laboratory procedures, etc. To minimize coding errors, it is advisable, if possible, that the meaning of any particular code remains constant throughout the data-collection form (e.g., a code of 9 should be given to the 'not known' answer of every question). Thirdly, a coding manual with all the coding values and rules should be compiled and given to field workers, data-coding and data-entry clerks. This manual should be updated if any changes in coding are made during the study.

Computer data entry

Once the data are coded, the information on the forms is ready to be entered into a computer. For each type of data-collection form, a computer file should be created to enter the data. It is possible to set up a data-entry programme so that the computer screen resembles the layout of the data collection form to minimize errors by data-entry clerks. The data-entry program is usually developed by using a database package. Most of these programs incorporate consistency and range checks so that the data are checked and edited in an interactive way. For instance, if an inadmissible value is entered, an error message appears on the screen and an audible warning alerts the data-entry clerk to the error. It is also important to design the data-entry program so that it does not allow data to be entered from records which were erroneously given the same identification number.

Each variable for which data are recorded must be given a name for use in computer processing. Variables may be identified by numbers (e.g., 'VAR001'), but it is better to use abbreviated names that easily identify the variables, such as 'sex', 'age', 'parity', 'fbirthag' (for age at first birth). The number of characters to be used in a variable name should not exceed the number allowed by the computer program (most packages do not allow the use of more than eight characters).

If data relating to the same individual may be obtained from different sources (e.g., interviewer-administered questionnaire, clinical notes and laboratory reports) or follow-up surveys conducted at different points in time, it is better to store the information from each source or survey in a separate file. It is relatively easy to link data from different database files using a common person-identifying code (i.e., the unique study number).

Each data-set collected in a study should be entered onto the computer twice. The second entry should be independent of the first and should be done by a different data-entry clerk. The two files of data should be compared using a specially written computer program (available in Epi Info). Any differences detected by this program should be checked against the original records and the incorrect file(s) edited. The program to compare the files should be run again and the editing process repeated until no differences between the files are found.

A manual with the names of the files where data from each form have been entered and with details of all the variables (what the variable is, meaning of codes, allowed values, etc.) should be compiled and distributed to all data-processing personnel. It should be updated on a regular basis, as necessary.

Data cleaning

Range and consistency checks should be run for each variable, either while they are being entered into the computer or after a whole batch has been entered. Range checks identify inadmissible values. For instance, if the variable sex was coded '1' for males and '2' for females, values other than 1 and 2 would be flagged as errors. Consistency checks cross-check the consistency of data for related variables. For example, males should not have a diagnosis of ovarian cancer.

In addition to checking for incorrect or unusual values, the distribution of each variable should be examined. Interim tabulations of the data and scatter plots of quantitative variables, such as height against weight, are effective in revealing unlikely outlying observations. These should be checked against the data collection forms, since they are unlikely but not necessarily impossible. In some cases, it may be possible to correct the data. In other cases, it will be necessary to insert a 'missing value' code, if it is certain that the data were in error (e.g., an impossible height).

Updating and storage

Back-up copies of the data should be made regularly (ideally on a daily basis, but if this is not possible, at least weekly). A minimum of two back-up copies of all data on computer should always exist. Some of the copies should be stored in a geographically separate location in a dry and relatively dust-free environment to guard against events such as fires, floods, robbery, etc. A complete and updated list should be made of what data are on all stored disks and tapes, and copies should be kept at more than one location.

The data collection forms should also be stored in a secure place to ensure confidentiality of the data. The forms should be filed in batches or in serial order (either by date of collection or by study identification number) to facilitate their retrieval for checking apparent errors detected in records on computer. Ideally, the forms should be kept well after the end of the study, but space restrictions may preclude this. In large studies, it may be worth considering the possibility of copying the data collection forms onto microfiches.

Preparing data for analysis

The variables entered into the computer files are not always the ones suitable for data analysis. Recoding and computing of new variables is likely to be necessary. For example, body mass index (BMI) may be calculated from height and weight, and age at the time of the survey from date of birth and date the interview was completed. Moreover, continuous variables are usually grouped for the 'classical' methods of analysis based on stratification. Some combination of groups may also be necessary for categorical variables with large numbers of categories or for categories in which there are no, or very few, cases.

It is preferable to keep a copy of the original file (as entered from the data-collection forms) and create new files for the new versions of the data. Preferably, the names of consecutive versions of the same file should be selected so that it is easy to recognize which one contains the latest version (e.g., STUD1, STUD2, STUD3, etc.). It is important to keep copies of the programs written to recode variables and compute new ones as a document of what exactly was done and to allow new versions of the data to be re-created from the original file if errors are detected.

Careful thought should be given to the planning of the analysis of the data (see Chapters 3, 4, 6 and 14). The steps given in Box 14.1 should be used as a general guideline.

18.4   Disseminating the results

Research projects are worthwhile only if their findings are properly disseminated to the scientific community. This usually involves publication of the findings in peer-reviewed scientific journals. Results may also be presented at scientific conferences and meetings. Depending on the aims and relevance of the study, it may also be appropriate to produce more detailed reports and/or reports written in lay language to be distributed to health authorities, community leaders, study subjects, etc.

18.4.1 Writing a paper

The process of writing a scientific paper has many similarities to that of writing a grant proposal. Thus, most of the issues presented in Box 18.1 are equally relevant to the preparation of scientific papers.

The first step is to identify journals that are likely to be interested in the topic of the study and are appropriate for the importance of the findings.

Box 18.7 lists some of the most important international journals of relevance to cancer epidemiologists. A useful way of choosing an appropriate journal is to see where most previous work on the same topic was published.

The journal's requirements—style, headings, referencing system, etc. must be followed closely. 'Instructions for Authors' are generally published in most issues of journals. The draft of the paper should be prepared exactly according to instructions. It is important to think carefully about how to illustrate the results (tables, figures, etc.) so that the main findings of the study are clearly presented to potential readers.

Most journals ask the authors to structure the paper into the following sections:

Title page

This page should include an informative and concise title for the paper; the name(s) of the author(s); the name of the institution in which the work was performed; the institutional affiliation of each author; and the name and address of the author to whom correspondence should be addressed.

Abstract

The abstract should summarize in no more than a few hundred words the reason for the study, the major findings, and the principal conclusions. Some papers (e.g., *British Medical Journal*) require a structured abstract which is divided into special sections. It is helpful to obtain some examples of abstracts published in the journal before attempting to write one. Some journals ask the authors to provide key words from the Medical Subject Headings of *Index Medicus* for indexing purposes.

Introduction

This section should include a description of the background of the investigation (citing only essential references) and the reason(s) for performing the study.

Data and methods

The methods (including the statistical approach) used should be described in enough detail that someone reading the paper could repeat the study. For research on human subjects, it is necessary to highlight any ethical issues that the conduct of the study might have raised, whether approval was obtained from the relevant ethical committees and how consent was obtained from the study participants.

Results

The findings should be presented in a clear and concise way. Repetition should be avoided by presenting data in only one format, that is, results displayed in a table should not be presented in the text.

Discussion

The discussion should cover the issues presented in Chapter 13: strengths and limitations of the study design, quality of the data, bias, confounding and chance. Finally, the findings of the study should be discussed in the light of previous work.

Acknowledgements

Contributions, including technical help or other assistance, and funding bodies that provided financial support for the study should be acknowledged.

References

The references should be written according to the specifications of the journal where the paper is going to be submitted.

Tables and figures

General rules for the preparation of tables and graphs were given in Section 3.4. Journals may have specific rules, which should be followed carefully.

Before submitting the paper, it is important to send a draft to all collaborators, as well as to colleagues who are successful at publishing articles and ask for their comments. If needed, the manuscript should be revised in the light of their comments before sending it to the journal

18.4.2 Review

If the editor thinks the journal might accept the paper, he/she will send it out to referees. The reports from these referees will then determine whether the paper is accepted or rejected. Papers are rarely accepted without alterations. Most commonly, it will be either rejected or accepted subject to modifications based on the referees' comments. The authors should submit a revised version of the paper which takes into account these comments, together with a covering letter to the editor explaining exactly how this was done.

Further reading

* The book by Smith & Morrow (1996) provides useful practical information on how to plan and conduct epidemiological studies. Although the book focuses on field trials, most of the issues presented are relevant to any type of epidemiological study.

Box 18.7. Some international journals of potential relevance to cancer epidemiologists	
American Journal of Epidemiology	International Journal of Cancer
British Journal of Cancer	International Journal of Epidemiology
British Medical Journal	Journal of Epidemiology and
Cancer	Community Health
Cancer Causes and Control	Journal of the National Cancer Institute
Cancer Research	Lancet
Epidemiology	Statistics in Medicine
European Journal of Cancer	

References

Acheson, E.D. (1967) *Medical Record Linkage*, Oxford, Oxford University Press

Alpha-Tocopherol, Beta Carotene Cancer Prevention Study Group (1994) The effect of vitamin E and beta carotene on the incidence of lung cancer and other cancers in male smokers. *New Engl. J. Med.*, **330**, 1029–1035

Altman, D.G. (1991) *Practical Statistics for Medical Research*, London, Chapman & Hall

American Cancer Society (1951) *Manual of Tumor Nomenclature and Coding*, first edition. Washington, DC

Andersen, L.P., Rosenstock, S.J., Bonnevie, O. & Jørgensen, T. (1996) Seroprevalence of immunoglobulin G, M, and A antibodies to *Helicobacter pylori* in an unselected Danish population. *Am. J. Epidemiol.*, **143**, 1157–1164

Anon. (1901) Verhandlungen des Comités für Krebsforschung. *Dtsch. Med. Wochenschr.*, suppl., 305–312

Aristizabal, N., Cuello, C., Correa, P., Collazos, T. & Haenszel, W. (1984) The impact of vaginal cytology on cervical cancer risks in Cali, Colombia. *Int. J. Cancer*, **34**, 5–9

Armitage, P. & Berry, G. (1994) *Statistical Methods in Medical Research*, third edition, Oxford, Blackwell Scientific Publications

Armstrong, B. & Mann, J.I. (1985) Diet. In: Vessey, M.P. & Gray, M. (eds), *Cancer Risks and Prevention*, Oxford, Oxford University Press, p. 71

Armstrong, B.K., White, E. & Saracci, R. (1992) *Principles of Exposure Measurement in Epidemiology* (Monographs in Epidemiology and Biostatistics, Vol. 21), Oxford, Oxford University Press

Ashley, J. & Devis T. (1992) Death certification from the point of view of the epidemiologist. *Population Trends*, **67**, 22–28

Baldwin, J.A., Acheson, E.D. & Graham, W.J. (eds.) (1987) *Textbook of Medical Record Linkage*, Oxford, Oxford University Press

Balzi, D., Buiatti, E., Geddes, M., Khlat, M., Masuyer, E. & Parkin, D.M. (1993) Summary of the results by site. In: Geddes, M., Parkin, D.M., Khlat, M., Balzi, D. & Buiatti, E. (eds.), *Cancer in Italian Migrant Populations* (IARC Scientific Publications No. 123), Lyon, International Agency for Research on Cancer, pp. 193–284

Bassett, M.T., Chokunonga, E., Mauchaza, B., Levy, L., Ferlay, J. & Parkin, D.M. (1995) Cancer in the African population of Harare, Zimbabwe, 1990–1992. *Int. J. Cancer*, **63**, 29–36

Beaglehole, R., Bonita, R. & Kjellström, T. (1993) *Basic Epidemiology*, Geneva, World Health Organization

Beasley, R.P., Hwang, L.-Y., Lin, C.-C. & Chien, C.-S. (1981) Hepatocellular carcinoma and hepatitis B virus. A prospective study of 22 707 men in Taiwan. *Lancet*, **ii**, 1129–1133

Belcher, D.W., Wurapa, F.K., Neumann, A.K. & Lourie, I.M. (1976) A household morbidity survey in rural Africa. *Int. J. Epidemiol.*, **5**, 113–120

Beral, V. (1974) Cancer of the cervix: a sexually transmitted infection? *Lancet*, **1**, 1037–1040

Beral, V., Chilvers, C. & Fraser, P. (1978) Does pregnancy protect against ovarian cancer? *Lancet*, **1**, 1083–1087

Beral, V., Chilvers, C. & Fraser, P. (1979) On the estimation of relative risk from vital statistical data. *J. Epidemiol. Community Health*, **33**, 159–162

Bergström, R., Adami, H.-O., Möhner, M., Zatonski, W., Storm, H., Ekbom, A., Tretli, S., Teppo, L., Akre, O. & Hakulinen, T. (1996) Increase in testicular cancer incidence in six European countries: a birth cohort phenomenon. *J. Natl. Cancer. Inst.*, **88**, 727–733

Bland, M. (1987) *An Introduction to Medical Statistics*, Oxford, Oxford University Press

Bland, J.M. & Altman, D.G. (1986) Statistical methods for assessing agreement between two methods of clinical measurement. *Lancet*, **1**, 307–310

Bleehen, N.M. & Stenning, S.P. (The Medical Research Council Brain Tumour Working Party) (1991) A Medical Research Council trial of two radiotherapy doses in the treatment of grades 3 and 4 astrocytoma. *Br. J. Cancer*, **64**, 769–774

Bone, M.R., Bebbington, A.C., Jagger, C., Morgan, K. & Nicolaas, G. (1995) *Health Expectancy and its Uses*, London, H.M.S.O.

Bosch, F.X., Muñoz, N., de Sanjosé, S., Izarzugaza, I., Gili, M., Viladiu, P., Tormo, M.J., Moreo, P., Ascunce, N., Gonzalez, L.C., Tafur, L., Kaldor, J.M., Guerrero, E., Aristizabal, N., Santamaria, M., Alonso de Ruiz, P. & Shah, K. (1992) Risk factors for cervical cancer in Colombia and Spain. *Int. J. Cancer*, **52**, 750–758

Bouchardy, C., Parkin, D.M., Khlat, M., Mirra, A.P., Kogevinas, M., de Lima, F.D. & de Cravalho Ferreira, C.E. (1993) Education and mortality from cancer in São Paulo, Brazil. *Ann. Epidemiol.*, **3**, 64–70

Bouwes Bavinck, J.N., Vermeer, B.J., van der Woude, F.J., Vandenbroucke, J.P., Schreuder, G.M.Th., Thorogood, J., Persijn, G.G. & Claas, F.H.J. (1991) Relation between skin cancer and HLA antigens in renal-transplant recipients. *New Engl. J. Med.*, **325**, 843–848

Breslow, N.E. & Day, N.E. (1980) *Statistical Methods in Cancer Research*. Volume I. *The Analysis of Case–Control Studies* (IARC Scientific Publications No. 32), Lyon, International Agency for Research on Cancer

Breslow, N.E. & Day, N.E. (1987) *Statistical Methods in Cancer Research*. Volume II. *The Design and Analysis of Cohort Studies* (IARC Scientific Publications No. 82), Lyon, International Agency for Research on Cancer

Breslow, N.E. & Enstrom, J.E. (1974) Geographic correlations between cancer mortality rates and alcohol–tobacco consumption in the United States. *J. Natl. Cancer Inst.*, **53**, 631–639

Broders, A.C. (1920) Squamous-cell epithelioma of the lip. A study of five hundred and thirty-seven cases. *J. Am. Med. Assoc.*, **74**, 656–664

Brothwell, D. (1967) The evidence for neoplasms. In: Brothwell, D. & Sandison, A.T. (eds.) *Diseases in Antiquity: A Survey of Diseases, Injuries and Surgery in Early Populations*, Springfield, IL, Charles C. Thomas, pp. 320–345

Buck, C., Llopis, A., Nájera, E. & Terris, M. (1988) *The Challenge of Epidemiology. Issues and Selected Readings*. Pan American Health Organization (PAHO) (Scientific Publication No. 505), Washington, DC, PAHO

Buell, P. & Dunn, J.E. (1965) Cancer mortality among Japanese Issei and Nisei of California. *Cancer*, **18**, 656–664

Buiatti, E., Palli, D., Amadori, D., Marubini, E., Puntoni, R., Avellini, C., Bianchi, S., Cipriani, F., Cocco, P., Decarli, A., Vindigni, C. & Blot, W. (1989a) Methodological issues in a multicentric study of gastric cancer and diet in Italy: Study design, data sources and quality controls. *Tumori*, **75**, 410–419

Buiatti, E., Palli, D., Decarli, A., Amadori, D., Avellini, C., Bianchi, S., Biserni, R., Cipriani, F., Cocco, P., Giacosa, A., Marubini, E., Puntoni, R., Vindigni, C., Fraumeni Jr, J. & Blot, W. (1989b) A case–control study of gastric cancer and diet in Italy. *Int. J. Cancer*, **44**, 611–616

Buring, J.E., Bain, C.J. & Ehrmann, R.L. (1986) Conjugated estrogen use and risk of endometrial cancer. *Am. J. Epidemiol.*, **124**, 434–441

Cameron, H.M. & McGoogan, E. (1981) A prospective study of 1152 hospital autopsies: I. Inaccuracies in death certificates. *J. Pathol.*, **113**, 273–283

Carpenter, L.M. (1987) Some observations on the healthy worker effect. *Br. J. Ind. Med.*, **44**, 289–291

Case, R.A.M. & Pearson, J.T. (1954) Tumours of the urinary bladder in workmen engaged in the manufacture and use of certain dyestuff intermediates in the British chemical industry. Part II. Further consideration of the role of aniline and of the manufacture of auramine and magenta (fuchsine) as possible causative agents. *Br. J. Ind. Med.*, **11**, 213–216

Case, R.A.M., Hosker, M.E., McDonald, D.B. & Pearson, J.T. (1954) Tumours of the urinary bladder in workmen engaged in the manufacture and use of certain dyestuff intermediates in the British chemical industry. Part I. The role of aniline, benzidine, alpha-naphthylamine, and beta-naphthylamine. *Br. J. Ind. Med.*, **11**, 75–104

Casley, D.J. & Lury, D.A. (1987) *Data Collection in Developing Countries*, second edition, Oxford, Clarendon Press

Chen, J., Campbell, T.C., Junkvao, L. & Peto, R. (1990) *Diet, Life-Style and Mortality in China. A Study of the Characteristics of 65 Chinese Counties*, Oxford, Oxford University Press

Chlebowski, R.T. & Grosvenor, M. (1994) The scope of nutrition intervention trials with cancer-related endpoints. *Cancer*, **74**, 2734–2738

Chuang, W.-L., Chang, W.-Y., Lu, S.-N., Su, W.-P., Lin, Z.-Y., Chen, S.-C., Hsieh, M.-Y., Wang, L.-Y., You, S.-L. & Chen, C.-J. (1992) The role of hepatitis B and C viruses in hepatocellular carcinoma in a hepatitis B endemic area. A case–control study. *Cancer*, **69**, 2052–2054

Cicchetti, D.V. & Feinstein, A.R. (1990) High agreement but low Kappa: II. Resolving the paradoxes. *J. Clin. Epidemiol.* **43**, 551–558

CIOMS (Council for International Organizations of Medical Sciences) and WHO (World Health Organisation) (1993) *International Ethical Guidelines for Biomedical Research Involving Human Subjects*, Geneva, CIOMS

Clarke, E.A. & Anderson, T.W. (1979) Does screening by "Pap" smears help prevent cervical cancer? A case–control study. *Lancet*, **2**, 1–4

Clayton, D. & Hills, M. (1993) *Statistical Models in Epidemiology*, Oxford, Oxford University Press

Clayton, D. & Schifflers, E. (1987a) Models for temporal variations in cancer rates. I. Age–period and age–cohort models. *Stat. Med.*, **6**, 449–467

Clayton, D. & Schifflers, E. (1987b) Models for temporal variations in cancer rates. II. Age–period–cohort models. *Stat. Med.*, **6**, 469–481

Cole, P & Morrison, A.S. (1978) Basic issues in cancer screening. In: Miller, A.B. (ed.) *Screening in Cancer* (A report of a UICC International Workshop, Toronto, Canada, April 24–27, 1978), Geneva, International Union Against Cancer, pp. 7–39

Collaborative Group on Hormonal Factors in Breast Cancer (1996) Breast cancer and hormonal contraceptives: collaborative reanalysis of individual data on 53 297 women with breast cancer and 100 239 women without breast cancer from 54 epidemiological studies. *Lancet*, **347**, 1713–1727

College of American Pathologists (1965) *Systematized Nomenclature of Pathology (SNOP)*, 1st edition, Skolkie, IL

College of American Pathologists (1977) *Systematized Nomenclature of Medicine (SNOMED)*, 1st edition, Skolkie, IL

COMMIT Research Group (1991) Community Intervention Trial for Smoking Cessation (COMMIT): summary of design and intervention. *J. Natl. Cancer Inst.*, **83**, 1620–1628

Cornfield, J. (1951) A method of estimating comparative rates from clinical data. Applications to cancer of the lung, breast, and cervix. *J. Natl. Cancer Inst.*, **11**, 1269–1275

Cottler, L.B., Zipp, J.F., Robins, L.N. & Spitznagel, E.L. (1987) Difficult-to-recruit respondents and their effect on prevalence estimates in an epidemiologic survey. *Am. J. Epidemiol.*, **125**, 329–339

Cox, D.R. & Snell, E.J. (1981) *Applied Statistics: Principles and Examples*, London, Chapman & Hall

Cramer, D.W. (1974) The role of cervical cytology in the declining morbidity and mortality of cervical cancer. *Cancer*, **34**, 2018–2027

Dawber, T.R., Meadors, G.F. & Moore, F.E., Jr. (1951) Epidemiological approaches to heart disease: the Framingham Study. *Am. J. Public Health*, **41**, 279–286

Day, N.E. & Boice, J.D., Jr (eds.) (1983) *Second Cancer in Relation to Radiation Treatment for Cervical Cancer* (IARC Scientific Publications No. 52), Lyon, International Agency for Research on Cancer

De Stavola, B. (transl.) (1987) Statistical facts about cancers on which doctor Rigoni-Stern based his contribution to the Surgeon's subgroup of the IV Congress of the Italian scientists on 23 September 1842. *Stat. Med.*, **6**, 881–884

Dey, P., Collins, S., Will, S. & Woodman, C.B.J. (1995) Randomised controlled trial assessing effectiveness of health education leaflets in reducing incidence of sunburn. *Br. Med. J.*, **311**, 1062–1063

Doll, R. (1955) Mortality from lung cancer in asbestos workers. *Br. J. Ind. Med.*, **12**, 81–86

Doll, R. & Hill, A.B. (1950) Smoking and carcinoma of the lung. Preliminary report. *Br. Med. J.*, **ii**, 739–748

Doll, R. & Hill, A.B. (1952) A study of the aetiology of carcinoma of the lung. *Br. Med. J.*, **ii**, 1271–1286

Doll, R. & Hill, A.B. (1954) The mortality of doctors in relation to their smoking habits. A preliminary report. *Br. Med. J.*, **i**, 1451–1455

Doll, R. & Peto, R. (1976) Mortality in relation to smoking: 20 years' observations on male British doctors. *Br. Med. J.*, **2**, 1525–1536

Doll, R., Payne, P. & Waterhouse, J.A.H. (1966) *Cancer Incidence in Five Continents*. Vol. 1. Geneva, UICC. Berlin, Springer

Doll, R., Gray, R., Hafner, B. & Peto, R. (1980) Mortality in relation to smoking: 22 years' observations on female British doctors. *Br. Med. J.*, **280**, 967–971

Doll, R., Peto, R., Wheatley, K., Gray, R & Sutherland, I. (1994a) Mortality in relation to smoking: 40 years' observations on male British doctors. *Br. Med. J.*, **309**, 901–911

Doll, R., Peto, R., Hall, E., Wheatley, K. & Gray, R. (1994b) Mortality in relation to consumption of alcohol: 13 years' observations on male British doctors. *Br. Med. J.*, **309**, 911–918

Dosemeci, M., Wacholder, S. & Lubin, J.H. (1990) Does nondifferential misclassification of exposure always bias a true effect toward the null value? *Am. J. Epidemiol.*, **132**, 746–748

Douglas, A.J., Omar, R.Z. & Smith, P.G. (1994) Cancer mortality and morbidity among workers at the Sellafield plant of British Nuclear Fuels. *Br. J. Cancer*, **70**, 1232–1243

Draper, G.J., Birch, J.M., Bithell, J.F., Kinnier Wilson, L.M., Leck, I., Marsden, H.B., Morris Jones, P.H., Stiller, C.A. & Swindell, R., (1982) *Childhood Cancer in Britain: Incidence, Survival and Mortality* (Studies in Medical and Population Subjects No. 37), London, H.M.S.O.

Enterline, P.E. (1965) Mortality among asbestos products workers in the United States. *Ann. N.Y. Acad. Sci.*, **132**, 156–165

Estève, J., Benhamou, E. & Raymond, L. (1994) *Statistical Methods in Cancer Research. Volume IV. Descriptive Epidemiology*, (IARC Scientific Publications No. 128). Lyon, International Agency for Research on Cancer

Farr, W. (1975) *Vital Statistics: A Memorial Volume of Selections from the Reports and Writings of William Farr* (The History of Medicine Series No. 46), Metuchen, NJ, Scarecrow Press.

Feinleib, M. (1984) Data bases, data banks and data dredging: the agony and the ecstasy. *J. Chron. Dis.*, **37**, 783–790

Feinstein, A.R. & Cicchetti, D.V. (1990) High agreement but low Kappa: I. The problems of two paradoxes. *J. Clin. Epidemiol.* **43**, 543–549

Ferlay, J. (1994) *ICD Conversion Programs for Cancer*, (IARC Technical Report No. 21), Lyon, International Agency for Research on Cancer

Fisher, R.A. & Yates, F. (1963) *Statistical Tables for Biological, Agricultural and Medical Research*, London, Longman

Fisher, B., Redmond, C., Fisher, E.R., Bauer, M., Wolmark, N., Wickerham, D.L., Deutsch, M., Montague, E., Margolese, R. & Foster, R. (1985) Ten-year results of a randomised clinical trial comparing radical mastectomy and total mastectomy with or without radiation. *New Engl. J. Med.*, **312**, 674–681

Flegal, K.M., Brownie, C. & Haas, J.D. (1986) The effects of exposure misclassification on estimates of relative risk. *Am. J. Epidemiol.* **123**, 736–751

Forman, D., Sitas, F., Newell, D.G., Stacey, A.R., Boreham, J., Peto, R., Campbell, T.C., Li, J. & Chen, J. (1990) Geographic association of *Helicobacter pylori* antibody prevalence and gastric cancer mortality in rural China. *Int. J. Cancer*, **46**, 608–611

Fukao, A., Komatsu, S., Tsubono, Y., Hisamichi, S., Ohori, H., Kizawa, T., Ohsato, N., Fujino, N., Endo, N. & Iha, M. (1993) *Helicobacter pylori* infection and chronic atrophic gastritis among Japanese blood donors: a cross-sectional study. *Cancer Causes Control*, **4**, 307–312

Gambia Hepatitis Study Group (1987) The Gambia Hepatitis Intervention Study. *Cancer Res.*, **47**, 5782–5787

Gardner, M.J. & Altman, D.G. (1986) Confidence intervals rather than P values: estimation rather than hypothesis testing. *Br. Med. J.*, **292**, 746–750

Geser, A., de Thé, G., Lenoir, G., Day, N.E. & Williams, E.H. (1982) Final case reporting from the Ugandan prospective study of the relationship between EBV and Burkitt's lymphoma. *Int. J. Cancer*, **29**, 397–400

Gilliand, F.D. & Samet, J.M. (1994) Lung cancer. In: Doll, R., Fraumeni, J.F., Jr & Muir, C.S. (eds.) *Trends in Cancer Incidence and Mortality*, *Cancer Surveys*, Vol. 19/20, New York, Cold Spring Harbor Laboratory Press, pp. 175–195

Gore, S.M. (1981) Assessing methods – survival. *Br. Med. J.*, **283**, 840–843

Greenland, S. & Morgenstern, H. (1989) Ecological bias, confounding, and effect modification. *Int. J. Epidemiol.*, **18**, 269–274

Greenland, S. & Robins, J.M. (1985) Estimation of a common effect parameter from sparse follow-up data. *Biometrics*, **41**, 55–68

Greenland, S. & Robins, J. (1994) Invited commentary: Ecologic studies – biases, misconceptions, and counterexamples. *Am. J. Epidemiol.*, **139**, 747–760

Greenland, S. & Thomas, D.C. (1982) On the need for the rare disease assumption in case–control studies. *Am. J. Epidemiol.*, **116**, 547–553

Grulich, A.E., Swerdlow, A.J., dos Santos Silva, I. & Beral, V. (1995) Is the apparent rise in cancer mortality in the elderly real? Analysis of changes in certification and coding of cause of death in England and Wales, 1970–1990. *Int. J. Cancer*, **63**, 164–168

Gupta, P.C., Bhonsle, R.B., Mehta, F.S. & Pindborg, J.J. (1984) Mortality experience in relation to tobacco chewing and smoking habits from a 10-year follow-up study in Ernakulam District, Kerala. *Int. J. Epidemiol.*, **13**, 184–187

Gupta, P.C., Mehta, F.S., Pindborg, J.J., Aghi, M.B., Bhonsle, R.B., Daftary, D.K., Murti, P.R., Shah, H.T. & Sinor, P.N. (1986) Intervention study for primary prevention of oral cancer among 36000 Indian tobacco users. *Lancet*, **i**, 1235–1239

Gupta, P.C., Mehta, F.S., Pindborg, J.J., Daftary, D.K., Aghi, M.B., Bhonsle, R.B. & Murti, P.R. (1990) A primary prevention study of oral cancer among Indian villagers. Eight-year follow-up results. In: Hakama, M., Beral, V., Cullen, J.W., Parkin, D.M. (1990) *Evaluating Effectiveness of Primary Prevention of Cancer* (IARC Scientific Publications No. 103), Lyon, International Agency for Research on Cancer, pp. 149–156

Haenszel, W., Loveland, D. & Sirken, M.G. (1962) Lung cancer mortality as related to residence and smoking histories. *J. Natl Cancer Inst.*, **28**, 947–1001

Hakama, M. (1982) Trends in the incidence of cervical cancer in the Nordic Countries. In: Magnus, K. (ed.), *Trends in Cancer Incidence. Causes and Practical Implications*, New York, Hemisphere, pp. 279–292

Hakama, M., Hakulinen, T., Pukkala, E., Saxén, E. & Teppo, L. (1982) Risk indicators of breast and cervical cancer on ecologic and individual levels. *Am. J. Epidemiol.*, **116**, 990–1000

Hakama, M., Miller, A.B. & Day, N.E. (eds.) (1986) *Screening for Cancer of the Uterine Cervix* (IARC Scientific Publications No. 76), Lyon, International Agency for Research on Cancer, p. 289

Hakulinen, T. & Pukkala, E. (1981) Future incidence of lung cancer: forecasts based on hypothetical changes in the smoking habits of males. *Int. J. Epidemiol.*, **10**, 233–240

Heasman, M.A. & Clarke, J.A. (1979) Medical record linkage in Scotland. *Health Bull.*, **37**, 97–103

Heasman, M.A. & Lipworth, L. (1966) *Accuracy of Certification of Cause of Death. A Report on a Survey Conducted in 1959 in 75 Hospitals of the National Health Service to Obtain Information on the Extent of Agreement Between Clinical and Post-mortem Diagnoses* (Studies on Medical and Population Subjects No. 20), London, H.M.S.O.

Henderson, M.M. (1995) Nutritional aspects of breast cancer. *Cancer*, **76** (suppl. 10), 2053–2058

Hennekens, C.H. & Eberlein, K. (Physicians' Health Study Research Group) (1985) A randomized trial of aspirin and β-carotene among U.S. physicians. *Prev. Med.*, **14**, 165–168

Hennekens, C.H., Buring, J.E., Manson, J.E., Stampfer, M., Rosner, B., Cook, N.R., Belanger, C., LaMotte, F., Gaziano, J.M., Ridker, P.M., Willett, W. & Peto, R. (1996) Lack of effect of long-term supplementation with beta carotene on the incidence of malignant neoplasms and cardiovascular disease. *New J. Engl. Med.*, **334**, 1145–1149

Herbst, A.L., Ulfelder, H. & Poskanzer, D.C. (1971) Adenocarcinoma of the vagina. Association of maternal stilbestrol therapy with tumor appearance in young women. *New Engl. J. Med.*, **284**, 878–881

Hill, A.B. (1965) The environment and disease: association or causation? *Proc. R. Soc. Med.*, **58**, 295–300

Hoffman, F.L. (1915) *The Mortality From Cancer Throughout the World*, Newark, NJ, Prudential Press

Howe, G.R., Burch, J.D., Miller, A.B., Morrison, B., Gordon, P., Weldon, L., Chambers, L.W., Fodor, G. & Winsor, G.M. (1977) Artificial sweeteners and human bladder cancer. *Lancet*, **2**, 578–581

IARC (International Agency for Research on Cancer) (1986) *IARC Monographs on the Evaluation of Carcinogenic Risks to Humans*. Vol. 38. *Tobacco Smoking*, Lyon, International Agency for Research on Cancer

IARC (International Agency for Research on Cancer) (1994a) *IARC Monographs on the Evaluation of Carcinogenic Risks to Humans*. Vol. 61. *Schistosomes, Liver Flukes and Helicobacter pylori*. Lyon, International Agency for Research on Cancer

IARC (International Agency for Research on Cancer) (1994b) *IARC Monographs on the Evaluation of Carcinogenic Risks to Humans*. Vol. 59. *Hepatitis Viruses*, Lyon, International Agency for Research on Cancer

Jensen, O.M., Parkin, D.M., MacLennan, R., Muir, C.S. & Skeet, R.G. (eds.) (1991) *Cancer Registration. Principles and Methods* (IARC Scientific Publications No. 95), Lyon, International Agency for Research on Cancer

Joint Iran–International Agency for Research on Cancer Study Group (1977) Esophageal cancer studies in the Caspian littoral of Iran: results of population studies – a prodrome. *J. Natl. Cancer. Inst.*, **59**, 1127–1138

Jolley, D (1993) The glitter of the *t* table. *Lancet*, **342**, 27–29

Jones, W.H.S. (transl.) (1923) *Hippocrates*, Vol. I, London, William Heinemann, pp. 71–137

Kaldor, J.M., Day, N.E., Bell, J., Clarke, E.A., Langmark, F., Karjalainen, S., Band, P., Pedersen, D., Choi, W., Blair, V., Henry-Amar, M., Prior, P., Assouline, D., Pompe-Kirn, V.,

Cartwright, R.A., Koch, M., Arslan, A., Fraser, P., Sutcliffe, S.B., Host, H., Hakama, M. & Stovall, M. (1992) Lung cancer following Hodgkin's disease: a case–control study. *Int. J. Cancer*, **52**, 677–681

Khlat, M., Vail, A., Parkin, M. & Green, A. (1992) Mortality from melanoma in migrants to Australia: variation by age at arrival and duration of stay. *Am. J. Epidemiol.*, **135**, 1103–1113

Kirkwood, B.R. (1988) *Essentials of Medical Statistics*, London, Blackwell Science

Kiviat, N.B., Koutsky, L.A., Critchlow, C.W., Galloway, D.A., Vernon, D.A., Peterson, M.L., McElhose, P.E., Pendras, S.J., Stevens, C.E. & Holmes, K.K. (1990) Comparison of Southern transfer hybridization and dot filter hybridization for detection of cervical human papillomavirus infection with types 6, 11, 16, 18, 31, 33, and 35. *Am. J. Clin. Pathol.*, **94**, 561–565

Kjaer, S.K., de Villiers, E.-M., Haugaard, B.J., Christensen, R.B., Teisen, C., Møller, K.A., Poll, P., Jensen, H., Vestergaard, B.F., Lynge, E. & Jensen, O.M. (1988) Human papillomavirus, herpes simplex virus and cervical cancer incidence in Greenland and Denmark. A population-based cross-sectional study. *Int. J. Cancer*, **41**, 518–524

Kubik, A., Parkin, D.M., Khlat, M., Erban, J., Polak, J. & Adamec, M. (1990) Lack of benefit from semi-annual screening for cancer of the lung: follow-up report of a randomised controlled trial on a population of high-risk males in Czechoslovakia. *Int. J. Cancer*, **45**, 26–33

Kurihara, M., Aoki, K. & Hisamichi, S. (eds.) (1989) *Cancer Mortality Statistics in the World 1950–1985*, Nagoya, University of Nagoya Press

Läärä, E. (1982) *Development of Cancer Morbidity in Finland up to the Year 2002* [in Finnish] (Health Education Series, Original Reports 3/1982), Helsinki, National Board of Health

Landis, J.R. & Koch, G.G. (1977) The measurement of observer agreement for categorical data. *Biometrics*, **33**, 159–174

Lane-Claypon, J.E. (1926) *A Further Report on Cancer of the Breast, with Special Reference to its Associated Antecedent Conditions* (Reports on Public Health and Medical Subjects No. 32), London, H.M.S.O.

Lantz, C.A. & Nebenzahl, E. (1996) Behavior and interpretation of the kappa statistic: resolution of the two paradoxes. *J. Clin. Epidemiol.*, **49**, 431–434

Last, J.M. (1995) *A Dictionary of Epidemiology*, third edition, Oxford, Oxford University Press

Lee, H.P., Day, N.E. & Shanmugaratnam, K. (1988) *Trends in Cancer Incidence in Singapore 1968–1982* (IARC Scientific Publications No. 91), Lyon, International Agency for Research on Cancer

Lee, H.P., Gourley, L., Duffy, S.W., Estève, J., Lee., J. & Day, N.E. (1991) Dietary effects on breast-cancer risk in Singapore. *Lancet*, **337**, 1197–1200

Levin, M.L., Goldstein, H. & Gerhardt, P.R. (1950) Cancer and tobacco smoking. A preliminary report. *J. Am. Med. Assoc.*, **143**, 336–338

Ley, C., Bauer, H.M., Reingold, A., Schiffman, M.H., Chambers, J.C., Tashiro, C.J. & Manos, M.M. (1991) Determinants of genital human papillomavirus infection in young women. *J. Natl. Cancer Inst.*, **83**, 997–1003

Lilienfeld, A.M. & Lilienfeld, D.E. (1979) A century of case–control studies: progress? *J. Chron. Dis.*, **32**, 5–13

Lippman, S.M., Lee, J.S., Lotan, R., Hittelman, W., Wargovich, M.J. & Hong, W.K. (1990) Biomarkers as intermediate end points in chemoprevention trials. *J. Natl. Cancer Inst.*, **82**, 555–560

Long, E.R. (1928) *A History of Pathology*, London, Baillière, Tindall & Cox

MacLennan, R. (1991) Items of patient information which may be collected by registries. In: Jensen, O.M., Parkin, D.M., MacLennan, R., Muir, C.S. & Skeet, R.G. (eds.) *Cancer Registration: Principles and Methods* (IARC Scientific Publications, No. 95), Lyon, International Agency for Research on Cancer, pp. 43–63

MacMahon, B., Cole, P., Lin, T.M., Lowe, C.R., Mirra, A.P., Ravnihar, B., Salber, E.J., Valaoras, V.G. & Yuasa, S. (1970) Age at first birth and breast cancer risk. *Bull. World Health Organ.*, **43**, 209–221

Malaty, H.M., Kim, J.G., Kim, S.D. & Graham, D.Y. (1996) Prevalence of *Helicobacter pylori* infection in Korean children: inverse relation to socioeconomic status despite a uniformly high prevalence in adults. *Am. J. Epidemiol.*, **143**, 257–262

Mantel, N. & Haenszel, W. (1959) Statistical aspects of the analysis of data from retrospective studies of disease. *J. Natl. Cancer Inst.*, **22**, 719–748

Mayans, M.V., Hall, A.J., Inskip, H.M., Lindsay, S.W., Chotard, J., Mendy, M. & Whittle, H.C. (1994) Do bedbugs transmit hepatitis B? *Lancet*, **343**, 761–763

McMichael, A.J. (1976) Standardized mortality ratios and the "healthy worker effect": scratching beneath the surface. *J. Occup. Med.*, **18**, 165–168

McMichael, A.J., Spirtas, R. & Kupper, L.L. (1974) An epidemiologic study of mortality within a cohort of rubber workers, 1964–72. *J. Occup. Med.*, **16**, 458–464

Meirik, O., Lund, E., Adami, H.-O., Bergström, R., Christoffersen, T. & Bergsjö, P. (1986) Oral contraceptive use and breast cancer in young women. A joint national case–control study in Sweden and Norway. *Lancet*, **2**, 650–654

Miettinen, O. (1976) Estimability and estimation in case–referent studies. *Am. J. Epidemiol.*, **103**, 226–235

Miettinen, O.S. & Wang, J.-D. (1981) An alternative to the proportionate mortality ratio. *Am. J. Epidemiol.*, **114**, 144–148

Møller, H., Knudsen, L.B. & Lynge, E. (1994) Risk of testicular cancer after vasectomy: cohort study of over 73 000 men. *Br. Med. J.*, **309**, 295–299

Morrison, A.S., Buring, J.E., Verhoek, W.G., Aoki, K., Leck, I., Ohno, Y. & Obata, K. (1984) An international study of smoking and bladder cancer. *J. Urology*, **131**, 650–654

Mould, R.F. (1983) *Cancer Statistics* (Medical Sciences Series), Bristol, Adam Hilger

Mueller, N., Evans, A., Harris, N.L., Comstock, G.W., Jellum, E., Magnus, K., Orentreich, N., Polk, B.F. & Vogelman, J. (1989) Hodgkin's disease and Epstein–Barr virus. Altered antibody pattern before diagnosis. *New Engl. J. Med.*, **320**, 689–695

Muir, C.S. & Percy, C. (1991) Classification and coding of neoplasms. In: Jensen, O.M., Parkin, D.M., MacLennan, R., Muir, C.S. & Skeet, R.G. (eds.) *Cancer Registration. Principles and Methods* (IARC Scientific Publications, No. 95), Lyon, International Agency for Research on Cancer, pp. 64–81

Muir, C., Waterhouse, J., Mack, T., Powell, J. & Whelan, S. (eds.) (1987) *Cancer Incidence in Five Continents*. Vol. V (IARC Scientific Publications, No. 88), Lyon, International Agency for Research on Cancer

Muñoz, N. & Day, N.E. (1996) Oesophageal cancer. In: Schottenfeld, D., Fraumeni Jr., J.F. (eds.) *Cancer Epidemiology and Prevention*, second edition. Oxford, Oxford University Press, pp. 681–706

Muñoz, N., Wahrendorf, J., Bang, L.J., Crespi, M., Thurnham, D.I., Day, N.E., Ji, Z.H., Grassi, A., Yan, L.W., Lin, L.G., Quan, L.Y., Yun, Z.C., Fang, Z.S., Yao, L.J., Correa, P., O'Conor, G.T. & Bosch, X. (1985) No effect of riblofavine, retinol, and zinc on prevalence of precancerous lesions of oesophagus. Randomised double-blind intervention study in high-risk population of China. *Lancet*, **2**, 111–114

Muñoz, N., Bosch, F.X., de Sanjosé, S., Tafur, L., Izarzugaza, I., Gili, M., Viladiu, P., Navarro, C., Martos, C., Ascunce, N., Gonzalez, L.C., Kaldor, J.M., Guerrero, E., Lörincz, A., Santamaria, M., Alonso de Ruiz, P., Aristizabal, N. & Shah, K. (1992a) The causal link between human papillomavirus and invasive cervical cancer: a population-based case–control study in Colombia and Spain. *Int. J. Cancer*, **52**, 743–749

Muñoz, N., Bosch, F.X., Shah, K.V. & Meheus, A. (eds.) (1992b) *The Epidemiology of Cervical Cancer and Human Papillomavirus* (IARC Scientific Publications, No. 119), Lyon, International Agency for Research on Cancer

Newton, R., Ferlay, J., Reeves, G., Beral, V. & Parkin, D.M. (1996) Effect of ambient solar ultraviolet radiation on incidence of squamous-cell carcinoma of the eye. *Lancet*, **347**, 1450–1451

Nomura, A., Stemmermann, G.N., Chyou, P.H., Kato, I., Perez-Perez, G.I. & Blaser, M.J. (1991) *Helicobacter pylori* infection and gastric carcinoma among Japanese Americans in Hawaii. *New Engl. J. Med.*, **325**, 1132–1136

OPCS (Office of Population Censuses and Surveys) (1970) *Classification of Occupations, 1970*. London, H.M.S.O.

OPCS (Office of Population Censuses and Surveys) (1978) *Occupational Mortality. The Registrar General's Decennial Supplement for England and Wales, 1970–72* (Series DS, No. 1), London, H.M.S.O.

OPCS (Office of Population Censuses and Surveys) (1981) *Cancer Statistics. Incidence, Survival and Mortality in England and Wales* (Studies on Medical and Population Subjects, No. 43), London, H.M.S.O.

OPCS (Office of Population Censuses and Surveys) (1983a, 1983b, 1985a, 1985b, 1986, 1988, 1990, 1991, 1993, 1994a, 1994b) *Cancer Statistics. Registrations* (Series MB1 Nos. 11–16, 18–22), London, H.M.S.O.

OPCS (Office of Population Censuses and Surveys) (1995) *Mortality Statistics. Review of the Registrar General on Deaths by Cause, Sex and Age, in England and Wales, 1993* (Series DH2 No. 20), London, H.M.S.O.

Omenn, G.S., Goodman, G.E., Thornquist, M.D., Balmes, J., Cullen, M.R., Glass, A., Keogh, J.P., Meyskens, F.L., Valanis, B., Williams, J.H., Barnhart, S. & Hammar, S. (1996) Effects of a combination of beta carotene and vitamin A on lung cancer and cardiovascular disease. *New. Engl. J. Med.*, **334**, 1150–1155

Orr, I.M. (1933) Oral cancer in betel nut chewers in Travancore. Its aetiology, pathology and treatment. *Lancet*, **ii**, 575–580

Parkin, D.M. & Hakulinen, T. (1991) Analysis of survival. In: Jensen, O.M., Parkin, D.M., MacLennan, R., Muir, C.S. & Skeet, R.G. (eds.) *Cancer Registration: Principles and Methods* (IARC Scientific Publications No. 95), Lyon, International Agency for Research on Cancer, pp. 159–176

Parkin, D.M. & Khlat, M. (1996) Studies of cancer in migrants: rationale and methodology. *Eur. J. Cancer*, **32A**, 761–771

Parkin, D.M., Muir, C.S., Whelan, S.L., Gao, Y.T., Ferlay, J. & Powell, J. (1992) *Cancer Incidence in Five Continents*. Vol. VI (IARC Scientific Publications No. 120), Lyon, International Agency for Research on Cancer

Parkin, D.M., Pisani, P. & Ferlay, J. (1993) Estimates of the world-wide incidence of eighteen major cancers in 1985. *Int. J. Cancer*, **54**, 594–606

Parkin, D.M., Chen, V.W., Ferlay, J., Galceran, J., Storm, H.H. & Whelan, S.L. (1994) *Comparability and Quality Control in Cancer Registration* (IARC Technical Reports No. 19), Lyon, International Agency for Research on Cancer

Parkin, D.M., Whelan, S.L., Ferlay, J., Raymond, L. & Young, J. (1997) *Cancer Incidence in Five Continents*. Vol. VII (IARC Scientific Publications No. 143), Lyon, International Agency for Research on Cancer

Pearce, N., Matos, E., Vainio, H., Boffetta, P. & Kogevinas, M. (eds) (1994) *Occupational Cancer in Developing Countries* (IARC Scientific Publications No. 129), Lyon, International Agency for Research on Cancer

Percy, C. L. (ed.) (1980) *Conversion of Malignant Neoplasms by Topography and Morphology from the* International Classification of Diseases for Oncology (ICD-O) *to Chapter II, Malignant Neoplasms*, International Classification of Diseases (ICD-8), *1965* (NIH Publication No. 80–2136), Bethesda, MD, US Department of Health, Education and Welfare

Percy, C. L. (ed.) (1981) *Conversion of Neoplasm Section, 8th Revision of* International Classification of Diseases (1965): *and 8th revision* International Classification of Diseases *Adapted for Use in the United States, to Neoplasm Section, 9th Revision of* International Classification of Diseases *(1975)* (NIH Publication No. 83–2448), Bethesda, MD, US Department of Health and Human Services

Percy, C.L. (ed.) (1983) *Conversion of Neoplasm Section, 9th Revision of* International Classification of Diseases *(1975): to* Neoplasm Section, 8th Revision of International Classification of Diseases *(1965) and 8th Revision of* International Classification of Diseases, *Adapted for Use in the United States* (NIH Publication No. 83–2638), Bethesda, MD, US Department of Health and Human Services

Percy, C.L., Berg, J.W. & Thomas, L.B. (eds.) (1968) *Manual of Tumour Nomenclature and Coding,* second edition. Washington, DC, American Cancer Society

Percy, C.L. & van Holten, V. (eds.) (1979) *Conversion of Neoplasms by Topography and Morphology from the* International Classifiction of Diseases for Oncology (ICD-O): *to Chapter II, Neoplasms, 9th Revision of the* International Classification of Diseases (NIH Publication No. 80–2007), Bethesda, MD, US Department of Health, Education and Welfare, Public Health Service

Percy, C., van Holten, V. & Muir, C. (eds.) (1990) *International Classification of Diseases for Oncology (ICD-O),* second edition. Geneva, World Health Organization

Peto, R., Pike, M.C., Armitage, P., Breslow, N.E., Cox, D.R., Howard, S.V., Mantel, N., McPherson, K., Peto, J. & Smith, P.G. (1976) Design and analysis of randomised clinical trials requiring prolonged observation of each patient. I. Introduction and design. *Br. J. Cancer,* **34**, 585–612

Peto, R., Pike, M.C., Armitage, P., Breslow, N.E., Cox, D.R., Howard, S.V., Mantel, N., McPherson, K., Peto, J. & Smith, P.G. (1977) Design and analysis of randomised clinical trials requiring prolonged observation of each patient. II. Analysis and examples. *Br. J. Cancer,* **35**, 1–39

Pike, M.C., Henderson, B.E., Krailo, M.D., Duke, A. & Roy, S. (1983) Breast cancer in young women and use of oral contraceptives: possible modifying effect of formulation and age at use. *Lancet,* **2**, 926–930

Pocock, S.J. (1983) *Clinical Trials: A Practical Approach,* Chichester, John Wiley

Polednak, A.P., Stehney, A.F. & Rowland, R.E. (1978) Mortality among women first employed before 1930 in the U.S. radium dial-painting industry. A group ascertained from employment lists. *Am. J. Epidemiol.,* **107**, 179–195

Potosky, A.L., Kessler, L., Gridley, G., Brown, C.C. & Horm, J.W. (1990) Rise in prostatic cancer incidence associated with increased use of transurethral resection. *J. Natl. Cancer Inst.,* **82**, 1624–1628

Pott, P. (1775) *Chirurgical Observations.* Vol. 3, London, Hawes, L., Clark, W, Collins, R., pp. 177–183.

Pottern, L.M., Stone, B.J., Day, N.E., Pickle, L.W. & Fraumeni, J.F., Jr (1980) Thyroid cancer in Connecticut, 1935–1975: an analysis by cell type. *Am. J. Epidemiol.,* **112**, 764–774

Powles, T.J., Jones, A.L., Ashley, S.E., O'Brien, M.E.R., Tidy, V.A., Treleavan, J., Cosgrove, D., Nash, A,G., Sacks, N., Baum, M., McKinna, J.A. & Davey, J.B. (1994) The Royal Mardsen Hospital pilot tamoxifen chemoprevention trial. *Breast Cancer Res. Treat.,* **31**, 73–82

Prince, A.M., Szmuness, W., Michon, J., Demaille, J., Diebolt, G., Linhard, J., Quenum, C. & Sankale, M. (1975) A case/control study of the association between primary liver cancer and hepatitis B infection in Senegal. *Int. J. Cancer,* **16**, 376–383

Puffer, R.R. & Griffith, G. W. (1967) *Patterns of Urban Mortality. Report of the Inter-American Investigation of Mortality* (Scientific Publication No. 151), Washington, DC, Pan American Health Organization

Qian G.-S., Ross, R.K, Yu, M.C., Yuan, J.-M., Gao, Y.-T., Henderson, B.E., Wogan, G.N. & Groopman, J.D. (1994) A follow-up study of urinary markers of aflatoxin exposure and liver cancer risk in Shanghai, People's Republic of China. *Cancer Epidemiol. Biomarkers Prev.,* **3**, 3–10

Rodrigues, L. & Kirkwood, B.R. (1990) Case–control designs in the study of common diseases: Updates on the demise of the rare disease assumption and the choice of sampling scheme for controls. *Int. J. Epidemiol.,* **19**, 205–213

Romieu, I., Willett, W.C., Colditz, G.A., Stampfer, M.J., Rosner, B., Hennekens, C.H. & Speizer, F.E. (1989) Prospective study of oral contraceptive use and risk of breast cancer in women. *J. Natl. Cancer Inst.,* **81**, 1313–1321

Rose, G. (1985) Sick individuals and sick populations. *Int. J. Epidemiol.,* **14**, 32–38

Rose, G. & Colwell, L. (1992) Randomised controlled trial of anti-smoking advice: final (20 year) results. *J. Epidemiol. Comm. Health,* **46**, 75–77

Ross, D.A. & Vaughan, J.P. (1986) Health interview surveys in developing countries: a methodological review. *Stud. Fam. Plann.,* **17**, 78–94

Ross, R.K., Yuan, J.-M., Yu, M.C., Wogan, G.N., Qian, G.-S., Tu, J.-T., Groopman, J.D., Gao, Y.-T. & Henderson, B.E. (1992) Urinary aflatoxin biomarkers and risk of hepatocellular carcinoma. *Lancet,* **339**, 943–946

Sackett, D.L. (1979) Bias in analytic research. *J. Chron. Dis.,* **32**, 51–63

Schatzkin, A., Freedman, L.S., Schiffman, M.H. & Dawsey, S.M. (1990) Validation of intermadiate end points in cancer research. *J. Natl. Cancer. Inst.,* **82**, 1746–1752

Schrek, R. & Lenowitz, H. (1947) Etiologic factors in carcinoma of the penis. *Cancer Res.,* **7**, 180–187

Schrek, R., Baker L.A., Ballard, G.P. & Dolgoff, S. (1950) Tobacco smoking as an etiologic factor in disease. I. Cancer. *Cancer Res.,* **10**, 49–58

Schwartz, D. & Lellouch, J. (1967) Explanatory and pragmatic attitudes in therapeutical trials. *J. Chron. Dis.,* **20**, 637–648

Scott, C. & Harpham, T. (1987) Sample design. In: Cleland, J. & Scott, C. (eds.), *The World Fertility Survey. An Assessment,* Oxford, Oxford University Press, pp. 309–324

Severson, R.K. (1990) Have transurethral resections contributed to the increasing incidence of prostatic cancer? *J. Natl. Cancer Inst.,* **82**, 1597–1598

Shapiro, S. (1977) Evidence on screening for breast cancer from a randomised trial. *Cancer,* **39** (suppl. 6), 2772–2782

Shapiro, S., Strax, P. & Venet, L. (1971) Periodic breast cancer screening in reducing mortality from breast cancer. *J. Am. Med. Assoc.*, **215**, 1777–1785

Shapiro, S., Goldberg, J.D. & Hutchison, G.B. (1974) Lead time in breast cancer detection and implications for periodicity of screening. *Am. J. Epidemiol.*, **100**, 357–366

Shimizu, Y., Schull, W.J. & Kato, H. (1990) Cancer risk among atomic bomb survivors. The RERF Life Span Study. *J. Am. Med. Assoc.*, **264**, 601–604

Shimizu H., Ross, R.K., Bernstein, L., Yatani, R., Henderson, B.E. & Mack, T.M. (1991) Cancers of the prostate and breast among Japanese and white immigrants in Los Angeles County. *Br. J. Cancer*, **63**, 963–966

Shu, X.O., Nesbit, M.E., Buckley, J.D., Krailo, M.D. & Robison, L.L. (1995) An exploratory analyis of risk factors for childhood malignant germ-cell tumors: report from the Childrens Cancer Group (Canada, United States) *Cancer Causes Control*, **6**, 187–198

Smith, P.G. & Day, N.E. (1984) The design of case–control studies: the influence of confounding and interaction effects. *Int. J. Epidemiol.*, **13**, 356–365

Smith, P.G. & Douglas, A.J. (1986) Mortality of workers at the Sellafield plant of British Nuclear Fuels. *Br. Med. J.*, **293**, 845–854

Smith, P.G. & Morrow, R.H. (eds.) (1996) *Field Trials of Health Interventions in Developing Countries: A Toolbox*, second edition. London, Macmillan Education

Smith, D.C., Prentice, R., Thompson, D.J. & Herrmann, W.L. (1975) Association of exogenous estrogen and endometrial carcinoma. *New Engl. J. Med.*, **293**, 1164–1167

Smith, P.G., Rodrigues, L.C. & Fine, P.E.M. (1984) Assessment of the protective efficacy of vaccines against common diseases using case–control and cohort studies. *Int. J. Epidemiol.*, **13**, 87–93

Smith, D.B., Newlands, E.S., Rustin, G.J.S., Begent, R.H.J., Howells, N., McQuade, B. & Bagshawe, K.D. (1991) Comparison of ondansetron and ondansetron plus dexamethasone as antiemetic prophylaxis during cisplatin-containing chemotherapy. *Lancet*, **338**, 487–490

Sparén, P. (1996) Early Detection and Screening for Cancer of the Cervix in Sweden during the 20th Century (Doctoral thesis. University of Uppsala, Sweden), Stockholm, Almqvist & Wiksell

Sriamporn, S., Black, R.J., Sankaranarayanan, R., Kamsa-AD, S., Parkin, D.M. & Vatanasapt, V. (1995) Cancer survival in Khon Kaen Province, Thailand. *Int. J. Cancer*, **61**, 296–300

Stadel, B.V., Rubin, G.L., Webster, L.A., Schlesselman, J.J. & Wingo, P.A. (1985) Oral contraceptives and breast cancer in young women. *Lancet*, **2**, 970–973

Stampfer, M.J., Buring, J.E., Willet, W., Rosner, B., Eberlein, K. & Hennekens, C.H. (1985) The 2×2 factorial design: its application to a randomzied trial of aspirin and carotene in U.S. physicians. *Stat. Med.*, **4**, 111–116

Strader, C.H., Weiss, N.S. & Daling, J.R. (1988) Vasectomy and the incidence of testicular cancer. *Am. J. Epidemiol.*, **128**, 56–63

Swerdlow, A.J. (1989) Interpretation of England and Wales cancer mortality data: the effect of enquiries to certifiers for further information. *Br. J. Cancer*, **59**, 787–791

Swerdlow, A.J., Marmot, M.G., Grulich, A.E. & Head, J. (1995) Cancer mortality in Indian and British ethnic immigrants from the Indian subcontinent to England and Wales. *Br. J. Cancer*, **72**, 1312–1319

Tabár, L., Fagerberg, C.J.G., Gad, A., Baldetorp, L. Holmberg, L.H., Gröntoft, O., Ljungquist, U., Lundström, B., Månson, J.C., Eklund, G., Day, N.E. & Pettersson, F. (1985) Reduction in mortality from breast cancer after mass screening with mammography. Randomised trial from the Breast Cancer Screening Working Group of the Swedish National Board of Health and Welfare. *Lancet*, **1**, 829–832

Thames Cancer Registry (1995) *Cancer in South East England 1992. Cancer Incidence, Prevalence, Survival and Treatment for Residents of the District Health Authorities in South East England*, Sutton, Thames Cancer Registry

Tomášek, L., Darby, S.C., Swerdlow, A.J., Plaček, V. & Kunz, E. (1993) Radon exposure and cancers other than lung cancer among uranium miners in West Bohemia. *Lancet*, **341**, 919–923

Tomášek, L., Swerdlow, A.J., Darby, S.C., Plaček, V. & Kunz, E. (1994) Mortality in uranium miners in West Bohemia: a long term cohort study. *Occup. Environ. Med.*, **51**, 308–315

Toniolo, P., Boffetta, P., Shuker, D.E.G., Rothman, N., Hulka, B. & Pearce, N. (1997) *Application of Biomarkers in Cancer Epidemiology* (IARC Scientific Publications No. 142), Lyon, International Agency for Research on Cancer

Trichopoulos, D., Tabor, E., Gerety, R.J., Xirouchaki, E., Sparros, L., Muñoz, N. & Linsell, C.A. (1978) Hepatitis B and primary hepatocellular carcinoma in a European population. *Lancet*, **ii**, 1217–1219

Tufte, E.R. (1983) *The Visual Display of Quantitative Information*, Cheshire, CT, Graphic Press

Tuyns, A.J. & Massé, L.M.F., (1973) Mortality from cancer of the oesophagus in Brittany. *Int. J. Epidemiol.*, **2**, 241–245

Tuyns, A.J. & Vernhes, J.C. (1981) La mortalité par cancer de l'oesophage dans les départements du Calvados et de l'Orne. *Gastroenterol. Clin. Biol.*, **5**, 257–265

Tuyns, A.J., Pequignot, G. & Jensen, O.M. (1977) Le cancer de l'oesophage en Ille-et-Vilaine en fonction des niveaux de consommation d'alcool et de tabac. Des risques qui se multiplient. *Bull. Cancer*, **64**, 45–60

Tuyns, A.J., Hu, M.X. & Pequignot, G. (1983) Alcohol consumption patterns in the department of Calvados (France) *Rev. Epidémiol. Santé Publique*, **31**, 179–197

United Nations (1987) *Fertility Behaviour in the Context of Development* (Population Studies No. 100), New York, United Nations, Department of International Economic and Social Affairs

Uppsala–Örebro Breast Cancer Study Group (1990) Sector resection with or without postoperative radiotherapy for Stage I breast cancer: A randomized trial. *J. Natl. Cancer Inst.*, **82**, 277–282

US Department of Health, Education, and Welfare (1969) *Use of Tobacco: Practices, Attitudes, Knowledge, and Beliefs. United States - Fall 1964 and Spring 1966,* Washington, DC, US Department of Health, Education, and Welfare

US Department of Health and Human Services (1991) *Smoking and Tobacco Control Monographs 1. Strategies to Control Tobacco Use in the United States: A Blueprint for Public Health Action in the 1990's* (NIH Publication No. 92–3316), Bethesda, MD, US Department of Health and Human Services, US Government Printing Office

US Surgeon General (1982) *The Health Consequences of Smoking: Cancer,* Bethesda, MD, US Department of Health and Human Services

Veronesi, U., Saccozzi, R., Del Vecchio, M., Banfi, A., Clemente, C., De Lena, M., Gallus, G., Greco, M., Luini, A., Marubini, E., Muscolino, G., Rilke, F., Salvadori, B., Zecchini, A. & Zucali, R. (1981) Comparing radical mastectomy with quadrantectomy, axillary dissection, and radiotherapy in patients with small cancers of the breast. *New Engl. J. Med.,* **305,** 6–11

Vineis, P. & Simonato, L. (1986) Estimates of the proportion of bladder cancers attributable to occupation. *Scand. J. Work Environ. Health,* **12,** 55–60

Vizcaino, A.P., Parkin, D.M. & Skinner, M.E.G. (1995) Risk factors associated with oesophageal cancer in Bulawayo, Zimbabwe. *Br. J. Cancer,* **72,** 769–773

Wagner, G. (1991) History of cancer registration. In: Jensen, O.M., Parkin, D.M., MacLennan, R., Muir, C.S. & Skeet, R.G. (eds.) *Cancer Registration: Principles and Methods* (IARC Scientific Publications, No. 95), Lyon, International Agency for Research on Cancer, pp. 3–6

Waldron, H.A. (1983) A brief history of scrotal cancer. *Br. J. Ind. Med.,* **40,** 390–401

Walter, S.D. (1991a) The ecologic method in the study of environmental health. I. Overview of the method. *Environ. Health. Perspect.,* **94,** 61–65

Walter, S.D. (1991b) The ecologic method in the study of environmental health. II. Methodologic issues and feasibility. *Environ. Health. Perspect.,* **94,** 67–73

Waterhouse, J.A.H., Doll, R. & Muir, C.S. (eds.) (1970) *Cancer Incidence in Five Continents.* Vol. II, Berlin, Springer

Waterhouse, J.A.H., Muir, C.S. & Correa, P. (eds.) (1976) *Cancer Incidence in Five Continents.* Vol. III (IARC Scientific Publications No. 15), Lyon, International Agency for Research on Cancer

Waterhouse, J.A.H., Muir, C.S., Shanmugaratnam, K. & Powell, J. (eds.) (1982) *Cancer Incidence in Five Continents.* Vol. IV (IARC Scientific Publications No. 42), Lyon, International Agency for Research on Cancer

Weinstock, M.A., Colditz, G.A., Willett, W.C., Stampfer, M.J., Rosner, B. & Speizer, F.E. (1991) Recall (report) bias and reliability in the retrospective assessment of melanoma risk. *Am. J. Epidemiol.,* **133,** 240–245

Whelan, S.L., Parkin, D.M. & Masuyer, E. (eds.) (1990) *Patterns of Cancer in Five Continents* (IARC Scientific Publications No. 102), Lyon, International Agency for Research on Cancer

WHO (World Health Organization) (1956) *Statistical Code for Human Tumours* (WHO/HS/CANC, 24.1 and 24.2, August 15, 1956), Geneva, WHO

WHO (World Health Organization) (1957) *Manual of the International Statistical Classification of Diseases, Injuries, and Causes of Death,* seventh revision, Geneva, WHO

WHO (World Health Organization) (1967) *Manual of the International Statistical Classification of Diseases, Injuries, and Causes of Death,* eighth revision, Geneva, WHO

WHO (World Health Organization) (1976) *International Classification of Diseases for Oncology (ICD-O),* first edition, Geneva, WHO

WHO (World Health Organization) (1977) *Manual of the International Statistical Classification of Diseases, Injuries, and Causes of Death,* ninth revision, Geneva, WHO

WHO (World Health Organization) (1983) *World Health Statistics Annual, 1983,* Geneva, WHO

WHO (World Health Organization) (1986) *World Health Statistics Annual, 1986,* Geneva, WHO

WHO (World Health Organization) (1992) *International Statistical Classification of Diseases and Related Health Problems,* tenth revision (ICD-10), Geneva, WHO

WHO Collaborative Study of Neoplasia and Steroid Contraceptives (1989) Combined oral contraceptives and liver cancer. *Int. J. Cancer,* **43,** 254–259

Willett, W.C., Stampfer, M.J., Colditz, G.A., Rosner, B.A., Hennekens, C.H. & Speizer, F.E. (1987) Dietary fat and the risk of breast cancer. *New Engl. J. Med.,* **316,** 22–28

Wright, W.C. (transl.) (1964) *Diseases of Workers,* by Ramazzini, B. (The History of Medicine Series No. 23), New York, Hafner

Wynder, E.L. & Graham, E.A. (1950) Tobacco smoking as a possible etiologic factor in bronchiogenic carcinoma. A study of six hundred and eighty-four proved cases. *J. Am. Med. Assoc.,* **143,** 329–336

Ziel, H.K. & Finkle, W.D. (1975) Increased risk of endometrial carcinoma among users of conjugated estrogens. *New Engl. J. Med.,* **293,** 1167–1170

Subject index